To my wife Susan and our two children Monica and Miriam

Published by
Futura Publishing Company, Inc.
P.O. Box 330, 295 Main Street
Mount Kisco, New York 10549

L.C.: 80-68262
ISBN: 0-87993-152-3

CONTRIBUTORS

Donna Bergen, M.D., Assistant Professor, Rush Medical College, Chicago, Illinois

John G. Brooks, M.D., Associate Professor, University of Rochester School of Medicine, Rochester, New York

James E. Carroll, M.D., Assistant Professor, Departments of Neurology, Neurosurgery (Neurology), and Pediatrics, Washington University School of Medicine, St. Louis, Missouri

Charles M. D'Angelo, M.D., Assistant Attending Surgeon, Department of Neurosurgery, Rush-Presbyterian-St. Luke's Medical Center; Assistant Professor of Neurological Surgery, Rush Medical College, Chicago, Illinois

Floyd A. Davis, M.D., Professor of Neurology, Rush Medical College, Chicago, Illinois

Larry E. Davis, M.D., Associate Professor of Neurology and Research, and Vice Chairman, Department of Neurology, University of New Mexico School of Medicine, Albuquerque, New Mexico

Christopher G. Goetz, M.D., Assistant Professor of Neurological Sciences, Rush-Presbyterian-St. Luke's Medical Center, Chicago, Illinois

Barbara Gothe, M.D., Assistant Professor of Medicine, Division of Pulmonary Medicine, Case Western Reserve University Hospitals, Cleveland, Ohio

Raj G. Gupta, M.D., F.C.C.P., Assistant Professor of Medicine, Director of Pulmonary Function Laboratory, University of Chicago, Michael Reese Hospitals, Chicago, Illinois

David L. Jackson, M.D., Ph.D., Associate Professor of Medicine and Co-Director, Division of Clinical Pharmacology and Critical Care Medicine, Case Western Reserve University Hospitals, Cleveland, Ohio

Harold L. Klawans, M.D., Associate Chairman, Department of Neurological Sciences, and Professor of Neurology and Pharmacology, Rush Medical College, Chicago, Illinois

William C. Koller, M.D., Ph.D., Department of Neurology, Harvard Medical School, Boston; Department of Medicine, Section of Neurology, Peter Bent Brigham Hospital, VA Medical Center, Brockton, Massachusetts

Jeffrey Kramer, M.D., Instructor of Neurology, Rush Medical College, Chicago, Illinois

Paul A. Nausieda, M.D., Assistant Professor, Departments of Neurology and Pharmacology, Rush-Presbyterian-St. Luke's Medical Center, Chicago, Illinois

Steven P. Ringel, M.D., Associate Professor of Neurology, University of Colorado Medical Center, Denver, Colorado

Dusan Stefoski, M.D., Assistant Professor of Neurology, Rush Medical College, Chicago, Illinois

Charles N. Swisher, M.D., Assistant Professor of Pediatrics and Neurology, University of Chicago Pritzker School of Medicine, and Director, Division of Pediatric Neurology, Michael Reese Hospitals and Medical Center, Chicago, Illinois

Caroline M. Tanner, M.D., Neuropharmacology Fellow, Department of Neurological Sciences, Rush-Presbyterian-St. Luke's Medical Center, Chicago, Illinois

S. Weber, Ph.D., Assistant Professor of Psychology, Department of Psychiatry and Sleep Center, Rush-Presbyterian-St. Luke's Medical Center, Chicago, Illinois

William J. Weiner, M.D., Associate Professor, Departments of Neurology and Pharmacology, Rush Medical College, Chicago, Illinois

INTRODUCTION

This book, which is concerned with the effect of neurologic dysfunction in the respiratory system, grew out of a neurology grand rounds presentation. In 1975, I had seen a patient with tardive dyskinesia who had, as part of her abnormal movement syndrome, irregularity of breathing–intermittent hyperventilation, gasping and grunting. This patient had a mild uncompensated respiratory alkalosis and when this patient was discussed, my pulmonary colleagues were unconvinced that the development of her respiratory complaints and findings could be explained on the basis of her movement disorder. The syndrome of respiratory dyskinesia has since become much more readily identifiable. It was, however, this initial interaction between neurologists and pulmonary internists regarding the effect of neurologic dysfunction on the respiratory system which serves as the focus of this text.

The following chapters were, with only two exceptions, written by clinical neurologists with varying areas of neurologic expertise. Each of the authors was asked to specifically address the questions of the importance, type, and mechanisms of respiratory dysfunction which they observed within their particular neurologic subspecialty. Their contributions, I hope, provide a unique text dealing with neurologists' views of respiratory dysfunctions in neurologic illness. I think it can serve as a source of information for neurologists dealing with specific clinical problems and, more importantly, it can serve as a source of information for primary care physicians and pulmonary specialists with regard to how broad categories of neurologic illness produce respiratory difficulties. Although there are portions of several chapters that deal with techniques of pulmonary function testing, this is not the main intent of this book. There are also several chapters in which the description of central respiratory anatomy may be overlapping and perhaps contradictory, but I feel that where this does occur it serves to emphasize the current state of the art.

William J. Weiner, M.D.
Chicago, Illinois

CONTENTS

Contributors iii

Introduction v

Chapter 1. Respiratory Neuroanatomy 1
Christopher G. Goetz, M.D.

Chapter 2. Respiratory Dysfunction in Movement Disorders 15
William J. Weiner, M.D., and Harold L. Klawans, M.D.

Chapter 3. Neurological Infections and Respiratory Dysfunction.............................. 41
Larry E. Davis, M.D., David L. Jackson, M.D., Ph.D., and Barbara Gothe, M.D.

Chapter 4. Respiratory Dysfunction in Motor Neuron Disease.. 71
Raj G. Gupta, M.D.

Chapter 5. Respiratory Dysfunction and Peripheral Neuropathy............................... 83
Caroline M. Tanner, M.D.

Chapter 6. Respiratory Complications of Neuromuscular Disease 113
Steven P. Ringel, M.D., and James E. Carroll, M.D.

Chapter 7. Respiratory Dysfunction in Cerebral Vascular Disease 157
Jeffrey Kramer, M.D.

Chapter 8. Respiratory Disease and Seizures 173
Donna Bergen, M.D.

Chapter 9. Central Disturbances of Respiration in Multiple Sclerosis 187
Dusan Stefoski, M.D., and Floyd A. Davis, M.D.

Chapter 10. Neurotoxins and Respiratory Dysfunction 197
Christopher G. Goetz, M.D.

Chapter 11. Respiratory Reflexes 211
William C. Koller, M.D., Ph.D.

Chapter 12. Respiratory Dysfunction in Pediatric Neurologic Disorders 243
John G. Brooks, M.D., and Charles N. Swisher, M.D.

Chapter 13. Respiratory Dysfunction in Neurosurgical Practice 267
Charles M. D'Angelo, M.D.

Chapter 14. Sleep Disorders and Respiratory Dysfunction 285
Paul A. Nausieda, M.D., and S. Weber, Ph.D.

Index 329

1

RESPIRATORY NEUROANATOMY

Christopher G. Goetz, M.D.

The neuronal nuclei ultimately responsible for respiratory control lie remote from the external environment and the tissues requiring oxygen supply. Afferent and efferent pathways converge on the central respiratory neurons where inputs are integrated and respiratory alterations are effected. The central and peripheral nervous systems are involved at multiple levels in this fundamental physiologic process.

The neuroanatomy of respiration is best understood when viewed from the perspective of the above three systems: the central respiratory centers; the afferent influences, both central and peripheral, that modify this primary respiratory pacing; and the efferent pathways that carry the integrated information from the central through the peripheral nervous system to the muscles of the thorax. Coordinated interaction between these three systems is prerequisite to normal physiologic respiration.

CENTRAL RESPIRATORY CENTERS

In contrast to the heart, the muscles of respiration possess no inherent rhythm and cannot function when separated from the central nervous system. Attempts to define central respiratory centers and connections began in 1812 with Legallois' demonstration that breathing continues

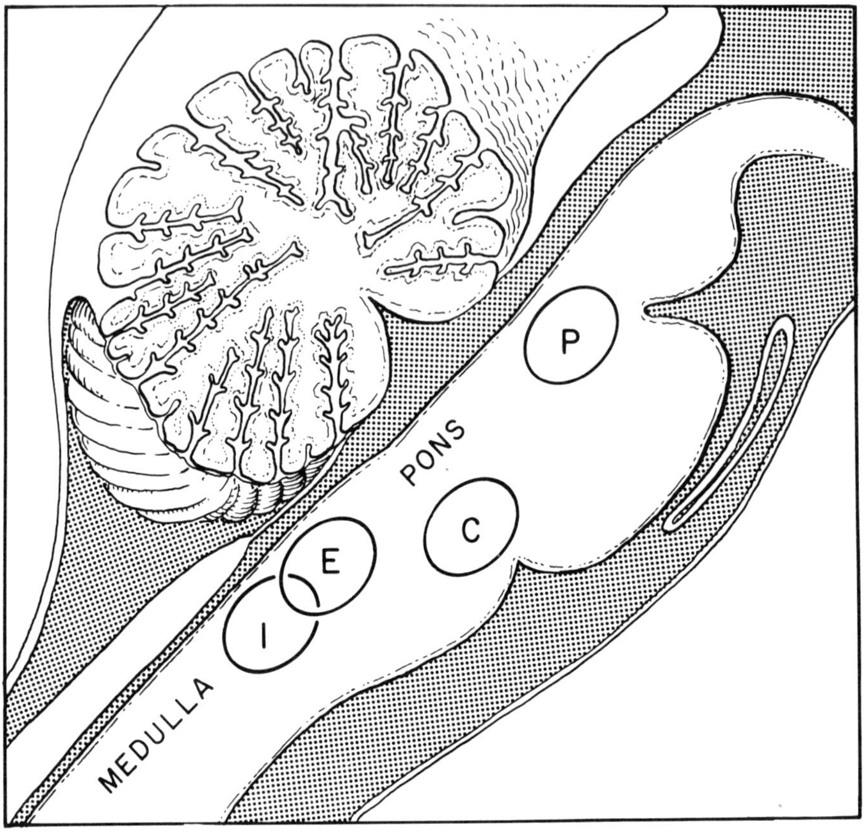

Figure 2. Sagittal diagram of brain stem with respiratory centers, identifying overlapping expiratory (E) and inspiratory (I) medullary centers, and the pontine pneumotaxic (P) and chemoreceptor (C) regions.

A third brain stem respiratory center, the apneustic center, was previously postulated, although it has now been concluded that apneustic breathing relates to excessive facilitation of the inspiratory medullary center rather than the activation of another specific brain stem nuclear group.[6,7]

AFFERENT MECHANISMS

While sustained respiration will be effected in an isolated brain stem preparation, normal respiratory function depends on intact afferent pathways. The neuronal connections to the primary brain stem centers are multiple. Neurons in both cerebral hemispheres, the hypothalamus and the brain stem reticular activating system, provide descending influences while peripheral inputs include the vagus and glossopharyngeal nerves and the tractus solitarus.[10,11] Voluntary control of respiration has been assumed to be evidence of cerebral hemispheral participation in respiratory organization.[12] Actual physiologic evidence includes expiratory apnea being produced when the anterior cingulate gyrus, subcollosal regions, ventral surface of the frontal lobe or the temporal pole are stimulated.[13] In contrast, an increased respiratory rate occurs with stimulation of the pyriform cortex.[3] Stimulation of other cortical regions induces rhythmic respiratory movements related to swallowing or vocalization.[2] The wide variety of respiratory disturbances seen with cortical dysfunction emphasizes the importance of corticomedullary integration. As already indicated, however, none of these cortical areas is essential to the maintenance of respiration. Respiratory periodicity persists even when the medulla is deprived of cortical and subcortical connections.

Studies on the respiratory afferent influences of the vagus nerve indicate that it participates in at least nine individual respiratory reflexes.[14] In addition to mediating the two Hering-Breuer reflexes, vagal fibers to the medullary respiratory center provide sensory innervation from the trachae and bronchi, irritation of which induces cough and active expiration. Stimulated afferent fibers from the aortic arch inhibit breathing, and fibers from the aortic body cause hyperpnea and elevated blood pressure when excited. The glossopharyngeal nerve provides additional afferent input from the carotid sinus region to the primary brain stem respiratory centers. In summary, peripheral neural influences on brain stem respiratory center activity can be divided into three basic afferent systems: first, somatic afferent fibers from mechanoreceptors of the respiratory muscles which influence brain stem ventilatory drive; second, the mechanoreceptors in the lungs themselves which activate neural afferants via the vagus nerve to form the basis of the Hering-Breuer reflexes; and third, afferent fibers originating from peripheral receptors not directly part of the respiratory system, being in the carotid sinus, aortic arch, or other usually vascular regions (Fig. 3).

These neural pathways provide the medullary center with information from peripheral baroreceptors and chemoreceptors. It is evident that stimulation of the baroreceptors exerts inhibitory influences on respiration. A rise in blood pressure activates these stretch receptors and causes an increase in their firing rates. This sequence inhibits sympathetic tone, exaggerates vagal cardiac effects and inhibits respiration.[11] The chemoreceptors, in contrast, have a positive effect on the medullary respiratory center and when stimulated will enhance respiratory drive. The influence of chemical changes at the carotid chemoreceptors increases respiratory frequency and depth, while the response to stimulation of the aortic chemoreceptors is primarily an increase in frequency only.[15]

In experiments involving electrical recordings from single chemoreceptor nerve fibers, enhanced firing is elicited by decreased pO_2, increased H^+, or increased pCO_2.[11,16] This suggests that the same receptor may be sensitive to all three stimuli. The precise mechanism of receptor activation is unclear, but it is not due simply to depolarization shifts, since lowered pO_2 depolarizes and increased pCO_2 hyperpolarizes nerve fibers.[17] It has been proposed that the nor-

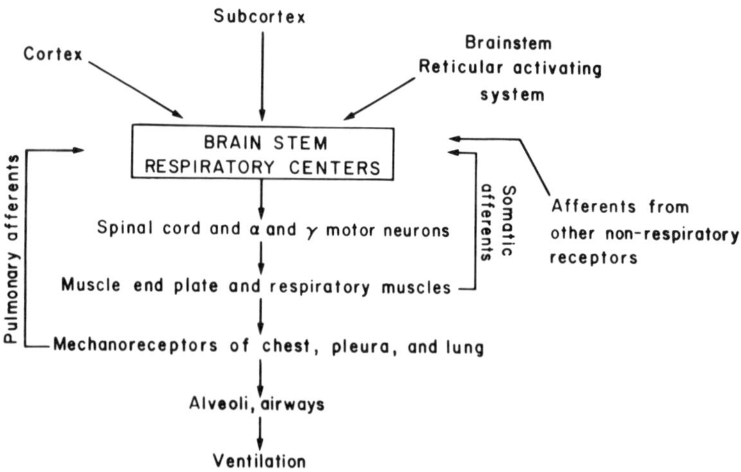

Figure 3. Outline of afferent and efferent paths converging on and leaving the brain stem respiratory centers.

mal physiologic mediator of chemoreceptor activation is acetylcholine, although there is no evidence that it plays the primary role.[18] Since the chemoreceptor is comprised of a number of different cell types, it is possible that acetylcholine plays a neurotransmitter role between one subunit and another, for instance from glomus or sustentacular cells to the firing neuron.[19]

When the vagus nerves are cut, the pneumotaxic center is freed and breathing characteristically becomes slower and deeper. The chest assumes a position of partial inspiration and the respiratory cycle is interrupted by pauses at the end of both inspiration and expiration. In spite of these effects, the actual morbidity of vagotomy relates mainly to aspiration, caused by poor swallowing coordination and the abolition of cough reflexes, rather than primary respiratory insufficiency.[20]

In addition to the neuronal connections already described, the respiratory centers receive important non-neural information via central chemoreceptors. Special receptors located on the lateral surface of the upper medulla appear sensitive to changes in central hydrogen ion concentration in the cerebrospinal fluid.[21] The relative contributions of the central and peripheral chemoreceptors to normal physiology and to pathologic conditions remain controversial although it is well established that the two inputs complement one another.[2,22] The enhanced ventilatory drive that results from increases in hydrogen ions at central receptors augments afferent signals due to hypoxia or increasing CO_2 from the periphery.[21] The situation is complicated, since CO_2 diffuses easily from arterial blood to cerebrospinal fluid and oxygen and hydrogen ions travel much slower. As a result, the central chemosensitive cells are exposed to levels of acid and oxygen quite different from the levels of these same factors in arterial blood.[23,24] This biochemical lag may be of specific pathophysiologic significance in the ventilatory abnormalities associated with metabolic encephalopathy and acidosis.[25]

EFFERENT MECHANISMS

The discussion has focused on the primary brain stem respiratory centers and the variety of converging afferent inputs that modulate this intrinsic system. Within the brain stem, the final integration of these contradictory excitatory and inhibitory impulses must occur with the result being a continually adjusting respiratory response. The efferent pathways for these alterations in respiratory response are directed from the brain stem towards the chest. The anatomy of these paths involves the spinal cord, the peripheral nervous system and the muscles of the thorax.

At the onset, it is wise to recall the observation of Hughlings Jackson that the term "respiratory muscles" suggests incorrectly an exclusive respiratory function.[26] Preferring the term "muscles of the thoracic cage" he emphasized the importance of these muscles not only for respiration, but for posture, volition, phonation and visceral-evoked acts like coughing, vomiting and defecating.

The principle inspiratory muscle is the diaphragm. It is innervated by the phrenic nerve, which is derived from cervical segments 5 through 6. Although this innervation is primarily efferent and the diaphragm is felt to have few proprioceptors, some afferent innervation is believed to exist. Through expansion and downward movement of the rib cage, the diaphragm is responsible for approximately three-fourths of normal tidal volume in man. It is not, however, the only important muscle related to inspiration, since complete diaphragmatic paralysis is not accompanied by immediate respiratory failure. The actions of the intercostals, scaleni, sternocleidomastoid, pectoralis minor and serratus posterior superior are able to maintain ventilation in resting conditions. Damage to the muscles or their peripheral nerves or roots will lead to compromised inspiratory function (Table I). In forced inspiration, the action of these muscles is further supplemented by additional muscles of the trunk, larynx, pharynx and face. Normal expiration is considered a predominantly passive act due to gravity and the elastic recoil of the lungs. In forced expiration, however, diminution in the size of the thorax may be accomplished in two ways: first, by forcing the diaphragm farther up into the thoracic cavity, a result of contracting the abdominal muscles, the external and internal oblique, the rectus and the transversalis; and second, by depressing the ribs, using the internal intercostals and triangularis sterni. In some

TABLE I
Muscles, Roots and Nerves Involved in the Phases of Respiration (Quiet expiration is felt to be muscularly passive and due to combined effects of gravity and elastic recoil of the lung tissue.)

MUSCLE	ROOT	PERIPHERAL NERVE
Quiet Inspiration		
Diaphragm	$C_{3\text{-}6}$	Phrenic
Intercostals (Ext.)	$T_{1\text{-}12}$	Intercostals
Scaleni	$C_{2\text{-}8}$	Cervical
Sternocleidomastoid	—	11th cranial nerve
Pectoralis minor	$C_{5\text{-}8}$	Anterior thoracic
Serratus p. superior	$T_{1\text{-}4}$	Intercostals
Forced Inspiration		
Intercostal (Int.)	$T_{1\text{-}12}$	Intercostals
Pectoralis major		
Facial muscles	—	7th cranial nerve
Forced Expiration		
Obliques (ext. and int.	$T_{8\text{-}11}$	Intercostals, subcostal, iliohypogastric
Transversus abdom.	$T_{8\text{-}11}$	Subcostal, iliohypogastric
Rectus abdom.	$T_{5\text{-}11}$	Subcostal
Quad. lumborum	$L_{1\text{-}4}$	Lumbar spinal nerves
Serratus p. inferior	$T_{7\text{-}11}$	Intercostal, subcostal
Triangularis sterni	$T_{7\text{-}11}$	Intercostals

cases, the iliocostalis, serratus posterior inferior and the quadratus lumborum are also recruited.[27]

Three groups of upper motor neurons converge on the anterior horn cell region.[28] The first of these originates in the inspiratory and expiratory medullary nuclei, has no apparent cortical representation, and is concerned with the mediation of involuntary rhythmic breathing. The fibers cross the midline in the region of the obex and descend in the lateral and ventral columns of the spinal cord respectively. The second group is concerned with voluntary breathing control and coordination, and lies in the corticospinal tract of the lateral columns, dorsal to the tract from the medullary centers. The cortical areas represented in this tract have been discussed. The third group is concerned with involuntary, nonrhythmic respiration reflexes (cough, hiccups) and does not appear to occupy a specific tract within the cord.[29]

Two types of cells form the lower motor neuron pool of the anterior horn. The thick α-motor neuron (12-20μm/diameter) passes through the ventral root directly to the neuromuscular junction. The γ-motor neuron has a thin efferent fiber (2-8μm/diameter) which also passes through the ventral root, but terminates in the intrafusal fibers of the muscle spindle. Coordination of these two efferent motor neurons systems is essential to normal physiologic respiratory patterns. The arc established by γ efferent-annulospiral afferent-α efferent systems provides an excellent mechanism for dealing with sudden changes in airway resistance. Compensations are made through this arc at the spinal level and operate within the duration of a single inspiration. This occurs long before changes in arterial blood gas tensions exert an effect.[30] The same spindle-servomechanisms typical of other skeletal muscles appear applicable to the respiratory system and provide unconscious data on muscle tension and stretch.[31-33]

CONCLUSIONS

It is clear that normal respiratory function depends on a nervous system whose central and peripheral circuitries are intact. While the primary brain stem respiratory centers control automatic respiration, integration occurs at multiple levels with cortical, brain stem, spinal and peripheral inputs. Coordination of impulses generates the rhythms of respiration with a continual feedback inhibition to alternating antagonistic nuclei and muscle groups. Disruption of this system in the form of neurologic disease can be effected at any level. Both structural disruption of functioning pathways and metabolic or toxic interference with neural integration can yield respiratory patterns that are therapeutically important to identify. The consequences of interrupting this integrated anatomy form the topics for the remaining chapters of this volume.

REFERENCES

1. Legallois, C.J.J.: *Experiences sur le principe de la vie.* Paris, D'Hautel, 1812.
2. Krogh, A.: *Comparative Physiology of Respiratory Mechanisms.* Philadelphia, University of Pennsylvania Press, 1959.
3. Gray, J.S.: *Pulmonary Ventilation and Its Physiological Regulation,* American Lecture Series 63. Springfield, Charles C. Thomas, 1950.
4. Lumsden, T.: Observations on the respiratory centers. *J. Physiol.* **57**: 354, 1922-1923.
5. Lumsden, T.: The regulation of respiration. *J. Physiol.* **58**: 81, 1923-1924.
6. Liljestrand, A.: Neural contral of respiration. *Physiol. Rev.* **38**: 691, 1958.
7. Wang, S.C., and Ngai, S.H.: Respiration coordinating mechanism of the brain stem: a few controversial points. *Ann. N.Y. Acad. Sci.* **109**: 550, 1963.
8. Wang, S.C. and Ngai, S.H.: General organization of central respiratory mechanisms: In Fenn, W.O., and Rahn, H. (eds.): *Handbook of Physiology.* Baltimore, Williams and Wilkins Co., 1964.
9. Pitts, R.F.: Organization of the respiratory center. *Physiol. Rev.* **26**: 609, 1946.
10. Cunningham, D.J.C., and Lloyd, B.B. (eds.): *Regulation of Hu man Respiration.* Oxford, Blackwell Scientific Publications, 1963.
11. Hesser, C.M.: Central and chemoreflex components in respiration during acid base displacement in the blood. *Acta Physiol. Scand.* **(Suppl. 64)**: 18, 1949.
12. Grodins, F.S.: Regulation of pulmonary ventilation. *Physiologist* **7**: 319, 1964.
13. Ingvar, D.H., and Bullow, K.B.: Respiratory regulation in sleep. *Ann. N.Y. Acad. Sci.* **109**: 870, 1963.
14. Widdicombe, J.G.: Respiratory reflexes. In Fenn, W.O., and Rahn, H. (eds.): *Handbook of Physiology.* Baltimore, Williams and Wilkins Co., 1964.
15. deBurgh-Daly, M., and Scott, M.J.: Cardiovascular responses to stimulation of carotid body chemoreceptors. *J. Physiol.* **165**: 179, 1963.
16. Biscoe, T.J., Purves, M.J., and Sampson, S.R.: Frequency of nerve impulses in single carotid body chemoreceptor afferent fibers. *J. Physiol.* **208**: 121, 1970.

17. Eyzaguirre, C., and Koyano, H.: Effects of hypoxia, hyperapnea, and pH on chemoreceptor activity. *J. Physiol.* **178**: 385, 1965.
18. Liljestrand, G.: Acetylcholine and respiration. *Acta Physiol. Scand.* **24**: 225, 1951.
19. Lambertsen, C.J.: Neurogenic factors in control of respiration. In Mountcastle, V.B. (ed.): *Medical Physiology,* Vol. 2. St. Louis, C.V. Mosby Co., 1974.
20. Tang, P.C.: Brain stem control of respiratory depth and rate in the cat. *Resp. Physiol.* **3**: 349, 1967.
21. Loescheke, H.H., and Mitchell, R.A.: Properties and localisation on intracranial chemosensitivity. In Cunningham, D.J.C., and Lloyd, B.B. (eds.): *The Regulation of Human Respiration.* Oxford, Blackwell Scientific Publications, 1963, pp. 243–256.
22. Gessell, R.: The regulation of respiration with special reference to metabolism of the respiratory center. *Am. J. Physiol.* **66**: 5, 1923.
23. Posner, J.B., and Plum, F.: Protection of CSF pH and of brain function during severe metabolic acidosis. *Trans. Am. Neurol. Assoc.* **91**: 38–43, 1966.
24. Fencl, V., Miller, T.B., and Pappenheimer, J.R.: Studies on respiratory response to disturbances of acid-base balance, with deductions concerning ionic composition of cerebral interstitial fluid. *Am. J. Physiol.* **210**: 459–472, 1966.
25. Posner, J.B., and Plum, F.: Spinal-fluid pH and neurologic symptoms in systemic acidosis. *N. Eng. J. Med.* **277**: 605–612, 1967.
26. Jackson, J.H.: Superior and subordinate centres of the lowest level. *Lancet* **1**: 476, 1895.
27. Newson Davis, J.: In Widdicombe, J.G. (ed.): *Control of the Muscles of Breathing in Respiratory Physiology.* London, Buttersworths, 1974.
28. Mitchell, R.A., and Berger, A.J.: Neural regulation of respiration. *Am. Rev. Resp. Dis.* **111**: 206–212, 1975.
29. Newsom Davis, J., and Plum, F.: Separation of descending spinal pathways to respiratory motoneurones. *Exp. Neurol.* **34**: 78, 1972.
30. Nunn, J.F.: *Applied Respiratory Physiology.* London, Buttersworths, 1977.
31. Granit, R.: *Receptors and Sensory Perception.* New Haven, Yale University Press, 1955.

32. Corda, M., von Euler, C., and Lennerstrand, G.: Proprioceptive innervation of the diaphram. *J. Physiol.* **178**: 161, 1965.
33. Aminoff, M.J., and Sears, T.A.: Spinal integration of segmental, cortical and breathing inputs to thoracic respiratory motoneurons. *J. Physiol.* **215**: 557–575, 1971.

2

RESPIRATORY DYSFUNCTION IN MOVEMENT DISORDERS

William J. Weiner, M.D. and
Harold L. Klawans, M.D.

Although extrapyramidal disease does not often produce clinically important respiratory dysfunction, abnormalities related to the respiratory system have been documented in several of these disorders. Diseases of the extrapyramidal system include Parkinson's disease, Huntington's disease, tardive dyskinesia and Wilson's disease. In addition, other movement disorders whose link to the traditional extrapyramidal system is less clear (Gilles de la Tourette's syndrome and stiff-person syndrome) have also occasionally been noted to produce respiratory dysfunction. Another idiopathic central nervous system degenerative disorder which includes extrapyramidal symptomatology is the Shy-Drager syndrome. The more widespread the central nervous system degenerative process the more likely that the brainstem respiratory centers will also be affected. Since there is no common pathophysiologic mechanism linking these widely different disorders, this chapter will review each syndrome separately with regard to the incidence, type, and mechanism of respiratory dysfunction observed.

PARKINSON'S DISEASE

The major clinical characteristics of Parkinson's disease include rigidity, tremor, bradykinesia and impaired postural reflexes. These symptoms are related to the degeneration of the substantia nigra and the subsequent loss of dopaminergic input to the striatum. Although respiratory function in Parkinson's disease has been more thoroughly investigated than respiratory dysfunction in other movement disorders, the clinical importance of respiratory dysfunction in Parkinson's disease is not a major issue. In fact, since the advent of levodopa therapy in 1969 the number of investigations reported in the medical literature related to respiratory dysfunction in Parkinson's disease has been negligible. This probably reflects the efficacy of dopaminergic therapy in ameliorating the motor symptoms of Parkinson's disease. Those reports that do exist reflect the new wave of interest in the toxicity of long-term dopaminergic therapy.

Descriptions of the respiratory problems seen in patients with Parkinson's disease often begin with a quote from the original essay on the shaking palsy wherein Parkinson described a single patient who "fetched his breath rather hard."[1] However, there was no further elaboration of this sign. It has been pointed out that several textbooks of neurology written by leading authorities (Denny-Brown,[2] Wilson,[3] Baker,[4] Grinker,[5] Brain,[6] and Merrit[7]) do not mention dyspnea as a symptom of the disease. On the other hand it is apparent in those clinical studies in which respiratory dysfunction in Parkinson disease is evaluated that there was almost always a significant percentage of patients who had abnormal respiratory function. Indeed, prior to the levodopa era it was commonly assumed that respiratory illness was one of the two major causes of death in patients with Parkinson's disease.

There have been a wide range of pulmonary dysfunction abnormalities reported in Parkinson's disease. These include lowered vital capacity, decreased forced expiratory volume, alterations in the spontaneous respiratory rhythm because the respirations are shallow or because normal deep sighing is absent, increase in total respiratory resistance, increases in the indices of poor distribution of ventilation, and weakening of cough mechanisms and unusual cough qualities.[8-12] In addition, minor alterations in arterial blood gas values have occasionally been reported, increased oxygen consumption at rest has been noted, and hypertonicity of intercostal accessory respiratory muscles has also been documented.[13-15] Despite these wide-ranging studies representing an overview of the type of pulmonary dysfunctions seen in Parkinson's disease, the actual clinical manifestation of these abnormalities is quite ill-defined.

In 1958, Nugent and colleagues[16] examined respiratory function in nine patients with Parkinson's disease after they were initially intrigued by the case of a 37-year-old woman with Parkinson's disease and dyspnea on exertion who had no pulmonary or cardiovascular disease. In their series, five of nine patients had dypsnea on mild exertion and no accompanying systemic illness to explain this symptom. There was no correlation of the dyspnea with degree of rigidity or tremor but the authors remarked that dyspnea is more common in those patients whose activities of daily living were the most impaired. Objective assessment of respiratory function in these patients revealed that the vital capacity and maximum breathing capacity in dyspneic patients was abnormal. Maximum breathing capacity in the symptomatic patients was 56 percent of predicted normal, while in the nondyspneic patients it was 92 percent of the predicted normal. The authors felt that the respiratory insufficiency was of a restrictive nature since physical examination, chest fluoroscopy, and spirograms revealed no evidence of obstruction to airflow. No anatomic evidence of abnormality in the thoracic cage or lungs was apparent to explain the restrictive deficit and they concluded that dynamic abnormalities of the respiratory musculature secondary to Parkinson's disease might contribute to the respiratory deficit. This was particularly emphasized since there was a marked contrast between high minute ventilation during exercise and limited maximum breathing capacity at rest, indicating that the restrictive deficit is not a simple mechanical problem. Mier[8] also emphasized that the pulmonary dysfunction in Parkinson's disease is a restrictive phenomenon. He also pointed out that if the restrictive element progresses, the patient may experience impairment of the cleansing function of the respiratory system and become more susceptible to infection. This tendency for repeated lower respiratory tract infection could lead to combined respiratory dysfunction with an element of obstructive emphysema appearing. Although tempted to lay the entire restrictive deficit on muscular rigidity, he also notes that patients with Parkinson's disease can perform respiratory movements quite quickly and that muscular rigidity may not explain the entire deficit. The progressive kyphosis seen in Parkinson's disease and the restrictive element that this produces is also considered a possible contributing factor to the restrictive pulmonary deficit observed.

In a further extensive evaluation of respiratory function in Parkinson disease, Neu and colleagues[9] investigated respiratory dysfunction in 23 parkinsonian patients without evidence of cardiopulmonary disease. These investigators examined ventilation at rest (tidal volume, rate, minute volume), maximal ventilatory efforts (expiratory reserve volume, inspiratory capacity, vital capacity, maximal inspiratory flow, maximal expiratory flow, maximal midtidal inspiratory pressure, maximal midtidal expiratory pressure, total range of maximal midtidal pressures), ventilatory mechanics-impedances (total respiratory resistance, total respiratory elastance), distribution of ventilation (single breath test-Fowler, time to equilibrium), inflationary tendencies (functional residual capacity, residual volume), and oxygen and carbon dioxide measurements (end-tidal CO_2 tension, arterial O_2 saturation), to evaluate respiratory function in nondyspneic Parkinson patients. The results of this investigation provided evidence that there are definite pulmonary function abnormalities present in parkinsonian patients who have no respiratory symptoms.[20,23] In addition, this study reconfirmed that there is a definite restrictive element to the pulmonary dysfunction. However, it also determined that the most widespread dysfunction was a reduction in maximal flows which was more consistently present and greater than the reduction simultaneously present in vital capacity and its subdivisions. This was interpreted as evidence of an obstructive ventilatory component to the respiratory dysfunction. In this study, degree of tremor and rigidity were closely correlated with abnormalities of vital capacity and flow rates. Although it is again tempting to correlate the restrictive elements to rigidity, the abnormalities in flow rates cannot be explained in this manner. The authors postulated that the obstructive element of the respiratory dysfunction in Parkinson's disease is the result of parasympathetic overactivity.

Lilker and Wool[10] studied pulmonary function in 21 patients with Parkinson's disease. They concluded that the major respiratory abnormalities in these patients consisted of impaired forced expiratory volume (1 second), impaired maximal midexpiratory flow rate, and impaired maximum voluntary ventilation. It was concluded that the respiratory dysfunction seen in this syndrome was related to several factors, including an abnormality of central control of respiration, a defect in extrapyramidal control of respiratory muscles, a defect in autonomic control of the tracheal bronchial tree, changes in respiratory tract secretions, and mechanical impairment of the abnormally shaped chest wall. This same study failed to find any correlation between objective assessment of pulmonary function and the degree of tremor and rigidity present. In addition, many of these patients underwent stereotaxic thalomotomy and significant improvement in degrees of tremor and rigidity were observed, but no associated improvement in pulmonary function was documented.

In the study of the effect of levodopa on respiratory function in 22 parkinsonian patients, Paulson and Tafrate[17] demonstrated that levodopa treatment results in a marked improvement in the minute ventilatory volume. They also pointed out that many parkinsonian patients have the ability to breath deeply once or twice voluntarily but that repetitive deep breathing appears to be a problem. This was relieved by levodopa administration. In this article it is noted that two patients developed a subjective feeling of shortness of breath which was associated with severe abdominal dyskinesias. This probably represents the first description of what has come to be a clear and defined syndrome of respiratory dyskinesias.[18,19] These will be discussed in more detail later in this chapter.

Postencephalitic Parkinson's Disease

Respiratory dysfunction in postencephalitic Parkinson's disease encompasses a wide range of alterations which are different than the previously described dysfunction in idiopathic Parkinson's disease. Although it may be that if patients with postencephalitic Parkinson's disease were studied in the manner just described, some of them would surely have had some of the restrictive and perhaps obstructive elements of respiratory impairment. The respiratory abnormalities described in patients who have had Von Economo's epidemic encephalitis were often of a dramatic nature and could be present in the presence or absence of postencephalitic parkinsonian features. Many of these disorders had a compulsive complex tic-like character. Woltman[20] described episodes of deep breathing, salaaming and breath holding. He cites particular instances of a child of seven who complained of being unable to "get his breath" and who at times was reported to breathe "hard and noisily," and of a child of ten whose respiratory trouble consisted of leaning backwards and taking six to ten deep breaths followed by breath holding until she became cyanotic and occasionally lost consciousness. Additional cases of hyperpnea followed by apnea, cyanosis, and loss of consciousness were reported by Wolff and Lennox.[21] Babinski and Charpentier[22] described a patient who episodically contracted the nares, breathed slowly, interrupted respiration in the inspiratory position and finally snored loudly as if dislodging a nasal plug. These dramatic descriptions of respiratory dysfunction in postencephalitic patients were also accompanied by many reports of lesser disturbances in respiratory dysfunction in these patients. In one attempt to assess the frequency of respiratory syndromes in these patients, Zeigler[23] reported that of 752 patients with epidemic encephalitis, respiratory syndromes were present in 9.3 percent. In contrast, postencephalitic Parkinson's disease was present in 78 percent.

Respiratory abnormalities were frequent enough in these postencephalitic patients that Turner and Critchley[24] were able to divide the types of respiratory disturbances into three broad categories: (1) disorders of respiratory rate, including tachypnea and bradypnea, (2) dysrhythmias, or disorders of respiratory rhythm, including breath holding, Cheyne-Stokes breathing, sighs, forced or noisy expirations and inversion of the inspiratory-expiratory ratio, (3) respiratory tics, including yawning, hiccups, spasmodic cough and sniffling. Since these early descriptions and recollections of the common respiratory sequelae of epidemic encephalitis there have been additional reports of respiratory dysfunction secondary to encephalitis in patients with postencephalitic Parkinson's disease. Kim[25] studied nine postencephalitic Parkinson's disease patients and defined a new abnormality in voluntary control of automatic respiratory function. He also noted that all the patients had rapid respiratory rates when compared to control subjects, and he observed that there was decreased variability of respiration in Parkinson's disease patients which was characterized by an absence of wavelike increases and decreases in the depth of respiration. However, the most striking abnormality which he described was the great difficulty that these patients had in voluntarily inhibiting respiratory rhythm on command. This was interpreted as indicating a degree of loss of higher control of the automatic reflex respiratory mechanisms that parallel a loss or restriction of other willed movements in Parkinson's disease.

The second category of long-term respiratory deficits in postencephalitic Parkinson's disease consists of a syndrome of hypoventilation. There have been multiple case reports similar to that reported by Garlind and Linderhold[26] in which they describe a patient with postencephalitic Parkinson's disease who developed minimal cyanosis and dyspnea on exertion. Extensive evaluation of pulmonary function revealed that the lung volume was normal, maximum breathing capacity was normal, mechanical properties of the lungs were normal, and that alveolar hypoventilation with low alveolar oxygen and high alveolar arterial CO_2 were found. In addition, inhalation of CO_2 (6.3 percent) failed to elicit a respiratory response or a sensation of dyspnea. On the other hand, a decrease in ventilation was found during 100 percent oxygen breathing and increased ventilation was found during low O_2 breathing. The case was summarized by the investigators as being an example of a postencephalitic parkinsonism with a hypoventilation syndrome characterized by arterial hypoxemia, polycythemia, hypoventilation and no or small ventilatory response to inhalation of carbon dioxide in spite of normal ability to ventilate the lungs and normal gas exchange. This disturbed regulation of ventilation was felt to be due to decreased or absent sensitivity of the chemoreceptors of the respiratory center with sparing of the remaining respiratory reflex. The etiology of this is presumed to be of a post-encephalitic nature.

Another example of respiratory dysfunction in parkinsonism occurs in the rare familial syndrome of mental depression, parkinsonism, and alveolar hypoventilation.[27,28] In the most recently reported family two identical twins were described as exhibiting lethargy, mental depression, progressive weight loss, mild parkinsonism (bradykinesia, cogwheel rigidity) and alveolar hypoventilation on a central basis.[29] Respiratory abnormalities included periods of ataxic respiration and apnea. Irregular tidal volumes and abnormal response to inhaled CO_2 were noted. Both died of respiratory failure within two years of the onset of the illness. Pathologic changes included degenerative changes in the substantia nigra, caudate nucleus, periaqueductal gray matter, pontine reticular formation, dorsal motor nucleus of X, nucleus tractus solitarius, lateral reticular formation, nucleus ambigus, and retroambigus. Both of these patients had failure of automatic ventilation with significant apnea, requiring the patients to remain alert most of the day and night. In view of the extensive area of brainstem focal gliosis, these authors postulated that the failure of automatic ventilation in these cases might be secondary to the observed pathologic changes.

HUNTINGTON'S DISEASE

Huntington's disease is a chronic degenerative disorder of the central nervous system characterized by choreiform movements and progressive mental deterioration. It commonly begins during adult life and is inherited in an autosomal dominant pattern. At autopsy there is degeneration of the small cells of the caudate nucleus and diffuse cortical atrophy.

Although the pathophysiology of the movement disorder appears to be related to altered sensitivity of striatal dopaminergic mechanisms,[30] there have been recent demonstrations that there are marked deficiencies in gama amino butyric acid (GABA) and glutamic acid decarboxylase activity in the basal ganglia of patients dying with Huntington's disease.[31,32] The exact interrelationship of basal ganglia neurotransmitter alterations in this disorder is unclear at this time. Although there are juvenile forms of the syndrome which present not with chorea but with rigidity and akinesia, there is little in the clinical literature to suggest that respiratory dysfunction is part of the clinical syndrome. There are isolated reports of juvenile Huntington's disease in which respiratory function is mentioned in relation to a discussion of dysarthria, with lack of adequate breath control (rhythm, rate) and abnormal nasal airflow being cited as contributing to decreased speech intelligibility.[33] Even the original description of the disorder by Huntington[34] does not describe any respiratory difficulty. In the first part of his essay when the discussion is focused on other types of chorea there is reference to two cases where "muscles of respiration were affected." However, clinical descriptions of Huntington's disease rarely contain any detailed description or study of pulmonary function in these patients. The description occasionally given is that the orderly sequence of innervation in breathing may be interrupted.[35] In fact, in the proceedings of a recent international symposium on Huntington's disease there was no mention at all of any respiratory dysfunction in this syndrome.[36]

There have been investigations into the cause of death in patients with Huntington's disease. The most recent survey of this type by Edmonds[37] indicated that respiratory deaths were more frequent in patients with Huntington's disease than in patients with dementia caused by other etiologies. In fact, 12 of 14 Huntington's disease patients died a respiratory death. It was proposed that the high incidence of respiratory demise was related to dysphagia and aspiration secondary to the involuntary movements affecting swallowing.

Another type of respiratory dysfunction occasionally described in anecdotal case reports are unusual episodes of apnea associated with the induction of anesthesia in patients with Huntington's disease. There appears to be nothing unusual about the clinical presentation of these patients and there is no common pharmacologic agent implicated. In one case the authors felt that thiopentone[38] was responsible, and in the other case succinylcholine,[39] for the pro-

The administration of neuroleptics occasionally induces acute dystonic posturing. This dramatic clinical syndrome is more commonly seen in adolescent and young adults early in the course of treatment. The clinical features can include opisthotonus, oculogyric crises, torticollis, retrocollis, fixed protruded tongue, inability to protrude the tongue, and axial and limb dystonic postures. The prominence and severity of the oral facial nuchal-dystonic reaction in these patients has raised speculation about whether or not this syndrome could ever produce respiratory embarassment. In fact, an early review of neuroleptic related side effects reported 23 cases of "hyperkinetic paroxysmal syndromes" which was an early descriptive term for the acute dystonic syndrome described above. These authors noted that there was often "protruding and swelling of the tongue, cyanosis, and bizarre torticollis-like cramps."[45] Other than mentioning that some of these patients became cyanotic there is no further comment on their respiratory function. In a later review of neuroleptic related neurologic syndromes it is noted that acute dystonic reactions secondary to neuroleptics may include "spasms of the respiratory muscles."[46] Recent case reports have focused on isolated laryngeal-pharyngeal dystonia as a cause of respiratory compromise. Flaherty and Lahmeyer[47] reported two patients who experienced acute respiratory distress early in the course of their treatment with haloperidol. In the first case, the patient was found "in bed making agonized gestures and noises and pointing to his throat." The patient is further described as having a normal respiratory rate, upper airway sounds, mild cyanosis and intraclavicular retractions. There was no evidence of dystonic posturing elsewhere. The second case was found "gasping in his bed, complaining that he could not breathe." He was further described as exhibiting intraclavicular retractions, stridor, and posterior neck muscle tightness. The authors felt that the acute respiratory dysfunction was related to laryngeal dystonia secondary to neuroleptic administration.

The possible role of respiratory dysfunction in the "sudden death" syndrome seen in otherwise physically healthy patients being treated with neuroleptics is the second category of respiratory dysfunction in tardive dyskinesia. Although many of these instances of sudden death remain unexplained, explanations advanced have included "sudden death" related to phenothiazines with more sedating properties, cardiac abnormalities, and asphyxiation. Since many of the autopsied cases of "sudden death" failed to reveal a cause of death, attention has focused on those cases in which asphyxiation and/or aspiration of food or gastric contents appears to be the primary finding. Plachta[48] reported seven autopsied cases of patients on neuroleptics whose sudden demise was characterized by dyspnea, apnea, cyanosis and collapse. In these cases, the common autopsy findings included gastric contents in the esophagus, pharynx, trachea, major bronchi and bronchioles. In addition, acute pneumonitis and bilateral pulmonary atelectesis was seen. It was postulated that the mechanism of aspiration and asphyxiation was related to drug-induced alterations in the function of the pharyngoesophageal and cricopharyngeal sphincters. Solomon[49] summarizes 17 additional cases of sudden death while patients were on phenothiazines in which aspiration was shown to be the cause of death at autopsy. He presents a single case of a 49-year-old male treated with fluphenazine who developed extrapyramidal symptomatology including acute dystonia followed by a parkinsonian syndrome. In addition, this patient was also reported to develop slurred nasal speech, drooling, dysphagia, and on examination was found to have absent gag reflexes, tongue deviation to the right, difficulty protruding the tongue, tongue fasiculations and absent jaw jerk. These signs were interpreted as an indication of a bulbar palsy related to the neuroleptic since the findings were transient (12 months) and disappeared entirely. This patient had considerable difficulty with choking on food, and this author postulated that this drug-related bulbar palsy might represent the mechanism of aspiration which is postulated to contribute to "sudden death" in patients on neuroleptics. It is of interest that in a very early report[50] on the clinical experience of using chlorpromazine it was noted that there was an alarming syndrome consisting of a "choking sensation in his throat, difficulty in swallowing and chewing, a thickness of the tongue and slurring speech, with occasional respiratory embarassment." No details of the neurologic examination are provided and it is unclear if these cases reported are similar to the phenothiazine-induced bulbar palsy reported by Solomon.[49] Of course it is not entirely clear that "sudden death" in patients on neuroleptics is definitely related to the neuroleptics.

The third category of respiratory dysfunction seen in tardive dyskinesia is related to actual dyskinetic movements of the face, tongue and axial musculature. This differs from the acute dystonic reactions since this form of movement disorder associated with neuroleptics is seen only after chronic exposure of the patient to these drugs. In 1971, Brandon, McClelland, and Protheroe,[46] in describing and classifying the type of facial dyskinesias seen in tardive dyskinesia, noted that the most severe cases have frequent movements which interrupt speech and respiration. The interruption of the latter may be severe enough to cause respiratory distress and cyanosis. In addition to this early report it has already been mentioned that Parkinson's disease patients treated with levodopa can also experience respiratory distress secondary to irregular respiratory muscle movements.[17] In 1978, Weiner and his colleagues[18] described four patients with respiratory dyskinesia. These four patients had acute dyspnea and chest pain due to primary neurologic disease, not cardiac or pulmonary disorders. They suffered from severe involuntary respiratory dyskinesias which resulted in an irregular respiratory rate, shortness of breath and chest discomfort. These respiratory dyskinesias occurred as one aspect of more generalized choreiform movement disorders. Three patients had neuroleptic-induced tardive dyskinesias and one had levodopa-induced dyskinesias. As a result of their ages and the nature of their complaints, some of these patients were originally thought to have cardiac and pulmonary disorders. All four of these patients with respiratory dyskinesias suffered from one of a group of choreiform disorders. This suggested that respiratory dyskinesias could be related to the same biochemical and physiologic mechanism as the choreic disorders themselves. It is generally thought that levodopa-induced dyskinesias, tardive dyskinesias and other phenomenologically similar movement disorders are related to the activity of dopamine at striatal dopamine receptor sites. In these four patients the striatum had already been altered by extrapyramidal disease, either as a primary degenerative process or secondary to drug administration and manifested by generalized abnormal movements. Respiratory dysfunction might be a different manifestation of the same pathophysiologic mechanism related to altered sensitivity of striatal dopamine receptors. This hypothesis formed the basis of the therapeutic trial in all the patients with agents known to decrease striatal dopminergic activity. Dopaminergic manipulation appeared successful in correcting the subjective discomfort and the respiratory abnormalities in all these patients. In three cases reserpine, which depletes central dopamine, was used and in one a lowered levodopa dosage was employed.

These patients all exhibited a respiratory alkalosis which was not fully compensated. In these patients metabolic compensation was not accomplished even though there was no evidence of renal disease. This lack of compensation was explained as a result of the character of the respiratory disorder. Extrapyramidal disorders, although chronic, show marked fluctuations in their severity throughout each 24-hour period. Variables that affect the degree of extrapyramidal dysfunction at any given time include therapeutic regimes, duration of the disease process and activity level. Abnormal movements related to extrapyramidal dysfunction disappear during sleep. Not unexpectedly, respiratory irregularities in these four patients fluctuated with dyskinetic body movements. When the movement was exacerbated, the respiratory abnormalities became worse. The breathing irregularity in one of these patients resolved completely during sleep. The fact that this breathing disorder is chronic but has intermittent severe exacerbations throughout the day may well account for the poor renal compensation. The importance of recognizing dyspnea and respiratory dyskinesias as a manifestation of dopaminergic striatal dysfunction was stressed in this report.

This seemingly unusual manifestation of choreatic disease is probably more frequent than first believed. There are large numbers of patients at risk for the development of this disorder and the diagnosis should be entertained in the appropriate patients who present with shortness of breath and chest discomfort. In fact, since our initial report of these four patients with respiratory dyskinesias we have seen numerous additional patients with levodopa-induced respiratory dyskinesia or respiratory dyskinesia as part of the syndrome of tardive dyskinesia.

In a dramatic and illustrative case report of a patient with severe respiratory and gastrointestinal disturbances secondary to tardive dyskinesia Casey and Rabins[51] described a potentially life-threatening dyskinesia in a 68-year-old woman. This patient, although never psychotic, was treated for many years with chlorpromazine. When the chlorpromazine was gradually reduced, severe oral facial dyskinesias, aerophagia, truncal rocking, grunting sounds, irregular respirations, and episodic retching appeared. Ten attempts to formally evaluate pulmonary function were unsuccessful because of irregular ventilatory movement patterns. Dyspnea was relieved with nasal oxygen, but the irregular breathing patterns continued. Severe retching and vomiting continued and the patient required parenteral fluid replacement. The respiratory dyskinesia and gastrointestinal disturbance were eventually controlled with the reinstitution of neuroleptic treatment. This treatment, although similar to that described previously as a treatment in respiratory dyskinesia in that it is antidopaminergic, is not usually recommended since it requires the use of the etiologic agent to treat the disorder it produces. However, in this case an unusual treatment was warranted since the respiratory and gastrointestinal disturbances were potentially life-threatening. When the patient was treated with haloperidol, a dose could be found which alleviated the severe axial chorea and at which the respiratory pattern was regular, normal blood gases were seen and no recurrent vomiting occurred. These authors concluded that tardive dyskinesia can present as respiratory distress and that the hypoxia seen in this patient was secondary to diaphragmatic dyskinesia and not to lung parenchymal disease, since blood gases became normal when the dyskinesias were controlled.

SHY-DRAGER SYNDROME

The Shy-Drager syndrome[52] is a progressive failure of autonomic function which is associated with signs of neurologic dysfunction. The syndrome includes orthostatic hypotension, anhidrosis, urinary incontinence, sexual impotence, and disturbances of voluntary movement including resting tremor, cogwheel rigidity, bradykinesia, and impaired postural reflexes. The most striking neuropathologic findings have included cell loss in the intermedolateral column of the spinal cord and multiple system atrophy of the olivo-ponto-cerebellar or striatonigral variety. Several striking respiratory difficulties have been seen in this disorder. Bannister and Oppenheimer[53] described four cases of Shy-Drager syndrome, two of whom had respiratory problems. The first case had attacks of nocturnal stridor and daytime episodes of periodic respiratory gasps resembling apneustic breathing. Their second case also had periodic inspiratory gasping. The first patient had evidence of widespread degeneration including changes in the striatum, substantia nigra, pontine nuclei, cerebellar cortex, inferior olive, and dorsal vagel nucleus; atrophy of the 9th and 10th cranial nerve nuclei; and medial vestibular nuclear loss. The second case had similar findings. They speculated that the locus ceruleus either is the so-called pneumotaxic center or is closely associated with it. They raised the possibility that the respiratory gasping that they observed is perhaps related to the degenerative pathology seen.

Lockwood[54] observed a single case of Shy-Drager in which, in addition to more typical symptoms and signs, irregular respiration and episodic dyspnea were prominent. Careful evaluation of the patient's respiratory pattern revealed that his respirations always occurred in clusters. The periods of apnea between the clusters became more prolonged during sleep (20 seconds awake to 40 seconds during sleep). The type of cluster breathing seen in this patient is said to be indicative of low pontine or high medullary destruction (infarction, bulbar poliomyelitis). In the course of studying this patient a normal ventilatory response to carbon dioxide was observed and Lockwood points out that this is in contradistinction to Plum's statement[55] that all cases of pontomedullary disease that affect respiratory patterns have a reduced response to carbon dioxide. Lockwood concludes that the abnormal respiratory pattern with normal chemoreceptor control of respiration indicates that two different populations of neurons subserve these functions and that they differ in their susceptibility to the Shy-Drager pathologic process.

An additional case with severe disturbance in respiratory rhythms in the Shy-Drager syndrome was described by Castaigne and colleagues.[56] The disturbance in respiratory rhythm consisted of multiple apneic episodes which did not appear until the Shy-Drager syndrome had been present for four years. The respiratory symptoms led to death in three months. It is of interest that pathologic study of this case revealed degenerative lesions in the substantia nigra, pontine nuclei, intermediolateral column of the spinal cord and, most intriguingly, in the locus ceruleus.

Another presentation of respiratory dysrhythmia in Shy-Drager was described by Chokroverty et al.[57] In four Shy-Drager patients who had normal respiratory patterns at rest, tilt-table studies demonstrated that as erect position was assumed, all four developed dysrhythmic breathing characterized by recurring apnea, ineffective ventilatory efforts and periods of normal respiration. In two patients the respiratory abnormalities appeared at a tilt of 30° and in the remaining two, abnormalities appeared at 60°. Apneic episodes lasted eight to 22 seconds. In addition one of the four patients had a mildly reduced ventilatory response to carbon dioxide inhalation. These authors concluded that although this newly described, periodically recurring, respiratory dysrhythmia in the erect posture might not be specific for Shy-Drager, it does reflect dysfunction of brain stem respiratory neurons.

A different mechanism of respiratory dysfunction in the Shy-Drager syndrome is reported by Israel and Marino.[58] They described a fifty-two-year-old woman with Shy-Drager syndrome who was hospitalized because of progressive dyspnea. At hospitalization the woman was described as being in moderate respiratory distress and utilizing accessory muscles of respiration. She had inspiratory wheezing over the entire thorax. Diagnostic tests revealed a flow-volume loop which showed an inspiratory plateau characteristic of upper airway obstruction and bronchoscopy revealed apposition of the vocal cords indicative of bilateral vocal cord paresis. This women developed acute respiratory failure and required emergency tracheostomy. Presumably the vocal cord paresis was secondary to brain stem degenerative changes.

The authors stressed that the clinical clues to upper airway obstruction include respiratory wheezing, stridor over the trachea, and a prolonged inspiratory phase of respiration. These unusual presentations of respiratory dysfunction in the Shy-Drager syndrome should alert physicians to be cautious of unusual sounding respiratory complaints in patients with this syndrome.

TOURETTE AND STIFF PERSON SYNDROME

The last two movement disorders in which respiratory dysfunction will be discussed are Gilles de la Tourette syndrome and stiff person syndrome. Both of these syndromes are not clearly related to extrapyramidal dysfunction. Tourette's syndrome is characterized by an age of onset between two and 15, multiple involuntary muscular and verbal tics, waxing and waning symptomatology, and chronic life-long symptoms. It is also associated with coprolalia, echolalia, and echopraxia. The role of central dopaminergic mechanisms in this disorder has received considerable attention since antidopaminergic agents (neuroleptics) are beneficial in ameliorating symptoms. In addition, there are several examples in which either chronic dopminergic antagonist treatment or chronic dopaminergic agonist treatment produced a Tourette-like syndrome.[59-61]

In an extensive review of Tourette's syndrome, Shapiro and colleagues[62] detailed the various symptomatic problems that patients experience. They noted that coughing, throat clearing and other throat noises occur in 62.4 percent of patients at some time in their illness. In addition, sniffling, snorting, expiratory hisses and noisy breathing occur in 58.6 percent of patients. They point out and caution that these symptoms are often misinterpreted as signs of allergic reaction and are frequently treated as such. However, no respiratory distress per se is indicated as being a major problem in this disorder despite the fact that stuttering and stammering reported in 22.1 percent of these patients is related by these authors to thoracic, abdominal, or diaphragmatic muscular contractions.

Stiff person syndrome is a rare clinical disorder characterized by increased muscular stiffness and involuntary spasms which was first described by Moersch and Woltman.[63] The disorder presented initially with symptoms of stiffness, tightness and rigidity of muscles and with intermittent spasms of the involved muscles. In almost all cases, there was a gradual onset with slow progression of signs and symptoms. Neurologic examination is normal except for the finding of a persistent marked increase in muscle tone. The muscle tone is most unusual and has been described as "feeling like stone." Superimposed on this increased tone are intermittent painful muscular spasms. These spasms may occur spontaneously or they may be associated with sudden noises, passive or active movement of the involved muscles, emotional upsets, or tactile stimuli. The spasms themselves are associated with increased tone, pain, tachycardia, and profuse sweating. The pattern of muscle involvement is generally proximal, usually beginning in the legs and back. The most severely affected muscles are the back and abdomen. Functional difficulties related to the increased muscle tone are reflected in severe problems of motor mobility. The face is usually spared although dysphagia may be a problem. There is no known familial incidence and the syndrome usually presents between the ages of 30 and 60. The etiology of the syndrome remains entirely unknown. Pharmacologic treatment has centered on the use of diazepam which in many instances has proven to be remarkably effective in relieving muscular spasms.

Respiratory dysfunction in these patients is not a prominent clinical problem. Moersch and Woltmann[63] in their original description of 14 cases mentioned two patients in whom spasms of thoracic muscles caused difficulty in breathing. Another patient was reported to complain of chest tightness, cough and dyspnea which was not related to exercise.[64] Another single case report also described spasms which "took the patient's breath away." In this patient clinical assessment of pulmonary function was normal.[65] Specific respiratory abnormalities reported include "spasms" of the diaphragm and lowered vital capacity, maximum breathing capacity and minute volume.[66-68] Gordon and colleagues summarized the respiratory abnormalities reported in stiff person syndrome by stating that "tonic rigidity of muscles of respiration may produce ventilatory restriction and dyspnea."[69] The suggestion has been made that with progression of the stiff person syndrome, respiratory difficulties become more prominent and become the source of fatalities in this illness.[70]

SUMMARY

This chapter has reviewed respiratory dysfunction in Parkinson's disease, Wilson's disease, Huntington's disease, tardive dyskinesia, Tourette's syndrome, stiff person and Shy-Drager syndrome. Additional comments on the effects of myoclonus on respiratory function can be found in the respiratory reflex chapter.

REFERENCES

1. Parkinson, J.: *An Essay on the Shaking Palsy.* London, Sherwood, Neel, and Janer, 1817.
2. Denny-Brown, D.: *Disease of the Basal Ganglia* (Oxford Loose-Leaf Medicine). New York, Oxford University Press, 1946.
3. Grinker, R.R., and Bucy, P.C.: *Neurology.* Springfield, Ill., Charles C Thomas, 1949.
4. Brain, W.R.: *Disease of the Nervous System.* London, Oxford University Press, 1951.
5. Wilson, S.A.K.: In Bruce, A.N. (ed.): *Neurology,* 2nd ed. Baltimore, Williams and Wilkins Co., 1955.
6. Baker, A.B.: *Clinical Neurology.* New York, Hoeber-Harper, 1955.
7. Merritt, H.H.: *A Textbook of Neurology,* 4th ed. New York, Lea and Febiger, 1967.
8. Mier, M.: Mechanisms leading to hypoventilation in extrapyramidal disorders with special reference to Parkinson's disease. *J. Am. Geriat. Soc.* **15**: 230–238, 1967.
9. Neu, H.C., Connolly, J.P., Schwestley, F.W., Lodwig, H.A., and Brody, A.W.: Obstructive respiratory dysfunction in parkinsonian patients. *Am. Rev. Resp. Dis.* **95**: 33–47, 1967.
10. Lilker, E.S., and Woolf, C.R.: Preliminary functions in parkinson syndrome. *Canad. Med. Assoc. J.* **99**: 752–757, 1968.
11. Bendall, M.J.: Parkinsonism with a bovine cough: on unusual presentations. *Br. Med. J.* **2** (2): 981–982, 1976.

12. Grewel, F.: Dysarthria in postencephalitic parkinsonism. *Acta Psych. Scand.* **32**: 440–449, 1957.
13. Mier, M., Boshes, B., and Canter, G.: Studies in parkinsonism. VIII. Arterial blood gas analysis: Some aspects of its relationship to clinical manifestations. *Quart. Bull. Northwestern Univ. Med. School* **34**: 226–231, 1960.
14. Richter, K., Hagemann, P., and Albert, M.: *Psychiat. Neurol. Med. Psychol. (Leipzig)* **13**: 125, 1961.
15. Delhez, L., and Petit, J.M.: *Rev. Franc. Etud. Clin. Biol.* **6**: 580, 1961.
16. Nugent, C.A., Hanes, H., Cohn, J., Smith, C.C., and Tyler, F.: Dyspnea as a symptom in parkinson syndrome. *Am. Rev. Tuberculosis Pub. Dis.* **78**: 682–691, 1958.
17. Paulson, G.D., and Tatrate, R.H.: Some "minor" aspects of parkinsonism, especially pulmonary function. *Neurology* **20**: 14–17, 1970.
18. Weiner, W.J., Goetz, C.G., Nausieda, P.A., and Klawans, H.L.: Respiratory dyskinesias: Extrapyramidal dysfunction and dyspnea. *Am. J. Intern. Med.* **88**: 327–331, 1978.
19. Weiner, W.J. and D. Bergen: Prevention and management of the side effects of levodopa. In Klawans, H.L. (ed.): *Clinical Neuropharmacology,* Vol. 2. New York, Raven Press, 1977.
20. Woltman, H.W.: Encephalitis: historical review and perspective. *Canad. Med. Ass. J.* **77**: 995–1000, 1957.
21. Wolf, H.F. and Lennox, W.G.: Encephalitic respiratory sequelae with periods of unconsciousness and convulsions. *J. Nerv. Ment. Dis.* **68**: 337–354, 1928.
22. Babinski, J., and Charpentier, A.: Syndrome parkinsonien fruste postencehpalitique: troubles respiratoires. *Rev. Neurol.* **38**: 1369–1377, 1922.
23. Ziegler, L.H.: Follow-up studies on persons who have had epidemic encephalitis. *J.A.M.A.* **91**: 138–141, 1928.
24. Turner, W.A., and Critchley, M.: Respiratory disorders in epidemic encephalitis. *Brain* **48**: 72–104, 1925.
25. Krum, R.: The chronic residual respiratory disorder in postencephalitic parkinsonism. *J. Neurol. Neurosurg. Psychiat.* **31**: 393–398, 1968.
26. Garlind, T., and Linderhold, H.: Hypoventilation syndrome in a case of chronic epidemic encephalitis. *Acta Med. Scan.* **102**: 333–349, 1958.
27. Perry, T.L., Bratty, P.J.A., Hansen, S., et al: Hereditary men-

tal depression and parkinsonism with taurine deficiency. *Arch. Neurol.* **32**: 108–113, 1975.

28. Perry, T.L.: Hereditary mental depression with taurine deficiency; further studies, including a therapeutic trial of taurine administration. In Huxtable, R., and Barbeau, A. (eds.): *Taurine.* New York, Raven Press, 1976.
29. Purdy, A., Hohn, A., Barnett, H.J.M., Bratty, P., Ahmad, D., Lloyd, K.G., McGeer, E.G., and Perry, T.L.: Familial fatal parkinsonism with alveolar hypoventilation and mental depression. *Ann. Neurol.* **6**: 523–531, 1979.
30. Weiner, W.J., and Klawans, H.L.: Cholinergic-monoaminergic interactions within the striatum. Implications for choreiform disorders. In Butcher, L. (ed.): *Cholinergic-Monoaminergic Interactions in the Brain: Basic Mechanisms and Clinical Implications.* New York, Academic Press, 1978, pp. 335–362.
31. Perry, L., Hansen, S., and Kloster, M.: Huntington's chorea—Deficiency of y-aminobutyric acid in brain. *N. Eng. J. Med.* **288**: 337–342, 1973.
32. Bird, E.D., and Iversen, L.L.: Huntington's chorea-postmortem measurement of glutamic acid decarboxylase, choline acetyltransferase and dopamine in basal ganglia. *Brain* **97**: 457–472, 1974.
33. Hansotia, P., Cleeland, C.S., and Chun, R.W.: Juvenile Huntington's chorea. *Neurology* **18**: 217–224, 1968.
34. Huntington, G.: On chorea. *Medical and Surgical Reporter* **26**: 317–321, 1872.
35. Wilson, S.K.: *Neurology.* London, Buttersworths and Co., 1940.
36. Chase, T.N., Wexler, N.S., and Barbeau, A. (eds.): *Huntington's Disease* (Advances in Neurology, Vol. 23). New York, Raven Press, 1979.
37. Edmonds, C.E.: Huntington's chorea, dysphagia and death. *Med. J. Anesthesiolog.* 273–274, 1966.
38. Davies, D.D.: Abnormal response to anesthesia in a case of Huntington's chorea. *Br. J. Anesth.* **38**: 490–491, 1966.
39. Gicolander, W., and Banbanti, G.: Un caso de apnea prolungota in corea de Huntington. *Acta Anaesth.* (Padova) **19**: 235–238, 1968.
40. Walshe, J.M. (Cambridge University, Cambridge, England): Personal communication, 1979.
41. Scheinberg, I.H. (Albert Einstein College of Medicine, N.Y.): Personal communication, 1979.

42. Cartwright, G.E. (University of Utah, Salt Lake City): Personal communication, 1979.
43. Steinlieb, I., Bennett, B., and Scheinberg, I.H.: D-penicillamine-induced Goodpasture's syndrome in Wilson's disease. *Ann. Intern. Med.* **82**: 673–676, 1975.
44. Klawans, H.L., and Weiner, W.J.: The pharmacology of choreatic movement disorders. In Kerkut, G.A., and Phillips, J.W. (eds.): *Progress in Neurobiology.* Oxford, Pergamon Press, 1975, pp. 1–32.
45. Hoefner, H., Heyden, B., and Kutreber, I.: Undesirable side effects and complications with the use of neuroleptic drugs. *Int. J. Neuropsychiat.* **1**: 46–58, 1965.
46. Brandon, S., McClelland, H.A., and Protheroe, C.: A study of focal dyskinesias in a mental hospital population. *Br. J. Psychiat.* **118**: 171–184, 1971.
47. Flaherty, J.A., and H.W. Lahmeyer: Laryngeal-pharyngeal dystonia as a possible cause of asphyxia with haloperidol treatment. *Am. J. Psych.* **135**: 1414–1415, 1978.
48. Plachta, A.: Asphyxia relatively inherent to tranquilization. *Arch. J. Psychiat.* **12**: 152–158, 1965.
49. Solomon, K.: Phenothiazine-induced bulbar palsy-like syndrome and sudden death. *Am. J. Psychiat.* **134**: 308–311, 1977.
50. Molitz, S., P.H. Hoch, and S. Lesse: A two year evolution of chlorpromazine in clinical research and practive. *Am. J. Psych.* **113**: 540–546, 1956.
51. Casey, D.E., and P. Robini: Tardive dyskinesia as a life-threatening illness. *Am. J. Psychiat.* **135**: 486–488, 1978.
52. Shy, G.M., and Drager, G.A.: A neurological syndrome associated with orthostatic hypotension. *Arch. Neurol.* **2**: 511–527, 1960.
53. Bannister, R., and Oppenheimer, D.: Degenerative diseases of the nervous system associated with autonomic failure. *Brain* **95**: 457–474, 1972.
54. Lockwood, A.H.: Shy-Drager syndrome with abnormal respiration and anti-diuretic hormone release. *Arch. Neurol.* **33**: 292–295, 1976.
55. Plum, F.: Neurological integration of behavioral and metabolic control of breathing. In Porter, R. (ed.): *Breathing: Hering-Breuer Centenary Symposium.* London, J. & A. Churchill, Ltd, 1970, pp. 159–181.
56. Castaigne, P., Laplane, D., Autret, A., Bousser, M.G., Gray, F., and Baron, J.C.: Syndrome du Shy et Drager avec troubles

de rythme respiratoire et de la vigilance. *Dev. Neurol.* **133**: 455–466, 1977.
57. Chokroverty, S., Sharp, J.T., and Barron, K.D.: Periodic respiration in erect posture in Shy-Drager syndrome. *J. Neurol. Neurosurg. Psychiat.* **41**: 980–986, 1978.
58. Israel, R.H, and Marino, J.M.: Upper airway obstruction in the Shy-Drager syndrome. *Ann. Neurol.* **2**: 83, 1977.
59. Golden, G.S.: Gilles de la Tourette's syndrome following methylphenidate administration. *Dev. Med. Child Neurol.* **16**: 76–78, 1974.
60. Klawans, H.L., Falk, D.K., Nausieda, P.A., and Weiner, W.J.: Gilles de la Tourette's syndrome after long-term chlorpromazine therapy. *Neurology* **28**: 1064–1068, 1978.
61. Bremner, A.B.: Methylphenidate-induced Tourette's syndrome. *Am. J. Psychiat.* **136**: 1334–1335, 1979.
62. Shapiro, A.K., Shapiro, E.S., Brun, R.D. and Sweet, R.D. (eds.): *Gilles de la Tourette's Syndrome.* New York, Raven Press, 1978.
63. Moersch, F.P., and Woltman, H.W.: Progressive fluctuating muscular rigidity and spasm (stiff-man syndrome). *Proc. Staff Meet. Mayo Clin.* **31**: 421, 1956.
64. Stuart, F.S., Henry, M., and Holley, H.L.: The stiff-man syndrome. Report of a case. *Arithrit. Rheumat.* **3**: 229, 1960.
65. Werk, E.E., Sholiton, L.J., and Marnell, R.T.: The stiff-man syndrome and hyperthyroidism. *Am. J. Med.* **31**: 647–653, 1961.
66. Brage, D.: Stiff-man syndrome. *Rev. Clin. Espan.* **72**: 30, 1959.
67. Howard, F.M.: A new and effective drug in the treatment of stiff-man syndrome. *Proc. Staff Meet. Mayo Clin.* **38**: 203, 1963.
68. Olafson, R.A., Mulden, D.W., and Howard, F.M.: Stiff-man syndrome. *Proc. Staff Meet. Mayo Clin.* **39**: 131, 1964.
69. Gordon, E.E., Jonuszko, D.M., and Kaufman, L.: A critical survey of stiff-man syndrome. *Am. J. Med.* **42**: 582–599, 1967.
70. Campbell, J.R.: Stiff-man syndrome and emphysema. *Arch. Neurol.* **36**: 387–388, 1979.

3

NEUROLOGICAL INFECTIONS AND RESPIRATORY DYSFUNCTION

Larry E. Davis, M.D., David L. Jackson, M.D., Ph.D., and Barbara Gothe, M.D.

INTRODUCTION

Infections of muscle and the nervous system not infrequently result in respiratory dysfunction. Many of these infections result in respiratory failure secondary to respiratory muscle weakness. Occasionally changes in lung parenchyma can be caused by a central nervous system infection. The etiological agents responsible for the respiratory dysfunction range from viruses to metazoites. Potential sites for pathologic involvement of respiratory function secondary to infection range from respiratory (skeletal) muscles through neuromuscular junction, peripheral motor nerves, spinal cord, to the brain itself. Table I outlines the pathological sites, giving examples of infections of the nervous system that cause damage at each of these sites. We will describe the pathological processes at each anatomical site and the different infections which are involved. Emphasis will be placed on clinical presentation, diagnostic methodology, pathogenetic mechanism, type of respiratory dysfunction encountered, and therapeutic approaches, both to the infection as well as the respiratory complications.

Supported by the Research Service Veterans Administration, U. S. Public Health Service.

TABLE I
Neurological Infections and Respiratory Dysfunction

ANATOMICAL SITE	INFECTIOUS AGENT	DISEASE
MUSCLE	Trichinella spiralis	Trichinosis
	Coxsackie A virus	Viral myositis
NEUROMUSCULAR JUNCTION	Clostridium botulinum	Botulism
	Dermacenter andersonii	Tick paralysis
PERIPHERAL NERVE	Corynebacterium diphtheriae	Diphtheritic polyneuritis
	Varicella-zoster virus	Diaphragmatic shingles
	Viral immunizations	Guillain Barré syndrome
SPINAL CORD	Poliovirus	Paralytic poliomyelitis
	Clostridium tetani	Tetanus
	Schistosoma mansoni	Spinal cord schistosomiasis
	Mycobacterium tuberculosis	Pott's paraplegia
BRAINSTEM AND	Poliovirus	Bulbar poliomyelitis
CEREBRAL CORTEX	St. Louis encephalitis virus	Encephalitis
	Influenza B virus	Reye's syndrome
	Neisseria meningitis	Noncardiac pulmonary edema

Respiratory dysfunction can be defined as any abnormality, with or without prior lung disease, that results in abnormalities in gas exchange, specifically oxygen transfer and/or changes in ventilation. The respiratory system consists of the upper and lower airways, the lungs, respiratory muscles, and a complex control system. Each of these structures can be affected directly or indirectly by neuromuscular disorders. Oxygen transport to the tissues and removal of CO_2 also require adequate circulation and sufficient hemoglobin in the red cells.

Gas exchange is not the only function of the lung. Nonrespiratory functions include protection of the organism from the potential adverse effects of inhaled noxious agents. The upper airways, particularly the nose, play an important role in cleaning and humidifying inhaled air. Cough reflex, mucociliary clearance system and humoral cellular defense systems are other protective mechanisms against damage or infection in the lung. The lower airways below the vocal cords are sterile under normal conditions as a result.

Respiratory complications in the course of infection of the nervous system result from primary injury to the lung, from disease of the respiratory muscles, or from a combination of both. Disorders of respiratory control may also occur, but seem less important clinically. At worst, respiratory or ventilatory failure occurs, characterized by hypoxemia and/or carbon dioxide retention requiring mechanical ventilation.

Infections of the neuromuscular system can damage the respiratory system at various sites, but most complications are directly or indirectly related to dysfunction of the respiratory muscles. Secondary changes of the lung may follow, such as atelectasis, shallow breathing pattern and ventilation-perfusion inequalities. Respiratory complications in neuromuscular disease may be caused by: (1) muscle weakness or paralysis leading to breathing pattern abnormalities, ineffective cough, ventilation/perfusion inequalities and hypoxemia; (2) dysfunction of the upper airway, i.e., loss of protective reflexes, such as the gag reflex, leading to recurrent aspiration; (3) loss of muscle tone of the upper airway (which is usually more pronounced during sleep) causing upper airway obstruction and apnea during sleep; (4) disturbances in coordination between respiratory movements of the chest wall and opening of the upper airway; and (5) disturbances in respiratory control. Breathing involves voluntary and automatic control mechanisms. Each may be disturbed and disorders may be consistently present or occur only during sleep or wakefulness.

EVALUATION OF RESPIRATORY DYSFUNCTION

Physical Examination

Clinical symptoms may be nonspecific and therefore early dysfunction of the respiratory system might not be recognized. Shortness of breath is a clue, but this may be absent at rest and present only during physical exertion. Other symptoms may be present and should be sought, such as morning headache (indicating respiratory difficulties during sleep), aspiration, cough, and postural dyspnea. Physical examination may also be quite nonspecific. Tachypnea is a common finding in many patients with respiratory dysfunction, but is not always present. Physical examination of the lungs is usually normal, unless underlying lung disease is present. Asynchrony of breathing movements is an important finding, when present. Strength of respiratory muscles can also be estimated at the bedside by measurement of tidal volume and forced vital capacity as well as cough and sniff maneuvers (see below).

Arterial Blood Gases

The single most important laboratory test is evaluation of an arterial blood gas sample. Hypoxemia or an increase in the oxygen (A-a) gradient are sensitive indicators of abnormal gas exchange. Hypoxemia is most often related to primary pulmonary disease, involving the airways, the pulmonary parenchyma and/or the pulmonary vascular bed. Respiratory muscle weakness can lead to decreased tidal volume and decreased functional residual capacity with progressive small airway collapse. This decrease in FRC leads to decreased compliance and thus a decreased tidal volume, initiating a potentially vicious cycle. This tendency is often more pronounced in the supine position. This sequence of events can lead to acute respiratory failure, with hypercarbia and respiratory acidosis.

Pulmonary Function Tests

Standard pulmonary function tests, PFT's (spirometry, lung volumes, diffusing capacity) can be used at the bedside or in the clinical laboratory to assess respiratory function. These tests, however, do not differentiate between abnormal lung function and abnormal respiratory muscle function. In addition, they require the cooperation and coordination by the patient. Weakness of the respiratory muscles leads to a decrease in vital capacity, maximum negative inspiratory force, and often total lung capacity. Position changes from sitting to supine may result in substantial differences in vital capacity and blood gases, particularly in patients with diaphragmatic paralysis. Maximal voluntary ventilation is often decreased with respiratory muscle weakness, but expiratory flow rates are normal unless airways or lung disease is present. At the bedside, the measurement of maximal negative inspiratory force is a useful estimate of muscle strength. Vital capacity, peak flow rates and maximal inspiratory pressure measurements are also easily done at the bedside and can be used to follow the clinical course of patients with respiratory muscle weakness secondary to CNS infection.

Other tests to assess respiratory muscle function, which are not routinely available but which can be useful in individual patients, are magnetometry, electromyogram (EMG) of the respiratory muscles, and determination of transdiaphragmatic pressures. Magnetometers are applied to the surface of the chest and abdomen to measure changes in diameter with breathing. They can be calibrated to translate diameter changes into lung volume changes. The advantages of this device or of strain gauges taped to the chest and abdomen are that breathing patterns can be monitored noninvasively and without use of a mouthpiece over long periods of time. They permit determination of those muscles primarily involved in generating the respiratory effort and pattern for a given patient. They can assess whether or not chest and abdominal respiratory movements are in synchrony. Applied during respiratory monitoring with magnetometers or strain gauges and thermistors at the nose or mouth they can obtain evidence of apneas during sleep.

The EMG can be measured with surface or needle electrodes. The record can be analyzed not only to detect respiratory muscle fatigue, but also to diagnose neuromuscular dysfunction.

Transdiaphragmatic pressure can be measured via small lumen balloon-tipped catheters placed in both the stomach and esophagus. Clinically, this determination is rarely necessary, but it may be extremely useful in certain patients.

Tests of Respiratory Control

Chemosensitivity is measured by determining the ventilatory response to changes in both pCO_2 and pO_2. The negative pressure generated by the inspiratory muscles against an occluded airway at the initiation of a breath is relatively independent of pulmonary mechanical factors and has been used as a measure of CNS respiratory drive and muscle strength. Assessment of respiratory control mechanisms can serve as an early warning sytem to detect or prevent adverse effects, when lung and/or respiratory muscle function are compromised by a physiological response to any stimulus that depresses respiratory activity.

Sleep Studies

Normally during sleep respiration is reduced. Arterial pCO_2 increases despite diminished CO_2 production and arterial pO_2 falls. When respiratory function is compromised during wakefulness, the additional reduction in ventilation with sleep may lead to overt respiratory failure. Worsening of respiratory function and significant changes in blood gases during sleep are often seen in patients with diaphragmatic paralysis. Monitoring of respiration, oxygen saturation and heart rate during sleep is therefore important. One can monitor electroencephalogram (EEG) temporal muscle eye movements, EMG (to determine sleep "stages"), oxygen saturation, breathing movements of chest and abdomen, airflow at the mouth, and EKG.

Management of Respiratory Complications

The management of respiratory complications during infections of the neuromuscular system depends on the cause and degree of respiratory dysfunction. Treatment of secondary infection of the lungs and airways includes selection of appropriate antibiotics, chest physiotherapy, and bronchodilator therapy. Judicious fluid balance, maintaining the patient relatively intravascularly volume depleted, is mandatory in the presence of neurogenic pulmonary edema. Adequate oxygenation should be maintained by correcting anemia, if present, and by supplemental oxygen to maintain oxygen saturation above 90 percent. Drugs which depress respiratory activity should be avoided when respiratory function is severely compromised. Ventilatory support is necessary, when vital capacity and maximal negative inspiratory force are rapidly falling, when arterial pO_2 cannot be maintained without toxic levels of inspired oxygen, when significant respiratory acidosis is present or when the patient seems exhausted from the work of breathing clinically.

SECONDARY CHANGES IN LUNG PARENCHYMA AND NONCARDIOGENIC PULMONARY EDEMA

The lung responds to a variety of insults with a nonspecific pathologic response pattern, the most serious complication being noncardiogenic pulmonary edema. Clinically, the onset may be rapid. Patients complain of dyspnea and may appear anxious with cyanosis. They are often tachypneic and tachycardiac. Bronchial breath sounds and rales are noted on physical examination. Arterial blood gases reveal hypoxemia and a respiratory alkalosis. The chest x-ray may show an alveolar filling pattern and may progress to a complete white-out of the lung with air bronchograms. The cardiac/thoracic ratio is normal. Central venous pressure is normal or low. Pulmonary artery pressure usually is low and pulmonary wedge pressure typically is normal or low, in sharp contrast to classical cardiogenic pulmonary edema. This clinical picture is the "final common pathway" of a wide variety of desperate processes, including shock, renal failure, trauma, and sepsis. Histopathologic studies show diffuse alveolar damage which can progress to frank necrosis of the alveolar and capillary membranes. An early change is an increase in interstitial fluid with a mild to moderate inflammatory cellular reaction. Whatever the inciting event, there is marked leakage of plasma into the alveolar space. The protein-rich edema fluid, which can be hemorrhagic, may appear in large airways or the mouth. Later in the course, one sees a proliferation of Type II alveolar epithelial cells, and fibrosis of the interstitium may follow. Permanent pulmonary damage may persist, although some patients recover completely and show no residual functional impairment. In some cases the pulmonary edema may be caused solely by primary central nervous system processes, i.e., "neurogenic" pulmonary edema. It has also been reported in patients with bacterial meningitis with sepsis.

The association between CNS damage (trauma) and pulmonary edema was first recognized clinically by Montier in 1918. Neurogenic pulmonary edema has been produced experimentally in animals by intracisternal injection of fibrin, blunt cranial trauma, electrolyte lesions in the hypothalamus and marked rapid increases in CSF pressure. Pretreatment of the animals with CNS depressants (phenobarbital, chloral hydrate, ether) or pretreatment with adrenergic blockers ameliorates the development of pulmonary edema. Increases in systemic blood pressure, central venous pressure and pulmonary arterial and venous pressures are seen. The rise in pulmonary arterial and venous pressure is transient and short-lived. It usually cannot be demonstrated in patients, although one recent case report seems to indicate that the same sequence of events seen in animal experiments can occur in man.

The available evidence suggests that the disorder is mediated by the sympathetic nervous system. The CNS triggers a massive activation of the sympathetic nervous system initially causing marked peripheral vasoconstriction. Adrenalectomy does not alter this sequence. Therefore, the increase in adrenergic activity appears to be centrally mediated within minutes of the inciting insult and the marked increase in systemic vascular resistance leads to a shift in blood volume from high (systemic) to low (pulmonary) resistance vascular beds. This in turn leads to an increase in hydrostatic pressure with damage/rupture of pulmonary capillaries. The resulting abnormal pulmonary capillary permeability persists and is responsible for the clinical picture of noncardiac pulmonary edema (Adult Respiratory Distress Syndrome).

PRIMARY ALTERATIONS IN SKELETAL MUSCLES

The primary respiratory muscles include the diaphragm and intercostal muscles. Accessory respiratory muscles include the sternocleidomastoid, scalenius, and abdominal muscles. A number of infectious agents directly affect skeletal muscles. In general, respiratory muscles are damaged in proportion to damage of other skeletal muscles. They are only infrequently involved to such an extent that there is interference with normal respiratory function. Nevertheless, occasionally diseases, like trichinosis, and rarely viruses, like Coxsackie A virus, may significantly alter the function of respiratory muscles.

Trichinosis

Most patients with trichinosis are asymptomatic. When overt illness occurs, there is usually a two to three day incubation period after ingestion of undercooked meat containing the encysted larvae. The early intestinal stage is marked by cramping abdominal pain, diarrhea, and fever. Several days later, muscle aches, weakness, periorbital and facial edema and headache may develop. Respiratory muscle infection commonly occurs. Patients may complain of pleuritic pain and rarely experience respiratory distress from weakness of respiratory muscles.

Trichinella spiralis is a helminth which is ingested as encysted larvae in the undercooked muscles of infected pigs, bears, and other carnivorous wild animals. In the United States, case clusters of trichinosis have been reported after ingestion of infected pork sausage and bear meat. On reaching the small intestine, larval *T. spiralis* rapidly grow and mate, producing offspring larvae. These larvae penetrate the mucosa of the small intestine giving rise to symptoms of the intestinal stage. The larvae become dispersed throughout the body via the blood stream and primarily invade skeletal muscles. Muscles of the diaphragm, chest, and limbs are those most commonly infected. Within the muscle, the larvae grow, cause an inflammation (myositis) and begin encysting after three weeks. By six to 12 months calcification of the cysts begins. Muscle biopsies often show pale swollen muscle fibers that microscopically demonstrate coiled worms within a muscle fiber surrounded by edema, lymphocytes, and eosinophils (Fig. 1).

Acutely, the typical patient presents with eosinophilia and elevated muscle enzymes (serum creatinine phosphokinase and aldolase). Three weeks into the clinical illness, positive serologic tests for trichinosis develop. Serologic tests include latex agglutination, bentonite flocculation, and complement fixation tests. Treatment with thiabendazole in dosage of 25 mg per kg, twice daily for seven days, has resulted in apparent improvement in severe cases and should be considered in patients who develop respiratory distress. Patients can develop angioedema, urticaria, and myocardial

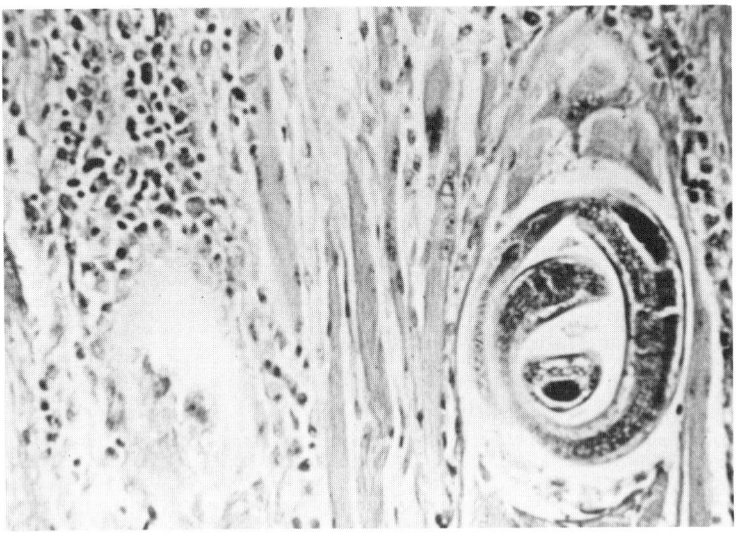

Figure 1. Muscle biopsy from a patient with severe trichinosis. Larva of *T. spiralis* is seen surrounded by inflammatory cells in adjacent muscle.

or central nervous system involvement. These patients may benefit from steroid therapy (prednisone 20 to 60 mg per day). Mild cases require no treatment, but analgesics often reduce the pain associated with breathing. Prevention of infection can be accomplished by heating the infected meat to 60°C or freezing it to −15° for 20 days.

INFECTIONS AFFECTING THE NEUROMUSCULAR JUNCTION

Blockage of synaptic transmission across the neuromuscular junction most commonly leads to clinical weakness of limb or eye muscles. However, as the synaptic transmission block progresses, dysphagia with bulbar weakness and respiratory muscle weakness develop. Two infectious agents, *Clostridium botulinum* and *D. andersonii,* commonly can cause respiratory muscle weakness which may require mechanically assisted respiration. In both entities, it is the toxin released by the organism, rather than the organism itself, that causes the neuromuscular blockade.

Botulism

In most instances, botulism is due to an intoxication following ingestion of preformed botulism toxin produced by the *C. botulinum.* One to several days after ingestion of the toxin, the patient complains of dizziness, dry mouth, diplopia, dysphonia, dysphagia, and weakness. Early in the clinical course, neurological examination will reveal loss of visual accommodation and weakness of the palatal, extraocular, and facial muscles. Later, weakness of the extremities and impairment of the muscles of respiration may occur (Fig. 2). Autonomic involvement can be seen with paralytic ileus and urinary retention reported in most reported epidemics. At least 50 percent of affected patients require mechanically assisted ventilation. Recovery is slow, and patients may require prolonged respiratory support.

Serotypes A, B, or E are most commonly involved in human outbreaks of *C. botulinum* illness. The organism is anaerobic. Most often the toxin is produced in improperly home-canned meats and vegetables that initially contained

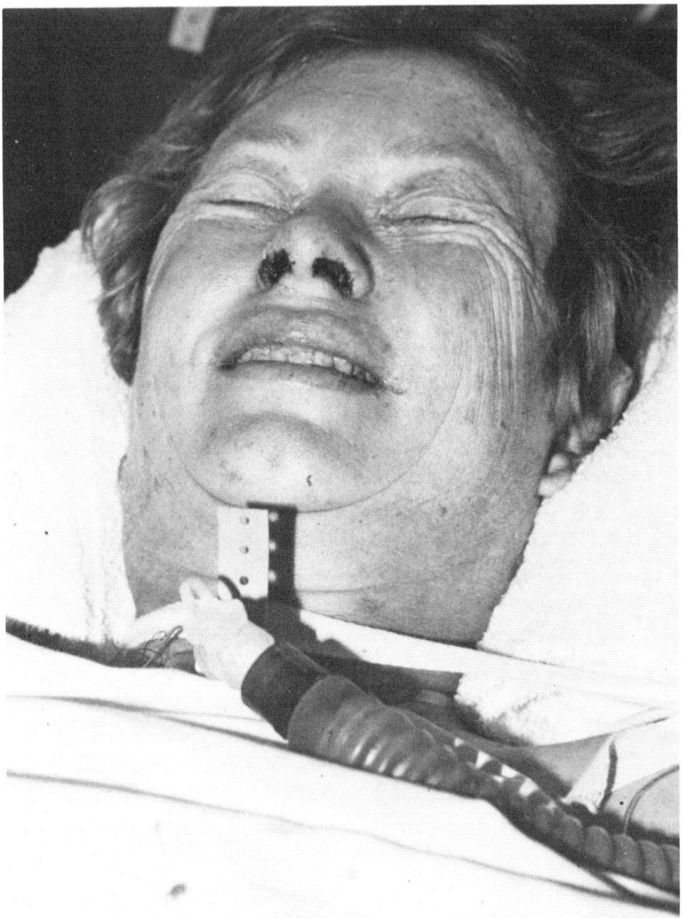

Figure 2. Woman with severe botulism type A poisoning. She is attempting to grimace and has weakness of facial, palatal, extraocular, and respiratory muscles. She required ventilatory assistance for several months before making a complete recovery.

the spores. Commercially canned foods have also been reported rarely to contain botulinum toxin. The toxin is both tasteless and odorless. It is unstable, and can be denatured by heating to 100°C for a few minutes or 60°C for 30 minutes. Thus, cooking contaminated foods usually destroys the toxin. In a few cases *C. botulinum* has been cultured from skin lesions. Children less than six months of age may develop an infection of the gastrointestinal tract with *in vivo* production and absorption of the toxin. These infants present as "floppy" infants with constipation.

The diagnosis of botulism is best made on clinical grounds and a history of eating home-canned foods should be vigorously sought. This diagnosis should be especially strongly considered, if several individuals present in rapid succession with descending weakness and respiratory difficulties. Confirmation of the diagnosis can often be made by submission of refrigerated, but not frozen, acute serum, stool specimens, and suspected food samples to the State Health Department or the Center for Disease Control (Atlanta, Ga.)

Treatment should be directed at removing unfixed toxin from the gastrointestinal tract by cathartics and inactivating circulating toxin with polyvalent type A, B, E botulism antitoxin. This can be obtained on request from any State Health Department. Penicillin should also be given to prevent replication of any viable *C. botulinum* organisms within the gastrointestinal tract that might have been ingested with the toxin. Any patient who develops significant difficulties in swallowing, clearing secretions, or breathing, should be intubated and placed on assisted respiration. Because of the long course of the respiratory paralysis, a tracheostomy is usually required.

Tick Paralysis

Tick paralysis is a disease occasionally seen in the southern and western parts of the United States during the spring and summer. It usually occurs in girls or males with long hair, where the tick can attach to the back of the head or neck and persist for several days unnoticed. The female wood tick, *Dermacenter andersonii,* is most commonly implicated in the United States, while *Iodes holocyclus* is the vector in Australia. The tick apparently releases an unidentified toxin that has been shown, for *I. holocyclus,* to block neuromuscular transmission. The involved individual typically develops a progressive motor weakness that leads to respiratory insufficiency. Clinically, the patients often resemble those with Guillain-Barré syndrome. Finding engorged ticks, usually in scalp hair, and their removal results in recovery within hours to a few days.

INFECTIONS THAT DAMAGE PERIPHERAL NERVE

There are several infections that can result in damage to peripheral motor nerves which can lead to respiratory muscle weakness. These infections usually cause generalized weakness as well as respiratory weakness. Accurate diagnosis and therapy usually result in total recovery.

Diphtheritic Polyneuropathy

This disease results in unimmunized individuals who develop oral, pharyngeal, or cutaneous infections with toxigenic *Corynebacterium diphtheriae.* Typically, patients develop an acute pharyngitis two to five days after exposure and colonization. As many as 50 percent of these patients will develop the classical finding of an adherent grayish pseudomembrane in the posterior pharynx. This pseudomembrane can cause acute upper airway obstruction requiring emergency tracheostomy.

The subsequent polyneuritic complications are a direct result of exotoxins produced by the toxogenic organisms. These complications are not clearly related to the severity of initial pharyngeal involvement. Most *C. diphtheritic* infections are due to non-toxin producers. These infections do not lead to motor weakness or respiratory failure. Neurologic and cardiac complications may occur as late as six weeks following the episode of acute pharyngitis. Characteristically, the patient's speech becomes nasal and he/she complains of dysphagia and clearing secretions. Facial weakness and varying degrees of limb and respiratory muscle weakness can be seen. Potentially lethal myocardial toxicity can also occur.

The occasional patient who develops a dermatological infection from *C. diphtheria* commonly presents with a picture similar to that seen with the Guillain-Barré syndrome. The exotoxin produced by *C. diphtheria* inhibits protein synthesis. The initial involvement of cranial nerves is likely due to the retrograde transport of the toxin along nerve fibers. The toxin causes demyelination of peripheral nerves (Fig. 3). Secondarily, conduction of nerve impulses are blocked. Since the axon itself is not destroyed, recovery occurs when the toxin is catabolized and remyelination restores the conduction of electrical impulses.

The diagnosis can be made in the acute pharyngitic stage by culture of *C. diphtheria* from the throat on special media, such as Loeffler's or tellurite. Cultures will occasionally (but less frequently) be positive in the diphtheric polyneuropathy stage. Treatment should be aimed at eradication of the organism with penicillin or erythromycin and neutralization of the toxin by administration of diphtheria

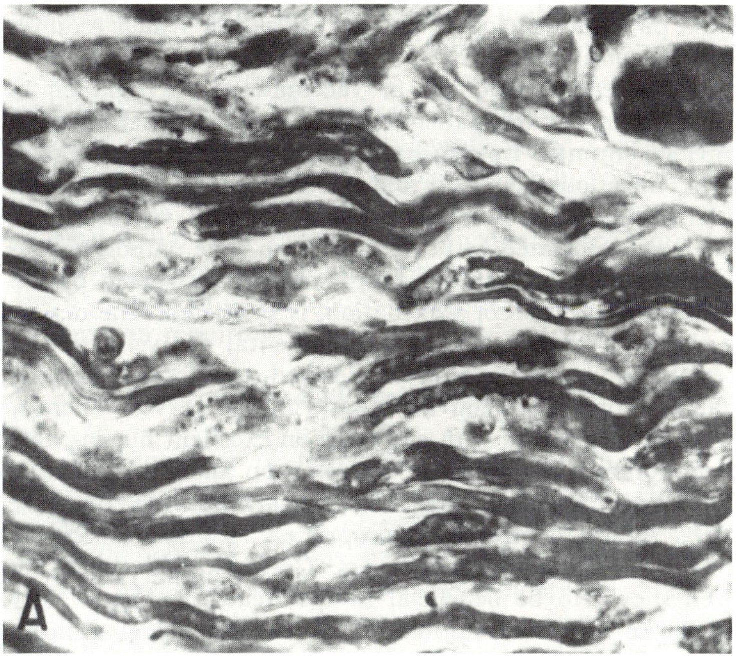

Figure 3. Lower cervical nerve from a patient with fatal diphtheric polyneuritis demonstrating active segmental demyelination with degenerating myelin sheaths. (Reproduced with permission from Fisher, C.M., and Adams, R.D.: Diphtheritic polyneuritis—a pathological study. *J. Neuropath. Exp. Neurol.* **15**:243–268, 1956.

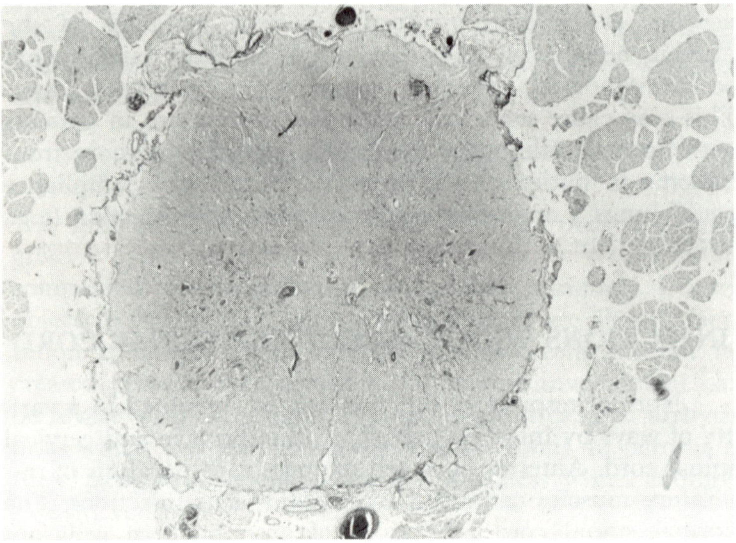

Figure 4. Histologic section of thoracic spinal cord from a patient with fatal poliomyelitis. The ventral horns show perivascular cuffing, edema, and marked loss of anterior horn neurons.

Infrequently in patients with respiratory dysfunction, only one or both sides of the thorax and/or diaphragm may be involved. Involvement of the abdominal muscle can result in a weak cough and difficulty in clearing pulmonary secretions. In bulbar poliomyelitis, involvement of the respiratory center in the medulla and paralysis of pharyngeal muscles can lead to aspiration and respiratory impairment. The latter causes upper airway obstruction from pooled secretions. Respiratory failure can develop rapidly in the course of poliomyelitis. Occasionally the vasomotor center is involved resulting in episodic hypertension, tachycardia, and even neurogenic pulmonary edema.

The diagnosis is based on clinical findings, an abnormal CSF (20 to 300 WBC/mm^3, elevated protein and normal glucose), and isolation of one of the three polio virus serotypes from the throat, stool, or, rarely, even CSF. There is no specific treatment for the viral infection. Efforts should be aimed at supporting respiration, circulation, and preventing subsequent complications. Patients with mild clinical involvement have an excellent chance for complete recovery. Patients with severe respiratory muscle weakness may never recover normal respiratory function and require mechanical respiratory assistance indefinitely.

A small group of patients who recover from severe poliomyelitis develop respiratory insufficiency years later. These patients often experience exertional dyspnea, respiratory tract infections, peripheral cyanosis to cold, headaches, depressions, and inability to concentrate. In one study, these patients tended to have kyphoscolioses and diaphragmatic paralysis. Pulmonary function studies typically demonstrated reduced vital capacity, normal FEV_1 values, normal arterial PO_2, elevated arterial pCO_2, and evidence of ventilation/perfusion imbalance.

Tetanus

Unlike the majority of infections of the nervous system that result in respiratory muscle dysfunction, tetanus causes not weakness, but rather severe forceful spasms of the respiratory muscles. This disrupts normal respiratory patterns and can cause respiratory failure. Early symptoms include irritability, headache, and low grade fever. In generalized tetanus, the patient develops spasms of the masseter muscles (lockjaw), spasms of facial muscles (risus sardonicus), spasms of somatic musculature (opisthotonos), board-like rigidity of the abdomen (Fig. 5), and respiratory muscle spasms. The spasms are acute, paroxysmal, widespread, repetitive, painful, and exhausting, as they often continue for many days.

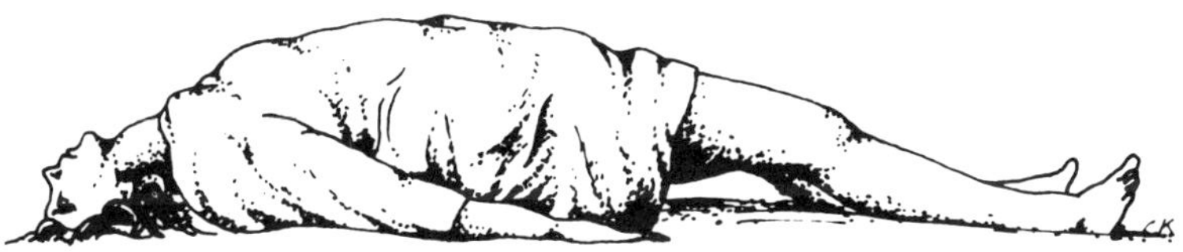

Figure 5. Drawing of opisthotonos in a patient with tetanus. Associated muscle spasms can cause respiratory insufficiency.

Hypoventilation, hypoxia, and even sudden death from respiratory arrest can follow a paroxysm of these spasms.

Tetanus results from production of tetanal toxin (tetanospasmin) by replicating *Clostridium tetani* organisms. This anaerobic organism is most often present in wound infections. The exotoxin acts on central nervous system by a mechanism similar to that of strychnine. It directly suppresses the inhibitory influences on motor neurons without directly enhancing synaptic excitatory activity. There is evidence that the toxin inhibits Renshaw cell activity in the spinal cord. This decrease in inhibitory influences on the alpha motor neuron pool leads to increased activity in these anterior horn cells.

The diagnosis is usually made on clinical grounds. In approximately one-third of clinically affected patients, *C. tetani* can be cultured from the suspected infection site. Treatment should be directed at removing the source of the tetanospasmin, neutralizing the circulating toxin and supporting the patient until the toxin that is fixed to the nervous system is metabolized. Thus, the wound should be adequately and thoroughly drained, debrided, and irrigated with three percent hydrogen peroxide. High-dose intravenous penicillin is the antibiotic of choice. Intramuscular administration of tetanal human immune globulin (3,000 units) should be given as soon as the diagnosis is clinically established. Supportive care is critically important. The patient should be placed in a quiet room with continuous nursing care. In severe cases, respiratory dysfunction from the frequent muscle spasms can significantly interfere with adequate respiration. These patients should be treated with muscle relaxants, such as diazepam or meprobamate. The optimal dosage required to minimize the spasms varies and must be titrated for each patient. Diazepam should be given intravenously, often requiring more than 100 mg over 24 hours to suppress the spasms. Supplemental oxygen, tracheostomy, and even assisted ventilation may be required to ventilate the patient adequately, especially if high doses of muscle relaxants cause respiratory depression.

Tetanus toxoid should also be administered to prevent future attacks. Tetanus only rarely develops in individuals who have received two or more injections of tetanus toxoid in the past.

Spinal Cord and Epidural Abscesses

Respiratory weakness occasionally results from localized infections involving the cervical and upper thoracic spinal cord. This can be caused either by direct parenchymal infection of the cord or secondarily by pressure effects from an extramedullary abscess. Throughout the world, tuberculosis of the vertebral column (Pott's disease) remains an important cause of kyphosis paraplegia and respiratory dysfunction. The lesion often starts as osteomyelitis of the thoracic vertebral body, sparing the disc space. Destruction of the vertebral body leads to collapse and secondary kyphosis. A paravertebral abscess can form, causing both spinal cord compression as well as a focal meningomyelitis. This combination can produce irreversible ischemic damage to the spinal cord. Occasionally bacteria, especially anaerobic species, can produce an acute epidural abscess or vertebral osteomyelitis (destroying disc space early) that can damage the spinal cord by similar mechanisms. Both of these infections are treatable, if therapy is begun before infarction occurs.

Primary parenchymal infections of the upper spinal cord are rare, but can be caused by a variety of organisms. Helminthic infections, such as cysticercosis and schistosomiasis, can cause cystic granulomas of the spinal cord. Primary spinal cord bacterial infections include tuberculosis (tuberculomas), syphilis (gummas), and anaerobic bacterial abscesses. Viral infections, such as varicella-zoster, can cause a myelitis that corresponds to the dermatomal involvement seen in shingles. Postinfectious myelitis has also been reported following rubeola, mumps, EB virus (infectious mononucleosis), and rabies vaccination.

These infections can cause respiratory dysfunction which varies with the level of spinal cord involvement. If the upper thoracic spinal cord is involved, intercostal muscle paralysis can result. If the upper cervical cord is affected, both diaphragmatic and intercostal muscles can be paralyzed, leading to acute respiratory failure. These lesions typically also cause limb paresis, spasticity, and sensory loss below the level of spinal cord involvement. Urinary and fecal incontinence is also common. Depending on the extent of the spinal cord injury, the impairment of these functions can be either partial or complete.

Diagnosis of spinal cord or epidural abscess must be made as rapidly as possible, as many lesions are reversible if treated early. The clinical signs and symptoms indicate the approximate level of the lesion. Spinal x-rays can suggest Pott's disease, etc. A myelogram more precisely localizes the lesion and can aid in distinguishing intramedullary spinal cord lesions from extramedullary lesions. Combining metrizamide contrast with computerized tomographic scanning of the vertebral column may provide an even more detailed picture of the anatomic localization of the lesion. Surgical decompression with appropriate cultures of the lesion is usually the indicated therapy for all early extramedullary lesions as well as certain intraparenchymal lesions. Appropriate antimicrobial therapy is also necessary. Prognosis from these lesions is often poor. However, functional recovery can occur, if surgical decompression is accomplished before the spinal cord is irreversibly damaged.

INFECTIONS WHICH AFFECT BRAINSTEM AND CEREBRAL CORTEX

Infections of the brainstem and cerebrum can potentially cause respiratory dysfunction through several different mechanisms. These include direct damage to the medullary respiratory center, paralysis of lower cranial nerves leading to aspiration pneumonia, coma with secondary respiratory depression and induction of noncardiac pulmonary edema.

The respiratory center is located in the reticular formation of the medulla and caudal pons. No infections have been recognized that selectively involve only this area. However, in epidemic encephalitis lethargica, described by Von Economo in 1917, it is likely that the respiratory center was involved, as many patients in the chronic stage had hiccups, respiratory tics, and disorders of respiratory rate and rhythm.

Infectious involvement of the brainstem can cause bulbar musculature weakness. Thus, patients with bulbar poliomyelitis have difficulties in swallowing and clearing secretions. This can lead to airway obstruction and aspiration pneumonia.

Infections of the cerebrum and meninges can produce coma with secondary respiratory depression. Coma can develop secondary to a diffuse parenchymal process (meningioencephalitis) or be related to an abscess with localized mass effect causing herniation with brainstem damage. Viral infections, such as western equine encephalitis, St. Louis encephalitis, herpes simplex encephalitis, etc., can cause diffuse parenchymal damage and inflammation sufficient to produce coma. Reye's syndrome is a postviral syndrome in children, occasionally seen following infections especially with influenza A, influenza B, and varicella-zoster viruses. The clinical setting is characterized by a combination of fatty liver degeneration, cerebral edema, and coma, often associated with respiratory insufficiency. In Reye's syndrome, respiratory function improves as intracranial pressure normalizes and consciousness returns. Therapy has generally been aimed at supporting vital functions, particularly respiration, and attempting to control the increased intracranial pressure until spontaneous recovery occurs.

Brain abscesses can be caused by many infectious organisms. They are often associated with either a distant primary infection (e.g., subacute bacterial endocarditis) or a parameningeal focus (e.g., otitis or sinusitis). They can create a sufficient mass effect to cause herniation of the brain through the tentorium or enough pressure on the brainstem from a posterior fossa/cerebellar mass to cause coma and respiratory depression. The abscess may contain aerobic bacteria (*Staphylococcus aureus, Proteus, Pseudomonas, Mycobacterium tuberculosis,* etc.), anaerobic bacteria (*Bacterioides, Clostridium, alpha streptococcus,* etc.), fungi (*actinomycetes, aspergillus,* etc.) or parasites (cysticercosis, echinococcosis, etc.). Such localized infections can also be found in the meninges. Subdural empyema occasionally produces coma by similar mechanisms. The diagnosis of a cerebral abscess, particularly in the posterior fossa, may be difficult. These patients will often present with headache and then develop focal neurological signs that can progress to coma with associated respiratory failure. The CAT scan and radionuclide brain scan have been shown to be sensitive tests for diagnosis and localization of brain abscess. Treatment most often requires surgical drainage of the abscess plus administration of appropriate antimicrobial agents. Recently there have been case reports of cure for cerebral abscesses by nonsurgical/medical therapy. If the mass effect of the abscess has caused herniation, the prognosis is obviously much worse.

Diffuse infections of the meninges, such as bacterial meningitis, can occasionally cause the syndrome of inappropriate antidiuretic hormone with fluid retention and dilutional hyponatremia. Such infections can also be complicated by noncardiac pulmonary edema (adult respiratory distress syndrome).

BIBLIOGRAPHY

I. *General*

1. Davis, J.N., Loh, L., and Casson, M.: The effects of respiratory muscle weakness on the pattern of breathing. *Acta Neurol. Belg.* **76**:291–292, 1976.
2. McCredre, M., Lovejoy, F.W., and Kaltreeder, N.: Pulmonary function in diaphragmatic paralysis. *Thorax* **17**:213–217, 1962.
3. Von Euler, C.: On the neural organization of the motor control of the diaphragm. *Rev. Resp. Dis.* **119**:45–50, 1979.
4. Newsom-Davis, J.: The diaphragm and neuromuscular disease. *Ann. Rev. Resp. Dis.* **119**:115–117, 1979.
5. Gibson, G.J., and Pride, N.B.: Lung mechanics in diaphragmatic paralysis. *Ann. Rev. Resp. Dis.* **119**:119–120, 1979.

II. *Trichinosis*

1. Brashear, R.E., Martin, R.R., and Glores, J.L.: Trichinosis and respiratory failure. *Am. Rev. Resp. Dis.* **104**:245–248, 1971.
2. Davis, M.J., Cilo, M., Plaitakis, A., and Yahr, M.D.: Trichinosis: Severe myopathic involvement with recovery. *Neurol.* **26**:37–40, 1976.
3. Most, H.: Trichinosis: Preventable yet still with us. *N. Engl. J. Med.* **298**:1178–1180, 1978.
4. Schantz, P.M., Juranek, D.D., and Schultz, M.G.: Trichinosis in the United States, 1975. *J. Infect. Dis.* **136**:712–715, 1977.

III. *Botulism*

1. Arnon, S.S., Midura, T.F., Clay, S.A., Wood, R.M., and Chen, J.: Infant botulism. Epidemiological, clinical and laboratory aspects. *J.A.M.A.* **237**:1946–1951, 1971.

2. Cherington, M.: Botulism, 10-year experience. *Arch. Neurol.* **30**:432–437, 1974.
3. Gangarosa, E.J., Donadio, J.A., Armstrong, R.W., et al.: Botulism in the United States, 1899–1969. *Am. J. Epid.* **93**:93–101, 1971.
4. Kao, I., Drachman, D.B., and Price, D.L.: Botulinum toxin: Mechanism of presynaptic blockade. *Science* **193**:1256–1258, 1976.
5. Koenig, M.G., Drutz, D.L., Mushlin, A.I., et al.: Type B botulism in man. *Am. J. Med.* **42**:208–219, 1967.

IV. *Tick Paralysis*

1. Abbot, K.H.: Tick paralysis I, II. *Proc. Staff Mayo Clinic.* **18**:39–45, 59–64, 1943.
2. Cherington, M., and Snyder, R.D.: Tick paralysis. Neurophysiologic studies. *N. Eng. J. Med.* **278**:95–97, 1968.
3. Cooper, B.J., and Spence, I.: Temperature-dependent inhibition of evoked acetylcholine release in tick paralysis. *Nature* **263**:693–695, 1976.
4. Stanbury, J.B., and Huyek, J.H.: Tick paralysis, a critical review. *Medicine* **24**:219–242, 1945.

V. *Diphtheritic Polyneuritis*

1. Fisher, G.M., and Adams, R.D.: Diphtheritic polyneuritis—a pathological study. *J. Neuropath. Exp. Neurol.* **15**:243–268, 1956.
2. Gaskill, H., and Korb, M.: Occurrence of multiple neuritis in cases of cutaneous diphtheria. *Arch. Neurol. Psych.* **55**:559–572, 1946.
3. McDonald, W.I., and Kocen, R.S.: Diphtheritic neuropathy. In Dyck, P.J., Thomas, P.K., and Lambert, E.H. (eds.): *Peripheral Neuropathy,* Vol. II. Philadelphia, W.B. Saunders Co., 1975, pp. 1281–1299.
4. Naiditch, M.J., and Bower, A.G.: Diphtheria: A study of 1433 cases observed during a ten-year period at the Los Angeles County Hospital. *Am. J. Med.* **17**:229–245, 1954.
5. Pleasure, D.E., Feldmann, B., and Prockop, D.J.: Diphtheria toxin inhibits the synthesis of myelin phospholipid and basic proteins by peripheral nerve *in vitro*. *J. Neurochem.* **20**:81–90, 1973.
6. Todesco, J.M.: Diphtheritic diaphragmatic analysis treated in box respirator. *Lancet* **1**:261, 1942.

VI. *Guillain Barré Syndrome*

1. Dowling, P.C., Menonna, J.P., and Cook, S.D.: Guillain Barré Syndrome in greater New York-New Jersey. *J.A.M.A.* **237**: 317–318, 1977.
2. Hewer, R.L.: Acute polyneuritis requiring artificial respiration. *Quart. J. Med.* **37**:479–491, 1968.
3. Palk, B.V.: Cardiopulmonary complications of Guillain Barré Syndrome. *Heart Lung* **5**:967–970, 1976.
4. Rice, D.: Landry-Guillain-Barré syndrome: Personal experience of acute ascending paralysis. *Br. Med. J.* **1**:1330–1332, 1977.
5. Rosen, A.D., and Vastula, F.F.: Clinical effects of cyclophosphamide in Guillain Barré polyneuritis. *J. Neurol. Sci.* **30**:179–187, 1976.

VII. *Varicella Zoster*

1. Anderson, J.P., and Keal, E.E.G.: Cervical herpes zoster and diaphragmatic paralysis. *Br. J. Dis. Chest* **63**:222–226, 1969.
2. Halpern, S.L., and Covner, A.H.: Motor manifestations of herpes zoster. Report of a case of associated permanent paralysis of phrenic nerve. *Arch. Int. Med.* **84**:907–916, 1949.

VIII. *Poliomyelitis*

1. Affeldt, J.E., Whittenberger, J.L., Mead, J., and Ferris, B.G.: Pulmonary function in convalescent poliomyelitic patients. II. The pressure-volume relations of the thorax and lungs of chronic respiratory patients. *N. Eng. J. Med.* **247**:43–47, 1952.
2. Bodian, D., and Horstmann, D.M.: Polio virus. In Horsfall, F.L., and Tamm, I. (eds.): *Viral and Rickettsial Infections of Man,* 4th ed., Philadelphia, J.B. Lippincott Co., 1965, pp. 430–473.
3. Bourdillon, R.B., Davis-Jones, E., Stoh, F.D., and Taylor, L.M.: Respiratory studies in paralytic poliomyelitis. *Br. Med. J.* **2**:539–547, 1950.
4. Faerber, J., Liebert, P.B., and Suskind, M.: Loss of functional residual capacity in poliomyelitis. *J. Appl. Physiol.* **17**:289–292, 1962.
5. Ferris, B.G., Whittenberger, J.L., and Cyfeldt, J.E.: Pulmonary function in convalescent poliomyelitic patients. I. Pulmonary subdivisions and maximum breathing capacity. *N. Eng. J. Med.* **246**:919–923, 1952.
6. Lane, D.J., Hazleman, B., and Nichols, P.J.R.: Late onset respiratory failure in patients with previous poliomyelitis. *Quart. J. Med.* **43**:551–568, 1974.

7. Lukas, D.S., and Plum, F.: Pulmonary function in patients convalescing from acute poliomyelitis with respiratory paralysis. *Am. J. Med.* **12**:388–396, 1952.

IX. *Tetanus*

1. Brooks, V.B., Curtis, D.R., and Eccles, J.C.: The action of tetanus toxin on the inhibition of motor neurones. *J. Physiol.* **135**:655–672, 1957.
2. Heurich, A.E., Brust, J.C.M., Richter, R.W.: Management of urban tetanus. *Med. Clin. N. Am.* **57**:1373–1381, 1973.
3. Tempero, K.F.: The use of diazepam in the treatment of tetanus. *Am. J. Med. Sci.* **5266**:5–12, 1973.
4. Weinstein, L.: Tetanus. *N. Eng. J. Med.* **289**:1293–1296, 1973.

X. *Spinal Cord Abscess*

1. Apt, W.L., Fierro, J.L., Calderon, C., Perez, C., and Mujica, P.: Vertebral hydatid disease. Clinical experience with 27 cases. *J. Neurosurg.* **44**:72–76, 1976.
2. Baker, A.S., Ojemann, R.G., Swartz, M.N., and Richardson, E.P.: Spinal epidural abscess. *N. Eng. J. Med.* **293**:464–468, 1975.
3. Bergofsky, E.H.: Mechanism for respiratory insufficiency after cervical cord injury. *Ann. Intern. Med.* **61**:435, 1964.
4. Cameron, G.S., Scott, J.W., Jousse, A.T., and Boterell, E.H.: Diaphragmatic respiration in the quadriplegic patient and the effect of position on his vital capacity. *Ann. Surg.* **141**:451, 1955.
5. Cheshire, D.J.: Respiratory and metabolic management of acute tetraplegia. *Paraplegia* **1**:1–23, 1966.
6. Fugl-Meyer, A.R.: Effects of respiratory muscle paralysis in tetraplegic and paraplegic patients. *Scand. J. Rehab. Med.* **3**:141, 1971.
7. Hancock, D.O.: A study of 49 patients with acute spinal extradural abscess. *Paraplegia* **10**:285–288, 1973.
8. Heusner, A.P.: Non-tuberculosis spinal-epidural infections. *N. Eng. J. Med.* **239**:845–853, 1948.
9. Hodgson, A.R., Skinsness, O.F., and Leong, C.Y.: The pathogenesis of Pott's paraplegia. *J. Bone Joint Surg.* **49**:1147–1156, 1967.
10. Kokkola, K., Moller, K., and Lehtonen, T.: Pulmonary function in tetraplegic and paraplegic patients. *Ann. Clin. Res.* **7**:76–79, 1975.
11. Marcial-Rojas, R.A., and Fiol, R.E.: Neurologic complications of schistosomiasis. *Ann. Int. Med.* **59**:215–230, 1963.

12. Roy, R.N., Bhattacharya, M.B., Chatterjee, B.P., and Pal, N.C.: Spinal cysticercosis. *Surg. Neurol.* **6**:129–131, 1976.
13. Slade, H.W., and Glazer, N.: Extramedullary spinal tuberculoma. *J. Pediat.* **46**:288–295, 1955.
14. Mortala, J.P., and Sant'Ambrogio, G.: Mechanics of breathing in tetraplegics. *Ann. Rev. Resp. Dis.* **119**:131–134, 1979.

XI. *Brainstem and Cerebral Cortex*

1. Black, P., ct al.: Penetration of brain abscess by systemically administered antibiotics. *J. Neurol. Sci.* **38**:705, 1973.
2. DeLouvois, H.V., Gortvai, P., and Hurley, R.: Bacteriology of abscesses of the central nervous system: A multicentre prospective study. *Br. Med. J.* **2**:981–983, 1977.
3. Editorial: Metabolic abnormalities in Reye's syndrome. *Lancet* **2**:183–184, 1976.
4. Farmer, T.W., and Wise, G.R.: Subdural empyema in infants, children and adults. *Neurol.* **23**:254–261, 1973.
5. Galbraith, J.G., and Barr, V.W.: Epidural and subdural empyema. *Adv. Neurol.* **6**:257–267, 1974.
6. Gode, G.R., Raju, A.V., Jay, A.L.A.K., Shomi, T.S., et al.: Intensive care in Ralxes Therapy. *Lancet* **2**:6–8, 1976.
7. Latovitzia, N., Abrams, G., Clark, C., et al.: Cerebral cysticercosis. *Neurol.* **28**:838–842, 1978.
8. Mickell, J.J., Cook, D.R., Reigel, D.H., et al.: Intracranial pressure—monitoring in Reye-Johnson syndrome. *Crit. Care. Med.* **4**:1–7, 1976.
9. Powell, K.E., and Blakey, D.L.: St. Louis encephalitis. *J. A. M. A.* **237**:2294–2298, 1977.
10. Van Alphen, H.A.M., and Dressen, J.J.R.: Brain abscess and subdural empyema. *J.N.N.P.* **39**:481–490, 1976.
11. Victor, M., and Banker, B.Q.: Brain abscess. *Med. Clin. N. Am.* **47**:1355–1370, 1963.
12. White, J.C., Sweet, W.H., and Richardson, E.P.: Cysticercosis cerebri—A diagnostic and therapeutic problem of increasing importance. *N. Eng. J. Med.* **256**:479–486, 1957.

XII. *Adult Respiratory Distress Syndrome: Non-Cardiac Pulmonary Edemas*

1. Gelb, A.F., and Klein, E.: Hemodynamic and alveolar protein studies in non-cardiac pulmonary edema. *Am. Rev. Resp. Dis.* **114**:831–835, 1976.
2. Hopewell, P.C., and Murray, J.F.: The adult respiratory distress syndrome. *Ann. Rev. Med.* **27**:343–356, 1976.

3. Robin, E.D.: Capillary leak syndrome with pulmonary edema. *Arch. Int. Med.* **130**:66–71, 1972.
4. Petty, T.: The adult respiratory distress syndrome (confessions of a "lumper"). *Am. Rev. Resp. Dis.* **111**:713–715, 1975.
5. Shanies, H.M.: Non-cardiogenic pulmonary edema. *Med. Clin. N. Am.* **61**:319–357, 1977.
6. Staub, N.C.: Pulmonary edema. *Physiol. Rev.* **51**:, 1974.
7. Stoler, B.S., and Davis, R.S.: Corticosteroids in postinfluenzal adult respiratory distress syndrome. *J. Ken. Med. Assoc.* **75**:367–371, 1977.
8. Teplity, C.: The core pathobiology and integrated medical science of adult acute respiratory insufficiency. *Surg. Clin. N. Am.* **56**:1091–1133, 1976.

XIII. *Diagnosis and Treatment of Respiratory Failure*

1. Aidinis, S.J., Lafferty, J., and Shapiro, H.M.: Intracranial responses to PEEP. *Anaesthesiol.* **45**:275–286, 1976.
2. Bone, R.C.: Compliance and dynamic characteristics curves in acute respiratory failure. *Crit. Care Med.* **9**:173–179, 1976.
3. Buscoe, W.A., Smith, J.P., Bergofsky, E., et al.: Catastrophic pulmonary failure. *Am. J. Med.* **60**:249–258, 1976.
4. Cotev, S., Peral, A., Katzenelson, R., et al.: The effect of PEEP on oxygenating capacity in acute respiratory failure with sepsis. *Crit. Care Med.* **4**:186–192, 1976.
5. Davis, H.L.: Acute respiratory insufficiency. *Adv. Intern. Med.* **19**:213–238, 1974.
6. Douglas, M.E., and Downs, J.B.: Pulmonary function following severe acute respiratory failure and high levels of positive end-expiratory pressure. *Chest* **71**:18–23, 1977.
7. Downs, J.B., Douglas, M.E., Ruiz, B.C., et al.: Comparison of assisted and controlled mechanical ventilation in anesthetized swine. *Crit. Care Med.* **7**:5–8, 1979.
8. Feely, R.W., and Hedley-Whyte, J.: Weaning from controlled ventilation and oxygen. *N. Eng. J. Med.* **292**:903–906, 1975.
9. Goldring, R.M., Heinemann, H.O., and Turino, G.M.: Regulation of alveolar ventilation in respiratory failure. *Am. J. Med. Sci.* **269**:160–170, 1975.
10. Hansen, J.E., and Simmons, D.H.: Error in the determination of blood pCO_2. *Am. Rev. Resp. Dis.* **115**:1061, 1063, 1977.
11. Henning, R.J., Shubin, H., and Weil, M.H.: The measurement of the work of breathing for the clinical assessment of ventilation dependence. *Crit. Care Med.* **5**:264–268, 1977.

12. Hodgkin, J.E., Bowser, M.A., and Burton, C.G.: Respirator weaning. *Crit. Care Med.* **2**:96–102, 1974.
13. Martin, L.: Respiratory failure. *Med. Clin. N. Am.* **61**: 1369–1396, 1977.
14. Mithofer, J.C., Bossman, O.G., Thibeault, D.W., et al.: The clinical estimation of alveolar ventilation. *Am. Rev. Resp. Dis.* **98**:868–871, 1969.
15. Nicotra, M.B., Stevens, P.M., Viroslav, J., et al.: Physiologic evaluation of positive end-expiratory pressure ventilation. *Chest* **64**:10–15, 1973.
16. Pierce, A.K.: Oxygen toxicity. *Basics of RD,* Vol. 1, No. 2, American Thoracic Society, 1972.
17. Rogers, R.M., and Jeurs, J.A.: Physiologic considerations in the treatment of acute respiratory failure. *Basics of RD,* Vol. 3, No. 5, American Thoracic Society, 1975.
18. Shoemaker, W.C., and Hauser, C.J.: Critique of crystalloid vs. colloid therapy in shock and shock lung. *Crit. Care Med.* **7**:117–124, 1979.
19. Suter, P.M., Fairley, H.B., and Isenberg, M.D.: Optimum and expiratory pressure in patients with acute pulmonary failure. *N. Eng. J. Med.* **292**:284–289, 1975.
20. Toung, T., Saharia, P., Permut, S., et al.: Aspiration pneumonia: Beneficial and harmful effects of positive end-expiratory pressure. *Surgery* **82**:279–283, 1977.
21. Wayne, K.S.: Positive and expiratory pressure (PEEP) ventilation: A review of mechanisms and actions. *J.A.M.A.* **236**:1394–1396, 1976.
22. Weil, M.H., Henning, R.J., and Puri, V.K.: Colloid oncotic pressure: Clinical significance. *Crit. Care Med.* **7**:113–118, 1979.
23. Zwillich, C.W., Pierson, D.J., Lakshominarayan, S.: Effect of sodium bicarbonate infusion in acute respiratory acidosis and acute metabolic acidosis. *Circ. Shock* **3**:39–43, 1976.

4

Respiratory Dysfunction in Motor Neuron Disease

Raj G. Gupta, M.D., F.C.C.P.

Charcot first described the clinical characteristics of motor neuron disease over a hundred years ago.[1] Although neurologists have recently been excited about possible new information shedding light on the syndrome's etiology,[2,3] respiratory physiologists have recently shown tremendous research interest in elucidating the respiratory dysfunction caused by neuromuscular weakness.[4,6] Clinicians, particularly pulmonary internists, are being increasingly confronted with management of respiratory failure in these patients. Fortunately, the availability of skilled respiratory therapy and intensive care facilities has facilitated the management and improved survival of patients with episodes of acute respiratory failure in neuromuscular disease.[7]

DEFINITION

Motor neuron disease is defined as an idiopathic degeneration of motor neurons at different levels of the central nervous system (CNS) from the anterior horn cell to motor cells in the cerebral cortex.

Although slow virus infection has been suggested as an etiology based on observations of clustering of ALS cases on the Island of Guam, the Kii Peninsula of Japan, and in the

Philippino population of Hawaii, there is no definite proof.[8] Intracellular inclusion bodies in notor neurons have been reported in a number of familial cases.[9] Investigations of environmental and hereditary causes have been unrevealing. An abnormality in the central nervous system's dopamine metabolism[10] has also been suggested based on the finding of low CSF homovanillic acid, but this has not been proven. A recent study demonstrated the high incidence of HLA-BW-35 histocompatibility antigen in ALS in the Guamanian population.[3]

In the U.S.A. there are estimated to be 8,000 to 12,000 patients with motor neuron disease. It occurs mainly in a sporadic form but six percent of the cases have a positive family history. The general clinical manifestation of the syndrome reflect those parts of motor neurons most involved at a particular time in the course of the illness. Progressive bulbar palsy occurs when the degenerative process involves the motor neuron of the brain stem whereas primary lateral sclerosis occurs when upper motor neurons are involved and anterior horn cells are spared. Progressive muscular atrophy is the result of involvement of the anterior horn cells with relative sparing of upper motor neurons. However, the most frequently occurring form of motor neuron disease is the form in which there are clinical manifestations of both upper and lower neuron dysfunction.

Usually the disease begins between 50 and 70 years of age. Males are affected twice as commonly as females. The disease is usually insidious in onset with slow progressive weakness and atrophy of peripheral muscles such as those of the hands. These symptoms are initially asymmetric but soon become bilateral. Since combined upper and lower motor neuron dysfunction is the form of disease in nearly two-thirds of the cases, combinations of weakness, spasticity, muscle atrophy, and exaggerated reflexes are observed. Sensory deficits do not develop but patients may complain of vague muscle pains and parasthesias. Fasciculations of the involved muscles suggest the diagnosis. Other important diagnostic features include preservation of intellect, sparing of extraocular muscles and sensory functions, and retention of sphincter control. Involvement of brain stem nuclei results in atrophy and fasciculations of the tongue and difficulty in chewing and swallowing which predisposes the patient to recurrent aspiration. Degeneration of corticobulbar fibers leads to emotional lability with uncontrolled episodes of crying or laughter.

Diseases reported to occur in association with motor neuron disease include acromegaly, hyperthyroidism, recurrent hypoglycemia, poliomyelitis and carcinoma. The clinical course is progressive with death in two to five years, usually from respiratory complications, either aspiration and pneumonia or respiratory failure or both.

PULMONARY MANIFESTATIONS

Respiratory dysfunction in motor neuron disease depends on (1) type of motor neuron disease, (2) degree of muscle weakness, (3) distribution of muscle weakness, for example, diaphragmatic paralysis versus other respiratory muscle paralysis, (4) secondary alterations in the mechanical properties of the lungs and chest wall.

In amyotrophic lateral sclerosis (ALS) exertional dyspnea is usually a late manifestation but, as reported by Miller et al.,[11] dyspnea and orthopnea may be initial, presenting symptoms mimicking cardiac or pulmonary disease. Respiratory failure generally occurs late in the disease but may be a presenting feature requiring mechanical ventilation.[12,13] In one study,[7] four out of five patients with acute respiratory failure complicating amyotrophic lateral sclerosis were successfully weaned from ventilators. Diaphragmatic paralysis occurs when there is involvement of the phrenic nerve nucleus in cervical segments C3 to C5. The diaphragm is the major inspiratory muscle and its importance in ventilation has been recently discussed.[14] Involvement of the diaphragm leads to marked alterations in pulmonary functions, alveolar hypoventilation and respiratory failure.[12,14] Patients with diaphragmatic paralysis develop orthopnea and prefer to sleep in semirecumbent positions. In these patients one observes epigastric retractions instead of protrusions on inspiration and the reverse on expiration. There are decreased breath sounds at the lung bases and tidal percussion fails to demonstrate variations in level of the diaphragm. Chest x-ray shows elevated diaphragms and fluoroscopy shows paradoxical movement or decreased excursions of the diaphragm. However, fluoroscopy may be misleading and paralysis of the diaphragm should be documented and quantified by transdiaphragmatic pressure measurements during maximal inspiratory efforts (ΔP_{Di}).[14-16] Patients in whom progressive bulbar palsy is the primary manifestation of the syndrome develop difficulty in chewing and swallowing and therefore develop recurrent aspiration pneumonias.

PULMONARY FUNCTION

Involvement of respiratory muscles in motor neuron disease affects various pulmonary function tests. Serial measurements of spirometry and lung volumes provide the clinician with objective and quantitative data concerning the progression of the disease as it affects the respiratory muscles secondary to the involvement of the cervical and thoracic motor neurons.[4,5] There have been recent studies of routine serial pulmonary function[4,5] and sophisticated studies of pulmonary mechanics in amyotrophic lateral sclerosis[16] and in other neuromuscular diseases.[15-17] The effect of ALS on various parameters of pulmonary function will be reviewed.

Spirometry

Vital capacity (VC) and maximum voluntary ventilation (MVV) are reduced in proportion to muscle weakness.[4,5] Fallat et al.[5] have recently reported pulmonary function tests in 218 patients with motor neuron disease and also carried out serial studies in 103 patients. This study showed the importance of spirometry in the early detection of muscle weakness because clinical evaluation alone missed up to 50 percent of reduction of forced vital capacity or MVV. Spirometry gives quantitative and objective data for serial studies. In addition, spirometry is of prognostic value in ALS because all of the fatal cases in the study of Fallat et al.[5] showed progressive deterioration in forced vital capacity and MVV. Effort-dependent flow rate, i.e., peak expiratory flow rate (PEFR) is reduced. Airway obstruction is not a prominent feature of ALS.

Static Pressures

Respiratory muscle weakness decreases the ability to increase pressures to normal levels at given lung volumes. Measurements of maximum static inspiratory pressure (P_I max) and maximum static expiratory pressure ($P_E$max) corrected for lung volumes are sensitive, accurate and simple methods of diagnosing respiratory muscle weakness even in the presence of co-existent pulmonary parenchymal disease.[18] These pressures are reduced even when vital capacity is normal. Quite often inspiratory muscles are less affected than the expiratory muscles, and therefore $P_E$max is decreased more severely than $P_I$max.

Flow Volume Loop

Muscular weakness results in decrease of inspiratory flow rates which are proportional to the decrease in pleural pressures generated by the inspiratory muscles. Since airway properties and lung elastic recoil rather than expiratory muscle effort determine air-flow rates during most of expiration, maximal inspiratory pressures may decline considerably before expiratory flow rates decrease. Therefore, in respiratory muscle weakness there is proportionally greater reduction in inspiratory flow rates then in expiratory flow rates, which can be easily measured in a flow volume loop generated during maximal inspiratory and expiratory maneuver. The ratio of maximum midinspiratory flow rate (MMIF) or $V_I$max 50 to maximum midexpiratory flow rate (MMEF) or $V_E$max 50 of less than 1 is seen in muscular weakness but can also be seen in extrathoracic variable obstruction.[19,20] Based on the shape of the maximal expiratory flow volume curve Kreitzer et al.[6] have identified patients with more severe expiratory muscle weakness. A flow-volume loop is a simultaneous plot of flow at a given lung volume. The initial portion of the flow volume loop is dependent on effort while the latter half is effort-independent and is governed by the mechanical properties of the lungs and airways. Muscle weakness must be of significant degree before affecting flows near the residual volume. As depicted in Figure 1, the patients with muscle weakness have a curve similar to Figure 1B showing the curve with

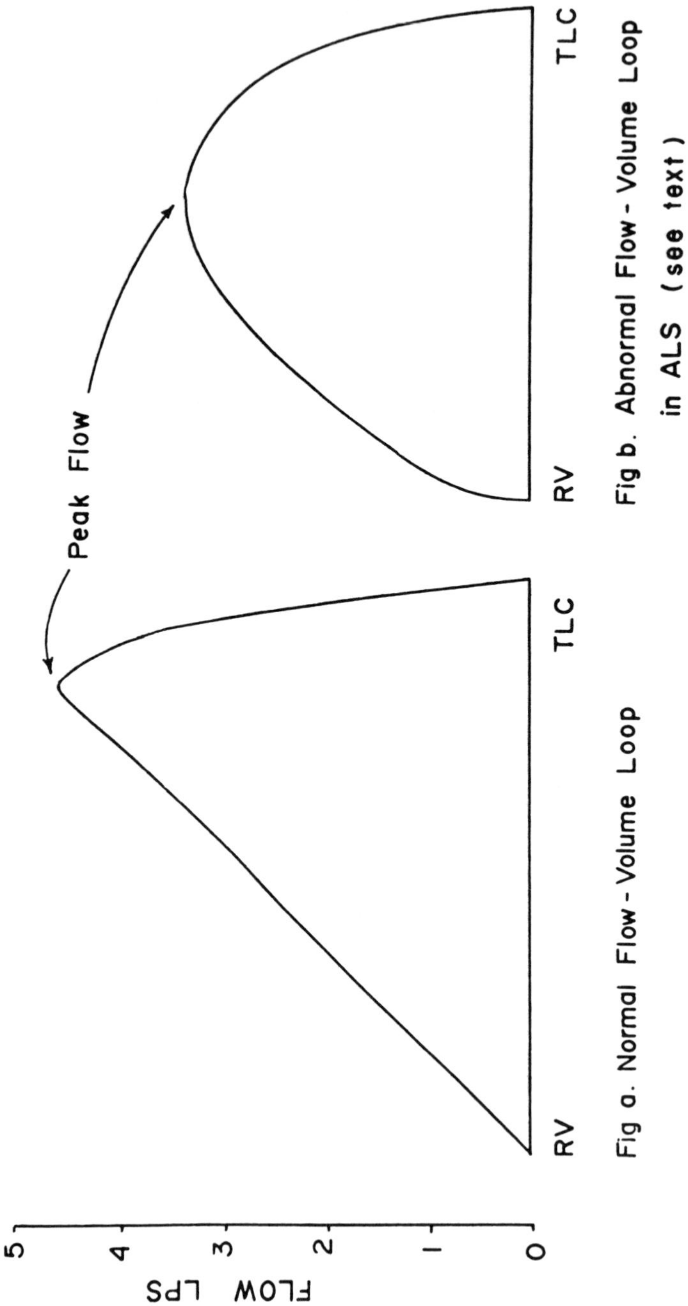
Peak Flow
FLOW LPS
0
1
2
3
4
5
RV
TLC
Fig a. Normal Flow - Volume Loop
RV
TLC
Fig b. Abnormal Flow - Volume Loop in ALS (see text)

Figure 1.

concavity toward the volume axis as residual volume is approached. Patients with this type of flow-volume curve showed marked changes in pulmonary function with added airway resistance, as may occur with minor respiratory infections. This may explain why these patients are prone to respiratory failure on exposure to added stress. Thus, flow volume loop pattern may be helpful for the clinician in assessing the degree of expiratory muscle weakness and identifying patients at risk of developing respiratory failure with any respiratory insult.

Lung Volumes

There is little or no change in the functional residual capacity (FRC) on serial testing.[4-6] In some studies total lung capacity is found to decrease progressively[4,5] while in another study total lung capacity (TLC) decreased only when the diaphragm was involved or in advanced disease.[6] Other factors such as parenchymal lung disease or lung fibrosis secondary to recurrent aspiration pneumonia or alterations in chest wall mechanics may lower the TLC.

Characteristically, in respiratory muscle weakness, residual volume and residual volume/total lung capacity (RV/TLC) ratio increases progressively in proportion to muscle weakness.[1-6] The increase in RV is generally explained by the impairment of the expiratory muscles, internal intercostals, and the abdominal wall. In the series of Fallat et al.[5] the RV was frequently elevated even in the presence of a normal TLC. The inability of the patients in this study to exhale to residual volume, despite repeated efforts, was often impressive. In some patients, a high residual volume and discoordination of expiratory efforts on flow-volume loop maneuver may be the early indicators of neurological involvement of the ventilatory system.

Pulmonary Mechanics

Measurements of static compliance, dynamic compliance and pulmonary resistance in 18 patients with amyotrophic lateral sclerosis showed no abnormalities.[6] This may be explained by relatively normal total lung capacity and diaphragm function in this group of patients. However, if secondary parenchymal lung changes such as fibrosis or microatelectasis occur or diaphragmatic paralysis develops then static compliance may be reduced.[16]

Blood Gases and Diffusing Capacity

Patients with muscle weakness have alveolar hyperventilation at rest but with progression of disease or with diaphragmatic paralysis they may develop respiratory failure requiring mechanical ventilation, particularly at the time of added respiratory insult.[6,7] The dead space to tidal volume ratio (V_D/V_T) ratio is increased. Arterial oxygen tension is normal while carbon dioxide tension is slightly decreased with mild respiratory alkalosis in uncomplicated cases.[6] With decrease in the expiratory reserve volume with diaphragm paralysis, ventilation/perfusion ($\dot{V}/\dot{Q}$) imbalance worsens. In one study,[4] steady-rate diffusing capacity was found to be below normal early in the course of the disease and also showed significant negative correlation over time on serial studies. This cannot be explained on the basis of neuromuscular weakness alone. Steady-state diffusing capacity is highly sensitive to $\dot{V}/\dot{Q}$ abnormalities which were present in the group of patients in this particular study and may not reflect alveolar capillary gas exchange abnormalities in the lung in patients with ALS.

Control of Ventilation

Tests of control of breathing and evaluation of respiratory center drive such as mouth-occlusion pressure during carbon-dioxide rebreathing have not been done in patients with ALS. However, these parameters may be difficult to evaluate in the presence of muscle weakness. It is conceivable that with bulbar involvement in this disease there may be disturbances in the regulation of ventilation which may lead to central hypoventilation.

Diaphragm Function

Clinical and fluoroscopic evaluation of diaphragm function are valuable but not confirmatory. Diaphragmatic paralysis occurs in this disease and therefore should be evaluated. Diaphragm electromyogram recordings, transdiaphragmatic pressure changes (ΔP_{Di}),[15,16] A-P diameter of the rib cage and abdomen with magnetometers[21,22] may be carried out to fully document diaphragmatic paralysis.

MANAGEMENT

There is no specific drug therapy for motor neuron disease. Because of neuromuscular weakness these patients have reduced ability to take deep breaths or to cough effectively and are therefore predisposed to recurrent aspiration pneumonias and pulmonary infections. Patients should be encouraged to keep active and carry out graded exercises in order to avoid superimposition of poor physical conditioning. What is to a normal person a trivial respiratory tract infection, may be lethal or near lethal to these patients, particularly those with severe involvement. Acute respiratory failure may be precipitated very suddenly and therefore these patients should be managed aggressively at the first sign of chest infection. Acute respiratory failure should be managed by usual methods including mechanical ventilation.[7] A volume-cycled ventilator should be used and when the patient recovers from the infection, he may be switched to rocking beds or pneumo-belts or even removed from ventilator support altogether. Chronic respiratory failure in these types of patients may require a cuirass-type respirator or a rocking bed and pneumo-belt. Attention should also be paid to the nutrition and feeding gastrostomy has been advocated for preventing aspiration and, at the same time, giving good nutrition to these patients. This aggressive management of respiratory failure may not be appropriate in all cases of ALS. The overall clinical situation and the patient's wishes should play a major role in these decisions.

REFERENCES

1. Charcot, J.M., and Joffroy, A.: Deux cas d'atrophe musculaire progressive avec lesions de la substance grise et des faisceaux anterolateraux de la moelle epiniere. *Arch. Physiol. Norm. Pathol.* **2**:354–367, 1869.

2. Murray, T.J., Pride, S., and Haley, G.: Motor neuron disease in Nova Scotia. Review article. *Can. Med. Assoc. J.* **110**:814–817, 1974.
3. Hoffman, P.M., Robbins, D.S., Nolte, M.T., Gibbs, C.J., and Gajdusek, D.C.: Cellular immunity in Guamanians with amyotrophic lateral sclerosis and Parkinsonism-dementia. *N. Eng. J. Med.* **299**:680–685, 1978.
4. Nakano, K.K., Bass, H., Tyler, H.R., and Carmel, R.J.: amyotrophic lateral sclerosis: A study of pulmonary function. *Dis. Nerv. Syst.* **37**(1):32–35, 1976.
5. Fallat, R.J., Jewitt, B., Bass, M., Kamm, B., and Norris, F.H.: Spirometry in amyotrophic lateral sclerosis. *Arch. Neurol.* **36**:74–80, 1979.
6. Kreitzer, S.M., Saunders, N.A., Tyler, H.R., and Ingram, R.H., Jr.: Respiratory muscle function in amyotrophic lateral sclerosis. *Am. Rev. Resp. Dis.* **117**(3):437–447, 1978.
7. O'Donohue, W.J., Jr., Baker, J.P., Bell, G.M., Muren, O., Parker, C.L., and Patterson, J.L., Jr.: Respiratory failure in neuromuscular disease—Management in a respiratory intensive care unit. *J.A.M.A.* **235**(7):733–735, 1976.
8. Kurland, L.T., and Mulder, D.W.: Epidemiologic investigations of amyotrophic lateral sclerosis. I. Preliminary report on geographic distribution, with special reference to the Marianas Islands, including clinical and pathologic observations. *Neurology (Minn.)* **4**:355–378, 1954.
9. Hirano, A., Malamud, N., Elizan, T.S., et al.: Amyotrophic lateral sclerosis and Parkinsonism-dementia complex on Guam. *Arch. Neurol.* **15**:35–51, 1966.
10. Mendell, J.R., Chase, T.N., and Ingel, W.K. Amyotrophic lateral sclerosis; metabolism of central monoamines and treatment with L-dopa. *Trans. Am. Neurol. Assoc.* **96**:284–286, 1972.
11. Miller, R.D., Mulder, D.W., Fowler, W.S., and Olsen, A.M.: Exertional dyspnea: A primary complaint in unusual cases of progressive muscular atrophy and amyotrophic lateral sclerosis. *Ann. Int. Med.* **46**(1):119–125, 1957.
12. Fromm, G.B., Wisdom, P.J., and Block, A.J.: Amyotrophic lateral sclerosis presenting with respiratory failure. Diaphragmatic paralysis and dependence on mechanical ventilation in two patients. *Chest* **71**(5):612–614, 1977.

13. Parhad, I.M., Clark, A.W., Barron, K.D., and Staunton, S.B.: Diaphragmatic paralysis in motor nueron disease. Report of two cases and a review of the literature. *Neurology* **28**:18–22, 1978.
14. Rochester, D.F., and Braun, N.M.T.: The respiratory muscles. Basics of respiratory disease. *Am. Thorac. Soc.* publication, Vol. 6, No. 4, March 1978.
15. Newsom-Davis, J., Goldman, M., Loh, L., and Casson, M.: Diaphragm function and alveolar hypoventilation. *Quart. J. Med.* New Series **XLV** (177):87–100, 1976.
16. Gibson, G.J., Pride, N.B., Newsome-Davis, J., and Loh, L.C.: Pulmonary mechanics in patients with respiratory muscle weakness. *Am. Rev. Resp. Dis.* **115**:389-395, 1977.
17. Keltz, H.: The effect of respiratory muscle dysfunction on pulmonary studies in patients with neuromuscular disease. *Am. Rev. Resp. Dis.* **91**:934–938, 1965.
18. Black, L.F., and Hyatt, R.E.: Maximum static respiratory pressures in generalized neuromuscular disease. *Am. Rev. Resp. Dis.* **103**:641-650, 1971.
19. Goldstein, R.L., Hyde, R.W., Lapham, L.W., Gazioglu, K., and de Papp, Z.G.: Peripheral neuropathy presenting with respiratory insufficiency as the primary compaint. Problem of recognizing alveolar hypoventilation due to neuromuscular disorders. *Am. J. Med.* **56**:443–449, 1974.
20. Kryger, M., Bode, R., Antic, R., and Anthonisen, N.: Diagnosis of obstruction of the upper and central airways. *Am. J. Med.* **61**:85–93, 1976.
21. Mead, J., Peterson, N., Grimby, G., and Mead, J.: Pulmonary ventilation measured from body surface movements. *Science* **156**:1383–1384, 1967.
22. Sharp, J.T.: Diaphragmatic function and respiratory failure (Editorial). *Chest* **71**(5):566, 1977.

5

RESPIRATORY DYSFUNCTION AND PERIPHERAL NEUROPATHY

Caroline M. Tanner, M.D.

The respiratory symptoms resulting from dysfunction of either pulmonary muscles or peripheral nerves are generally expressions of the same basic pathophysiology, that of weakness of pulmonary respiratory musculature, and as such are often symptomatically identical. Despite major differences in pathophysiology, the clinical presentation of respiratory disorders caused by a wide range of other disease states may be deceptively similar. This chapter will review the mechanism of pulmonary dysfunction secondary to peripheral nerve or muscle disease, the methods of differentiating these problems from intrinsic lung disease and the appropriate approach to therapy. The first section will discuss general considerations in pathophysiology and diagnosis. Following this, the clinical presentation of injuries to specific anatomic areas will be considered. In the last section, specific disorders of peripheral nerves as they affect pulmonary function will be considered.

PATHOPHYSIOLOGY AND DIAGNOSIS

General Considerations

In most neuromuscular disease, the underlying dysfunction of the respiratory system is that of respiratory muscle weakness, particularly that of the diaphragm. Cinically, this may manifest as resting or exertional dyspnea with hypoxia and hypercarbia and thus mimic the symptomatology of intrinsic lung disease. The basic pathophysiology of the two disorders is distinctly different, however, for patients with intrinsic lung disease suffer from a primary disorder of expiratory flow. The opposite is true in neuromuscular disease, where the major deficit is inspiratory. The hallmark of neuromuscular respiratory disease is hypoxemia, the result of inspiratory insufficiency and resultant alveolar hypoventilation. Intercostal muscle weakness results in a decreased resting lung volume, ultimately with airway closure, atelectasis and progressive decrease in alveolar ventilation with secondary hypercapnia. Abdominal muscle weakness results in impaired cough and retention of secretions compounds the dysfunction.[1-3] Abnormalities of brainstem motor neurons or bulbar musculature increase the likelihood of aspiration and subsequent infection, and weaken accessory respiratory muscles with a resultant increased inspiratory deficit.[4,5] Abnormalities of the autonomic nervous system and neuromuscular-based chemoreceptor responses may further complicate the picture of primary inspiratory deficit.[6]

Routine pulmonary function testing may often differentiate patients with intrinsic lung disease from those with primary dysfunction of respiratory nerves or muscles. In patients with neuromuscular respiratory insufficiency, the predominantly inspiratory deficit with resultant alveolar hypoventilation leads first to a decreased pO_2, with hypercarbia following as dysfunction becomes more severe. Pulmonary function deficits are those of vital capacity (VC), functional residual capacity (FRC), residual volume (VR), and total lung capacity (TLC), and are generally worsened by assumption of supine posture, as is arterial oxygenation.[7-10] But in other patients with neuromuscular disorders, routine pulmonary function tests may fall within the normal range or be nondiagnostic. Since most pulmonary function tests are designed specifically for the evaluation of patients with intrinsic lung disease, inspiratory deficits are often overlooked.

In respiratory insufficiency caused by neuromuscular disease, the primary disorder is that of inspiratory weakness. The tests of pulmonary function which are of most use in initial diagnosis and subsequent follow-up are those which provide some estimate of respiratory muscle strength. Two such tests are maximal voluntary ventilation (MVV) and maximal midinspiratory and midexpiratory flow rates (MMIF and MMEF). MVV evaluates respiratory function over time, and rapid fatiguing of abnormal respiratory muscles will be an early finding here. Although changes in MVV are not specific to neuromuscular disease, in the absence of expiratory abnormalities suggesting intrinsic lung disease, neuromuscular dysfunction may be suspected. In the case of documented neuromuscular respiratory insufficiency, MVV is a useful monitor of respiratory impairment.[9] The spirometric evaluation of maximal midinspiratory and midexpiratory flow values may show significant inspiratory impairment in patients with neuromuscular disease while those with intrinsic lung disease characteristically show abnormalities of expiratory flow in the presence of normal inspiratory values.[11] A third determination frequently abnormal in neuromuscular disease is that of maximal static inspiratory and expiratory respiratory pressures ($P_I$max and $P_E$max). These parameters provide a specific measurement of pulmonary muscle strength, and can easily be determined at the bedside. Intrinsic lung disease does not result in abnormalities of these values, and accompanying weakness of oral musculature does not generally preclude accurate determinations. An excellent description of this technique and tables of normal values have been published by Black and Hyatt[12,13] and the reader is referred to their work for additional information. The simplicity and specificity of $P_I$max and $P_E$max determinations may qualify this as the single most useful respiratory parameter in patients with neuromuscular disease.

Specific Abnormalities

Diaphragm

Abnormalities of the above tests suggest that respiratory insufficiency may relate to the class of neuromuscular disorders. To delineate the disorder more precisely, additional investigation is required. Since the diaphragm is the principal inspiratory muscle, it is especially important to determine whether diaphragmatic compromise plays a role in respiratory insufficiency.

Radiographic evaluation is the mainstay of traditional diagnostic methods. One expects to see elevated diaphragmatic leaves, poor movement with fluoroscopic visualization and the classic paradoxical movement on sniffing. However, purely radiographic analysis of diaphragmatic disease has several disadvantages. X-ray studies in patients with bilateral disease may appear to be normal. Fluoroscopic examination has also been found to have frequent false negatives, and six percent of normal subjects may show paradoxical movements with the sniff maneuver.[14] Routine pulmonary function testing may show the expected decrease in VC and FRC, but this is frequently not the case. In this situation, determination of values in the supine posture, nocturnal ABG measurements, and the previously described determinations of MMIF and MMEF, MVV and maximal static respiratory pressures ($P_I$max and $P_E$max) may be of diagnostic value.

Additional clues may be provided by history or physical examination which suggest diaphragmatic dysfunction. In the patient with diaphragm dysfunction, the downward inspiratory movement of the diaphragm may be a passive phenomenon in the erect posture, where the abrupt relaxation of functioning abdominal muscles at end-expiration increases the abdominal anteroposterior diameter and, with the assistance of gravitational forces, permits downward diaphragmatic excursion.[15] This movement is opposed by gravity in the supine posture, and effective respiration is impaired.[2,16] A patient thus afflicted may have essentially normal waking respiration, but nocturnal blood gases show significant hypoxia and hypercapnia. Complaints of daytime sleepiness, headache on awakening and poor sleep may be misinterpreted as primary alveolar hypoventilation. Exertional dyspnea or the presence in long-standing dysfunction of pulmonary hypertension and right heart disease may further complicate the picture.[11,16-18] During the physical examination, the patient with diaphragmatic disease is best observed in the supine posture. A paradoxical inward movement of the abdominal musculature during inspiration is strongly suggestive of diaphragmatic paralysis.

When phrenic nerve dysfunction is considered as an etiology of diaphragmatic failure, the measurement of phrenic nerve conduction velocity may be a valuable determination. The technique is noninvasive, and affords minimal discomfort to the patient. In this procedure, the phrenic nerve is stimulated in the neck and the compound diaphragmatic muscle action potential is recorded via a surface electrode over the lateral chest wall. A range of normal values has been established and slowing of conduction time consistent with phrenic nerve dysfunction has been shown in patients with peripheral neuropathy including the phrenic nerve as well as in those with isolated phrenic nerve lesions from invasive, compressive, or traumatic destruction. Difficulty in interpreting this test arises when diaphragmatic response is not elicited. Such a finding is consistent either with complete loss of phrenic nerve function, or merely with technical difficulty in locating the appropriate stimulation site.[19] Despite these potential false negatives, this relatively innocuous, noninvasive procedure should be considered in the evaluation of many patients with suspected phrenic neuropathy.

Another means of evaluating diaphragmatic function is the measurement of transdiaphragmatic pressure changes with respiration. Simultaneous measurement of gastric and esophageal pressures during maximal inspiration is obtained using balloons whose pressures are recorded by an electromanometer. Pressure changes are presented against rib cage diameter on an oscilloscope and recorded on Polaroid film for analysis. Patients with normal vital capacities and fluoroscopic studies but symptoms suggestive of diaphragmatic dysfunction were found to have significant decrease or absence of transdiaphragmatic pressure changes using this technique.[16] The disadvantages of this procedure are two-fold. Intraesophageal technique provides more patient discomfort than other methods of evaluation. Also, correct positioning may be difficult, and allow for difficulty in interpreting test results. A similar evaluation, that of intraesophageal electrode placement for the determination of diaphragmatic EMG, is subject to the same difficulties.

Recently, some investigators have performed direct EMG recording from the diaphragm using a percutaneous insertion technique. This evaluation is specifically useful in differentiating neuropathic from myopathic dysfunction of the phrenic nerve and diaphragm. When clinically indicated, this test has proven to be less noxious and considerably more reliable than EMG determination using intraesophageal electrodes, since difficulties in electrode placement, electrocardiographic artifact, and other technical difficulties are nearly eliminated in this technique. Morbidity has been small in the cases reported. The interested reader is referred to more technical descriptions of the procedure.[20,21]

The use of specific evaluations of diaphragm function is critical in patients with otherwise minimal neuromuscular disease. In such cases the clinical presentation of arterial hypoxia and hypercapnia may be misinterpreted as primary alveolar hypoventilation. The fact that many of these patients can voluntarily correct blood gas abnormalities with hyperventilation and have no underlying lung disease makes diagnosis even more difficult, and requires careful evaluation using techniques described above in all symptomatic patients with diagnosed or suspected neuromuscular disease.[11,22,23]

Intercostal Muscles

Isolated dysfunction of the intercostal muscles is not frequently reported, and in general the degree of respiratory impairment in such a situation will not be overwhelming. As in the more common problem of combined diaphragmatic and intercostal paresis, alveolar hypoventilation is the underlying disorder. A suggestion of the specific pathologic process contributed by intercostal paralysis is presented by studies in normal subjects under halothane anesthesia. In this situation, depression of spinal respiratory motor neurons is much greater than phrenic nerve depression. Patients anesthetized with halothane show a paradoxical retraction of intercostal muscles during inspiration. Inspiratory rib cage stabilization is lost, and there is no chemoreceptor recruitment of rib cage expansion.[24] Thus, tidal volume is decreased, and falls in arterial oxygenation and resting lung volume may supervene. Although similar studies have yet to be performed on patients with pathology of intercostal nerves and muscles, similar pathophysiologic mechanisms are likely to be identified in these disease states.

Although isolated intercostal weakness is likely to lead to profound respiratory insufficiency, the frequently observed combined weakness of intercostal and diaphragmatic musculature presents a significant clinical problem, and recognition of the added impairment of intercostal function may be important to management. The selective effect of halothane anesthesia on intercostal function is an important consideration when evaluating patients with neuromuscular disease for surgical procedures, as concomitant diaphragmatic impairment, although insignificant in normal conditions, may lead to serious recovery room difficulty.[24] Similar immediate postoperative respiratory distress has been reported with other general anesthetics in patients with neuromuscular disease, affecting not only inspiratory capacity but also impairing cough and clearing of secretions via suppression of abdominal muscle function.[25,26]

Several methods are available for diagnosis of intercostal dysfunction, and in patients with suspected combined intercostal/diaphragmatic dysfunction they may be preferable to the more complicated techniques of diaphragmatic evaluation in differentiating neuropathic from myopathic disease. The clinical observation of poor expansion of the fourth to seventh intercostal spaces during inspiration may lead to the suspicion that the intercostals are impaired, as other respiratory muscles will have little activity here. Similarly, decreased rib excursion in the coronal plane at fluoroscopy provides a coarse estimate of intercostal disease.[27] However, the most valuable and specific tests are those of intercostal muscle biopsy and electromyography. Both tests are well described, carry little clinical risk, and may provide valuable information.[18,20] One recent study has shown intercostal muscle biopsy to have equivalent diagnostic value with less morbidity than limb muscle biopsy in assessing patients with neuromuscular disease.[28]

Abdominal Muscles

Rarely would isolated abdominal muscle disease present with primary respiratory symptomatology. The significance of dysfunction in these muscles is most commonly that created by difficulties in the effective clearing of secretions, especially in patients with underlying problems of respiration. Clinical suspicion of abdominal neuromuscular disease is suggested to the examiner by the observation of poor cough or in more severe cases by observation of impaired volitional muscle contraction. In the absence of central nervous system disease or local surgical trauma, the loss of abdominal reflexes may suggest a disorder of peripheral abdominal nerves or an intrinsic disorder of muscle. However, in the absence of more definitive evidence, impairment of abdominal reflexes alone cannot be considered a reliable test of abdominal muscle function. Positive diagnosis of abdominal neuromuscular disease may be easily obtained with electromyographic and biopsy evaluation.[27]

Bulbar Muscles

Disease states affecting muscles of the larynx and pharynx can also contribute to respiratory insufficiency, and are not uncommon in disorders of the vagus nerve.[29] Symptoms may include dysphonia and dysphagia, and the examiner may note impaired gag reflexes and paresis of palatal movement. The danger of aspiration, with subsequent infection superimposed on an already compromised respiratory system, is significant. A further problem arises in those patients requiring mechanical ventilation. It has been observed that some patients with chronic neuromuscular disease requiring respiratory assistance with cuirass or tank-type ventilators are unable to maintain adequate nocturnal ventilation.[30] Recently, specific evaluation of laryngeal muscle function in these patients has revealed passive inspiratory vocal cord closure which is most prominent during sleep, with subsequent decrease in tidal volume and inspiratory flow. Stridor is a frequent accompaniment. Diagnosis can be made by direct visualization with fiberoptic bronchoscopy.[31]

Disorders of the eleventh cranial nerve may lead to weakness of accessory respiratory musculature. Although weakness of trapezii and sternocleidomastoids alone never contribute to clinical symptoms of respiratory insufficiency, in combination with other respiratory muscle dysfunction this weakness may add to an already unstable respiratory state.

Autonomic Nervous System

Isolated dysfunction of pulmonary autonomic nerves is not well described but in the presence of widespread autonomic neuropathy such abnormalities should be suspected. The effects of the autonomic nervous system are complex, and of these the most clearly defined is that of vagal afferent influence on central respiratory mechanisms (See Chapter 1, this volume). Recent experimental studies have also shown an independent sensitivity of spinal respiratory motor neurons to alterations of arterial CO_2 that is apparently also mediated by peripheral chemoreceptors. The clinical significance of this finding remains to be studied, but experimentally observed alterations in tidal volume and inspiratory and expiratory duration suggest that synchronous spinal motor neuron firing during respiration is a summation of central and peripheral input, and may be affected by either.[32-34]

The function of pulmonary smooth muscle and glandular secretion is also under autonomic control, and abnormalities here should be suspected in the presence of autonomic neuropathy. Upper thoracic sympathetic fibers mediate bronchiolar dilatation, while vagal parasympathetic influence results in bronchiolar constriction and increased glandular secretion.[35,36] Surfactant release is stimulated by both vagal parasympathetic and beta-adrenergic systems, and significant decreases in pulmonary compliance may result from impaired autonomic function.[37]

Pulmonary vascular tone is also under complex autonomic control. In animal studies two pharmacologically distinct postganglionic sympathetic systems as well as a parasympathetic, probably vagal, system have been identified. Both parasympathetic and sympathetic fibers mediate vasodilatation, while a distinct set of sympathetic fibres mediates vasoconstriction.[37] It also appears that both sympathetic and parasympathetic systems carry afferent information from pulmonary vasculature which mediates reflex alteration of respiratory rate.[38]

To date, there is little clinical data specifically describing the effects of isolated autonomic neuropathies on respiration. It is possible that such disorders are much less prominent in their symptomatology than concurrent dysfunction in other organ systems. Neurophysiologic evidence, however, suggests that disorders of compliance, respiratory reflexes and pulmonary vasculature probably do occur. Knowledge of this may be of future help in the diagnosis and rational treatment of patients suffering from autonomic neuropathies.

Impaired CO_2 Response

A final respiratory disorder observed in neuromuscular disease is a blunted sensitivity to elevated arterial CO_2 which has been noted in many patients with chronic myopathy but minimal respiratory muscle weakness.[39,40] The pathophysiology of this disorder is not known, but a similar blunted CO_2 response is seen in some patients with chronic lung disease.[41] One postulate is that prolonged abnormal proprioceptive input from diseased respiratory muscle may alter the central ventilatory response to CO_2.[40] The Read rebreathing test, used in conjunction with direct measurement of pulmonary function ($P_E$max, $P_I$max and diaphragmatic pressure gradients), will help to differentiate this problem from frank diaphragmatic dysfunction.[10,42,43] As treatment may differ in the two conditions, such a distinction is significant.

SPECIFIC DISORDERS OF PERIPHERAL NERVES

Introduction

Disease of the peripheral nerve by definition includes that portion of the nervous system wherein neuronal elements are associated with the characteristic satellite cell, the Schwann cell, rather than the glial cells characteristic of spinal cord, brainstem and cortex. Peripheral nerve dysfunction may be the result of any number of etiologic processes, including tumors, trauma, carcinomatous invasion, multisystem disorders, toxins, metabolic derangements, hereditary disorders, infectious disorders and deficiency states. With the exception of isolated dysfunction of the phrenic nerve, most peripheral nerve problems causing respiratory dysfunction fall into the category of polyneuropathies. Such clinical states are characterized by symmetric distal weakness with flaccid musculature and absent tendon reflexes. Pathophysiologically, peripheral nerve disease may be divided into those characterized primarily by a loss of normal myelination of peripheral nerve fibers, or demyelinating neuropathies, and those characterized by degeneration of the neural axon itself, with only secondary loss of myelin. The former are distinguished by markedly delayed nerve conduction velocities, while the latter may have variable results to electrophysiologic testing, ranging from normal to absent nerve conduction velocities.

The peripheral neuropathic problems which include prominent dysfunction of motor neurons are those most commonly associated with clinical respiratory dysfunction. This section will identify the most common of these disorders of peripheral nerve without attempting to list every peripheral nerve disease which may occasionally include some respiratory impairment. In general, the clinical picture and respiratory pathophysiology will be similar for many types of motor neuropathy. Consequently, this discussion will focus on acute inflammatory polyradiculoneuropathy, perhaps the most common peripheral neuropathy to frequently include severe respiratory dysfunction. Other motor neuropathies, such as diphtheria, alcohol, herpes and idiopathic or isolated phrenic neuropathies, will be discussed in less detail.

Acute Inflammatory Polyradiculoneuropathy

Acute inflammatory polyradiculoneuropathy, or the Guillain-Barré-Strohl syndrome, is one of the commonest forms of acute polyneuritis. In one recent series, the mean incidence was shown to be about 1.6 per 100,000 population.[44] Acute inflammatory polyradiculoneuropathy (AIPN) occurs most commonly in young adulthood and early middle age, preceded in about half the patients by an antecedent infectious illness whose symptoms have generally cleared by the onset of neurologic dysfunction.[45] Although AIPN may be classified as a demyelinating neuropathy, the pathophysiology is not known. It is believed that some as yet unidentified allergen is responsible for this inflammatory demyelinating process, and experimental evidence has demonstrated a similar condition after the injection of peripheral nerve tissue into experimental animals.[46-49]

The characteristic presenting complaint is weakness, generally first manifesting in the lower extremities and progressing over a period of days to weeks to involve trunk, arms and cranial nerves. The pattern of involvement is symmetric: a period of stabilization usually follows progression to maximal involvement and a slow recovery is in most cases completed within six months.[47] Although the severity of the clinical picture may vary, life-threatening respiratory involvement has been reported in as many as 20 percent of all AIPN patients.[50-53] Prior to the advent of mechanical ventilation, respiratory failure was the major source of mortality in AIPN.[54] Modern techniques of respiratory intensive care have improved this picture, and complete recovery has been reported in patients requiring respiratory support for as long as 266 days.[47] The potential for complete recovery in nearly all of these patients emphasizes the importance of meticulous respiratory evaluation and treatment from the onset of symptoms. Although many variations are observed from the typical course, a recent ad hoc committee of NINCDS requires progressive symmetric motor weakness with absent deep tendon reflexes to allow the diagnosis of AIPN.[55]

Morbidity and mortality in AIPN is usually of cardiopulmonary etiology, although the original dysfunction lies in the innervation of these organ systems. Primary respiratory embarrassment is caused by weakness or paralysis of intercostal and diaphragmatic muscles when the phrenic nerve and respiratory motor neurons are affected. The underlying pathophysiology is one of progressive alveolar hypoventilation. Debilitation may be slowly progressive or fulminant, and the lack of clinical signs or symptoms of respiratory distress cannot be considered a basis for neglecting vigorous monitoring of respiratory function once the diagnosis of AIPN is suspected. Abrupt and life-threatening respiratory deterioration within minutes of minimal respiratory symptomatology is commonly observed in patients suffering from AIPN. The routine management parameters used in intrinsic lung disease, that is, the determination of arterial blood gases and vital capacity measurements, are frequently not adequate measures of respiratory function, and may present a misleading picture of respiratory compensation in the face of impending disaster.[56]

As in all cases of diaphragmatic dysfunction, the supine posture places the patient at the greatest disadvantage in maintaining respiration. Determination of MMEF and MMIF values in this position may provide early clues to respiratory paresis, but this position should otherwise be avoided in favor of a semi-sitting position when possible. At least every four hours, monitoring of respiratory function should be carried out in all patients with AIPN, and in those patients with more rapidly progressive disease more frequent evaluation and intensive care unit monitoring is mandatory.[54] An important neurologic warning signal may be provided by the presence of facial diplegia. This sign has been noted in about half of all cases of AIPN,[47] and of this group roughly half develop respiratory difficulties requiring mechanical ventilation.[58] It should be stressed, however, that the absence of facial diplegia does not indicate safety from respiratory impairment.

The careful monitoring of respiratory muscle strength in AIPN should be supplemented with meticulous pulmonary care. Patients with abdominal muscle weakness will have ineffectual cough, and appropriate modalities to ensure mobilization of secretions should be employed. Routine testing of gag reflexes will provide a rough clinical index of pharyngeal function and observation of vocal tone will assist in assessment of laryngeal musculature. The potential for aspiration should be remembered in patients with impaired bulbar musculature, and prophylactic measures such as nasogastric tube feeding or parenteral hyperalimentation should be instituted when appropriate. The danger of pulmonary infection is high in patients with impairment of abdominal, thoracic and pharyngeal muscles, and careful monitoring and early intervention with appropriate antibiotic therapy are critical.

Intervention with mechanical respiratory assistance should be instituted at the earliest signs of possible respiratory embarrassment. As ventilatory assistance may be necessary for prolonged periods, meticulous respiratory care protocols, preferably in a respiratory intensive care unit, should be followed. One author suggests aseptic atraumatic suctioning of the tracheostomy at least every hour, with alternate day tracheostomy replacement. The respirator and nebulizer should be carefully decontaminated. Weaning should begin when respiratory parameters approach normal values. In making this determination attention again should be directed to those specific tests which assess the function of respiratory musculature. As the majority of patients stricken with AIPN are in otherwise good health, meticulous respiratory care can result in total recovery, even after months of mechanical ventilation, in a large number of patients.[59-62]

The most serious threat to survival from AIPN today results from dysfunction of the autonomic nervous system. Mechanical ventilatory assistance has made death from respiratory failure a relative rarity in AIPN. Death now more commonly occurs in patients receiving adequate ventilatory assistance as a sudden event whose pathophysiology is poorly understood. Although Osler[63] as early as 1892 attributed death in AIPN to be the result at times of cardiac dysfunction, the syndrome of autonomic dysfunction in AIPN has only recently been studied. Advanced intensive-care unit technology has allowed the identification of autonomic disorders separate from those occurring as a result of anoxia. Such symptoms have been found to be common occurences in AIPN, and are often associated with a poor prognosis. Although these autonomic symptoms are most prominently cardiovascular, the implications raised in the pulmonary care of patients suffering such symptoms merits their discussion here.

The symptoms of autonomic dysfunction in AIPN do not appear to correlate with the degree of clinical weakness. Patients with apparently mild muscle paresis may nonetheless be at risk for life-threatening autonomic changes. Characteristically, such changes are paroxysmal, and do not follow a predictable clinical pattern. Symptoms may be those of excess or of deficit in either the sympathetic or parasympathetic nervous system, and commonly show dizzying fluctuations from one pathologic state to another. The most common abnormalities of autonomic dysfunction are those of heart rate and blood pressure. In a study of 50 fatal cases of AIPN, Haymaker and Kernohan[45] found transient tachycardia and hypertension to be extremely common.

Similar disorders of vasomotor tone and heart rate have been reported by other authors.[64-68] In these and other studies, transient abnormalities of the electrocardiogram and of cardiac rhythm have also been reported.[69-71]

Such reports prompted a recent study by Lichtenfeld[71] which examined specific autonomic dysfunction in 28 patients with AIPN. In his study, 61 percent of patients showed transient hypertensive episodes and 43 percent showed postural hypotension. In two patients, postural hypotension was the presenting complaint. Bradycardia was present in 21 percent of patients, persistent sinus tachycardia was seen in 50 percent, and facial flushing was observed in 25 percent. In some cases clinical response was seen to such maneuvers as carotid massage or atropine administration in treatment of the observed arrhythmias, while in others no response was noted. Fifty-seven percent of patients showed symptomatic hypotension in response to Valsalva-like maneuvers such as cough or straining at stool, and sedative administration resulted in severe hypotension in one. A few patients reported loss of their normal "fear" response. Sixty-four percent of patients showed EKG abnormalities in the absence of anoxia or clinical suspicion of heart disease. Of these, T wave abnormalities, S-T segment depression, QRS voltage changes and prolonged QT intervals were most common. Atrial fibrillation and atrial tachycardia were also observed. Similar EKG findings are reported in another study.[72]

These observations of extreme autonomic dysfunction have several implications in the management of patients with AIPN. Since autonomic dysfunction may occur in the absence of severe paralysis, specific monitoring of autonomic function should be routine in all patients. Those patients not requiring respiratory assistance should be cautioned against frequent Valsalva or rapid postural change, and frequent blood pressure determinations in supine and standing or sitting positions should be made by nursing staff. Daily EKG monitoring may be of value in even the least affected patients, as in some cases EKG changes were the harbinger of subsequent autonomic dysfunction.[71] In those patients requiring mechanical ventilation, pressures should be carefully monitored to prevent Valsalva-like effects. Cardiac monitoring should be instituted in any patient with signs suggestive of autonomic dysfunction, and staff should be alert to the possibility of cardiac arrhythmia occurring without previous EKG abnormality. Although the effect of autonomic dysfunction on surfactant regulation, bronchiolar dilatation and pulmonary blood supply has not to date been studied, the clinician should remember the possibility of such abnormalities in patients with AIPN and autonomic neuropathy.

The general approach to treatment of autonomic dysfunction in AIPN should be predicated on the observations that autonomic symptoms are often paroxysmal and widely fluctuating, and that extreme responses to chemotherapeutic intervention are not uncommon. The institution of any therapeutic measure should be done cautiously, preferably with short-acting and easily reversible compounds and under conditions of careful clinical monitoring. Treatment of hypotension should first be attempted with volume replacement. Cardiac arrhythmias may be controlled with the assistance of a temporary pacemaker. Careful and continuous monitoring should be the mainstay of treatment in any state of autonomic instability.

In addition to the above observations, those patients with AIPN should of course receive the careful nursing and respiratory therapist care which is critical to all paretic patients. Effective clearing of respiratory secretions, frequent changes in position and passive movement of the extremities in order to avoid the sequelae of prolonged immobilization are invaluable in determining the recovery of these patients. As has been stressed by many authors, the careful and meticulous care of a patient with AIPN may be one of the most rewarding in medicine, resulting in the full recovery of a healthy young person.

AIPN-Like Syndromes

Disease entities clinically indistinguishable from AIPN have been reported in association with a number of specific disorders (Table I). The clinical presentation and course of the syndrome in these cases is not significantly different from that in classic AIPN. Management considerations will of course involve treatment of coexisting disease processes, but will otherwise not differ from AIPN.

TABLE I
Other Neuropathies Which May Include Respiratory Dysfunction

ETIOLOGY	NERVES AND MUSCLES INVOLVED	FREQUENCY OF RESPIRATORY SYMPTOMS	MAY OCCUR AS AN ISOLATED FINDING	PROGRESSION	CAUSE OF DEATH
1. Beriberi (94)	Vagus: larynx and pharynx Phrenic: diaphragm	Common	No	Slow	No
2. Alcohol (95)	Vagus	Rare	No	Slow	No
3. Herpes zoster (96)	Phrenic: diaphragm	Rare	Yes	Weeks	No
4. *Metabolic disorders:* uremia, hepatic dysfunction, macroglobulinemia, post-tetanus toxoid, lymphoma, multiple myeloma, and others (97-101)	AIPN-like syndromes — Clinical picture not distinguishable from AIPN				

Diphtheria

Corynebacterium diphtheriae infections are relatively uncommon events in the United States, yet the specific tendency of the bacterial toxins to produce neuropathy resulting in respiratory dysfunction merits a brief discussion here. Neuropathy follows infection in about 10 to 20 percent of cases,[73] the result of bacterial toxins which create demyelination in the ganglia of peripheral nerves.[74] Prior to the advent of mechanical respiratory support, mortality was virtually 100 percent if phrenic neuropathy ensued.[75,76] The clinical course of faucial diphtheria follows a characteristic pattern in the majority of cases, and the severity of neurologic involvement seems to correlate with the severity of initial infection and the time of antitoxin administration, those cases receiving antitoxin within the first 48 hours showing the best prognosis.[77] The acute infection is followed in two to three weeks by paralysis and sensory loss of the soft palate, manifesting clinically as dysphagia and nasal voice associated with fatiguing of ocular accommodation.[78] These symptoms alone present no threat to the patient, but herald the possibility of more serious toxin-produced abnormalities.

The life-threatening neuropathies associated with diphtherial toxins are of two types. The first is the result of damage to the vagus nerve and ganglion as well as to the intracardiac conduction system, and results in cardiac arrhythmias. This neuropathic change follows shortly after the onset of bulbar symptoms and is characteristically self-limited, lasting for only a few weeks and not recurring. The second serious neuropathy affects the phrenic nerve and other peripheral nerves, and results in respiratory failure. This more generalized paralysis occurs after the resolution of the cardiac symptoms, about four to six weeks after the onset of illness. A complete paralysis of truncal and extremity musculature may occur, and changes in sensory as well as motor function in the areas involved are the rule.[79]

The characteristic clinical pattern of diphtheritic neuropathy, in association with the distinctive picture of previous diphtheria infection, does not usually present diagnostic difficulty. The neuropathic involvement of peripheral and autonomic nerves is demyelinating, and the pathophysiology of resultant cardiac and respiratory dysfunction is similar to that described for AIPN. The two conditions differ in that diphtheritic neuropathy follows a characteristic clinical progression, involving peripheral nerves of first the palate, then the heart and autonomic nervous system, and finally the diaphragm and other respiratory muscles. This orderly clinical progression is quite at variance with the precipitous deteriorations often seen in AIPN. Since the advent of mechanical respiratory support, the most dangerous aspect of diphtheritic neuropathy is abnormalities of cardiac rate and rhythm. In a recent report, a number of patients who were observed to survive this stage and to then require mechanical respiratory assistance were observed to have no further cardiac abnormalities. In these patients, paralysis resolved over several months, and residual pulmonary and cardiac damage was not observed.[79]

The general approach to the treatment of diphtheritic pulmonary and cardiac dysfunction is similar to that described for AIPN. The more predictable clinical course, without the precipitous changes so common to AIPN, allows the development of a rational treatment plan. Careful clinical monitoring, anticipation of cardiac and respiratory decompensation, and early intervention should be the mainstays of therapy. Prognosis for those patients surviving the initial phase of cardiac arrhythmias, when provided with meticulous respiratory care, is excellent.

Disorders of Porphyrin Metabolism

The hereditary hepatic porphyrias (acute intermittent porphyria, hereditary coproporphyria and variegate porphyria) may result in peripheral neuropathy with respiratory impairment that is clinically quite similar to that seen in AIPN. The pathophysiology of the peripheral nerve dysfunction remains a matter of investigation, but current evidence suggests that the primary abnormality is of the axonal type, with secondary demyelination contributing to the process.[80,81] The underlying metabolic disorder of porphyrin metabolism results clinically in attacks of abdominal pain, psychiatric syndromes and neuropathy, occurring either singly or in combination. The most common of these disorders, acute intermittent porphyria, classically presents early in adult life and is more common in females than in males. Onset may be precipitated by ingestion of a number of drugs, most characteristically barbiturates, sulfas and alcohol. Administration of these agents during an attack may aggravate existing symptoms.[82]

The neuropathy may be the presenting complaint or may occur after the presentation of either abdominal symptoms or psychiatric difficulties ranging from mild disorders of mood to acute psychosis. Pain is a frequent precursor to frank motor disability. Although the classic picture is that of a symmetric, progressive and predominantly motor neuropathy, asymmetric presentations and atypical distributions of sensory deficit are not uncommon. Respiratory disturbance may be precipitous, or the patient may suffer a slowly progressive course of muscle weakness over a period of weeks, which finally terminates in frank respiratory deterioration. Alterations of voice may herald impending respiratory dysfunction. When clinical respiratory distress is evident, bilateral diaphragmatic weakness is always the primary dysfunction, although weakness of other respiratory muscles may add to this impairment. Central nervous system dysfunction is also a frequent accompaniment to attacks, most commonly presenting as toxic states and seizures.[83] In some cases, disorders of central respiratory control have also been reported, with resultant central neurogenic hyperventilation.[84] An autonomic neuropathy is also a frequent problem in acute intermittent porphyria. Hypertension and resting tachycardia are the most common clinical abnormalities. As in other disorders of peripheral nerve where modern respiratory support has prevented death from respiratory arrest, death from cardiac arrest and arrhythmia is becoming a more frequent problem in porphyria.[85]

Treatment of the porphyrias is supportive, and vigorous care is indicated, as the possibility of complete or near complete recovery exists in this disorder. Early management should include careful monitoring of respiratory and cardiac status, in most cases within an intensive care unit. Drugs which are known to cause a deterioration in the porphyrias, including barbiturates, sulfonamides, various anesthetic agents, hydantoin and succinamides, and methyldopa should be avoided. A number of experimental therapeutic regimens have been reported by some authors to be of benefit to the underlying metabolic disturbance, and their administration should be considered.[86,87]

Respiratory monitoring should follow the pattern outlined for AIPN, and tracheostomy and respiratory support should be instituted promptly, when respiratory distress appears. Lengthy respiratory support is again indicated, and good recovery has been recorded after prolonged maintenance by artificial ventilation. The hypertension and tachycardia commonly present have been reported to respond to beta-adrenergic blocking agents such as propranolol. It has been suggested that an attack of porphyria should not be considered to have subsided unless the resting heart rate has returned to normal.[88]

Idiopathic Phrenic Neuropathy

Unilateral phrenic nerve dysfunction is generally of identifiable etiology, either from traumatic interruption, inflammatory involvement, or infiltrating, usually neoplastic disease. The condition itself is usually asymptomatic, although some patients may report exertional dyspnea. When unilateral phrenic neuropathy is present, the most important task for the physician is to detect the underlying pathology. A number of cases, however, have been reported with an apparently idiopathic etiology, in several cases despite exploratory thoracotomy in search of etiologic cause. In general, these patients seem to do well, and do not progress to suffer further neuromuscular respiratory disorders.[89-91]

A more unusual disorder is bilateral phrenic neuropathy presenting as the first manifestation of polyneuropathy. The few reported cases describe the onset in adults of progressive respiratory impairment characterized by orthopnea and, in some cases, exertional dyspnea. In several cases, intrinsic cardiac or pulmonary disease was diagnosed and treated without relief of symptoms. Respiratory complaints were always the predominant cause of patient discomfort, although subsequent neurologic evaluation sometimes revealed either an apparently long-standing peripheral motor neuropathy or documented progression of the presenting disorder to include more extensive peripheral neuropathy after several weeks. In all cases, the diagnosis of neuromuscular rather than primary cardiopulmonary dysfunction was determined by the use of specific tests of respiratory muscle function, as described in the first section of this chapter. Although reports of such cases are few, their existence emphasizes the importance of clinical suspicion and appropriate diagnostic evaluation in atypical or poorly responsive cases of apparent intrinsic cardiac or pulmonary disease.[11,17,18,92,93]

Other Peripheral Neuropathies

A number of other disorders of peripheral nerve have been found occasionally to include disorders of respiration during the course of the disease process. In general, respiratory dysfunction in these entities has been mild and slowly progressive in nature, and has usually not been responsible for significant disability or death. A summary of some of these neuropathies is presented in Table I. It should be remembered, however, that this list is not exhaustive, and the appropriate evaluation of any patient presenting with respiratory difficulty in the absence of clearly defined cardiopulmonary pathology should include an evaluation of respiratory nerve and muscle function.

A final disorder of peripheral nerve which may result in respiratory symptoms is Isaac's syndrome. The clinical picture of myokymia, generalized muscle stiffness and depressed tendon reflexes was described in 1961.[102] This syndrome is the result of continuous neural activity originating in the peripheral motor nerve, rather than in central nervous system structures or peripheral muscle. In those cases reported, the most common pulmonary abnormalities are secondary to the decreased compliance of chest wall musculature and to kyphosis induced by persistent hypertonicity of truncal musculature.[103] Prominent decreases of forced expiratory volume (one second), vital capacity, and maximum breathing capacity are documented in untreated cases.[104] In one recent report,[105] a patient who presented with exertional dyspnea and hoarseness was found to have additional physical findings and electrodiagnostic studies consistent with Isaac's syndrome. Pulmonary function studies in this case were consistent with an extrathoracic obstructive abnormality presumably the result of laryngeal spasm. Treatment with phenytoin and/or carbamazepine is effective in relieving symptoms in most cases of Isaac's syndrome.[103,105,106]

SUMMARY

The first section of this chapter describes techniques available for diagnosis and clinical monitoring of patients suffering respiratory distress secondary to dysfunction of peripheral nerve and respiratory musculature. The most important of these abnormalities is dysfunction of the phrenic nerves or diaphragm, and particular attention is paid to this area.

The second section describes those peripheral neuropathies which most commonly present significant respiratory distress in association with the neuropathy. Acute inflammatory polyradiculoneuropathy serves in many ways as a prototype for the pathophysiologic respiratory mechanisms underlying all of these disorders. AIPN is also the most common peripheral neuropathy to cause respiratory failure, and is therefore discussed more extensively than other neuropathic processes. Important distinguishing points between AIPN and other neuropathies causing respiratory impairment are clarified in the sections describing other neuropathic processes.

Central to all these pathologic processes, however, is the importance of early recognition and intervention. The coordinated interplay between neurologist, respiratory physician and respiratory support personnel is essential to maximize recovery. Clearly, prompt and careful management of these often self-limited but temporarily devastating diseases has dramatically changed the long-term prognosis for these conditions.

REFERENCES

1. Hall, W.J.: Respiratory failure as a complication of neuromuscular disease. In Griggs, R.C., and Moxley, R.T. (eds.): *Advances in Neurology*, Vol. 17. New York, Raven Press, 1977, p. 317.

2. Agostoni, E., and Mead, J.: Statics of the respiratory system. In Fenn, W.O., and Rahn, H. (eds.): *Handbook of Physiology,* Sec. 3. Baltimore, Waverly Press, 1964, p. 387.
3. Mead, J., and Agostoni, E.: Dynamics of breathing. In Fenn, W.O., and Rahn, H. (eds.): *Handbook of Physiology,* Sec. 3. Baltimore, Waverly Press, 1964, p. 411.
4. Jones, J.G.: The chest wall–tone and movement. *Anesthesiology* **47**: 325–326, 1977.
5. Sears, T.A.: Pathways of supraspinal origin regulating the activity of respiratory motor neurons. In Grant, R. (ed.): *Nobel Symposium I: Muscular Afferents and Motor Control.* New York, John Wiley and Sons, 1966, pp. 187.
6. Von Euler, C.: Proprioceptive control in respiration. In Grant, R. (ed.): *Nobel Symposium I: Muscular Afferents and Motor Control.* New York, John Wiley and Sons, 1966, pp. 197.
7. Lindall, A., Medina, A., and Grisiner, J.T.: A reevaluation of normal pulmonary function measurement. *Am. Rev. Resp. Dis.* **95**: 1061, 1967.
8. Harrison, B.D.W., Collins, J.V., Brown, K.G.E., et al.: Respiratory failure in neuromuscular disease. *Thorax* **26**: 579–584, 1971.
9. Keltz, H.: The effect of respiratory muscle dysfunction on pulmonary function; Studies in patients with neuromuscular disease. *Am. Rev. Resp. Dis.* **91**: 934, 1965.
10. Burrows, B., Kasik, J.E., and Niden, A.H.: Clinical usefulness of the single breath pulmonary diffusing capacity test. *Am. Rev. Resp. Dis.* **84**: 789, 1961.
11. Goldstein, R.L., Hyde, R.W., Lapham, L.W., Gazioglu, K., and de Papp, Z.G.: Peripheral neuropathy presenting with respiratory insufficiency as the primary complaint. Problem of recognizing alveolar hypoventilation due to neuromuscular disorders. *Am. J. Med.* **56**: 443–449, 1974.
12. Black, L.F., and Hyatt, R.E.: Maximal static respiratory pressures in generalized neuromuscular disease. *Am. Rev. Resp. Dis.* **99**: 696–702, 1969.
13. Black, L.F., and Hyatt, R.E.: Maximal respiratory pressures: normal values and relationship to age and sex. *Am. Rev. Resp. Dis.* **99**: 696, 1969.
14. Alexander, C.: Diaphragm movements and the diagnosis of diaphragmatic paralysis. *Clin. Radiol.* **17**: 79, 1966.
15. Agostini, E.: Action of respiratory muscles. In Fenn, W.O.,

and Rahn, H. (eds.): *Handbook of Physiology,* Sec. 3. Baltimore, Waverly Press, 1964.

16. Davis, J.N., Goldman, M., Loh, L., et al.: Diaphragm function and alveolar hypoventilation. *Quart. J. Med.* **177**: 87–100, 1976.
17. Spitzer, S.A., Korczyn, A.D., and Kalaei, J.: Transient bilateral diaphragmatic paralysis. *Chest* **64**: 355–357, 1973.
18. Schmalsteig, E.J., Peters, B.H., Schochet, S.S., and Findly, S.R.: Neuropathy presenting as prolonged dyspnea. Case report and a review of the literature. *Arch. Neurol.* **34**: 473–476, 1977.
19. Davis, J.N.: Phrenic nerve conduction in man. *J. Neurol. Neurosurg. Psychiat.* **30**: 420–426, 1967.
20. Taylor, A.: The contribution of the intercostal muscles to the effort of respiration in man. *J. Physiol.* **151**: 390–402, 1960.
21. Fink, B.R.: Electromyography in general anesthesia. *Br. J. Anaesth.* **33**: 555, 1961.
22. Rhoads, G.G., and Brody, J.S.: Idiopathic alveolar hypoventilation: Clinical spectrum. *Ann. Intern. Med.* **71**: 271, 1969.
23. Mellin, R.B., Balfour, H.H., Jr., Turino, G.M., and Winters, R.W.: Failure of automatic control of ventilation (Ondine's curse). *Medicine* **49**: 487, 1970.
24. Tusiewiczk, K., Bryan, A.C., and Froese, A.B.: Contributions of changing rib cage-diaphragm interactions to the ventilatory depression of halothane anesthesia. *Anesthesiology* **47**: 327–337, 1977.
25. Gilliam, P.M.S., Heat, P.J.D., Kaufman, L., and Lucas, B.G.B.: Respiration in dystrophia myotonia. *Thorax* **19**: 112–120, 1964.
26. Kaufman, L.: Anaesthesia in dystrophia myotonia. A review of the hazards of anaesthesia. *Proc. Roy. Soc. Med.* **53**: 183, 1960.
27. Campbell, E.J.M., Agostini, E., and Davis, J.N.: *The Respiratory Muscles: Mechanics and Neural Control.* London, Lloyd-Luke, 1970.
28. Stern, L.Z., Gruener, R., and Anderson, R.M.: External intercostal muscle biopsy. *Arch. Neurol.* **32**: 779–780, 1975.
29. Eyzaguirre, C., Sampson, S., and Taylor, J.R.: The motor control of intrinsic laryngeal muscles in the cat. In Grant, R. (ed.): *Nobel Symposium I: Muscular Afferents and Motor Control.* New York, John Wiley and Sons, 1966, p. 209.

30. Elam, J.O., Hemingway, A., Gulliekson, G., and Visscher, M.B.: Impairment of pulmonary function in poliomyelitis. *Arch. Intern Med.* **81**: 649, 1948.
31. Scharf, S.M., Feldman, N.T., Goldman, M.D., Haut, H.Z., Bruce, E., and Ingram, R.H., Jr.: Vocal cord closure: A cause of upper airway obstruction during controlled ventilation. *Am. Rev. Resp. Dis.* **117**: 391, 1978.
32. Eldridge, F.L.: Central nervous system and chemoreceptor factors in control of breathing. *Chest* **73** (2) Suppl.: 256, 1978.
33. Sears, T.A.: The respiratory motoneuron and apneusis. *Fed. Proc.* **36**: 2412–2420, 1977.
34. Gabella, G.: *Structure of the Autonomic Nervous System.* New York, John Wiley and Sons, 1976, pp. 158.
35. Brodal, A.: *Neurological Anatomy in Relation to Clinical Medicine,* 2nd Ed. New York, Oxford Press, 1969.
36. Oyarzun, M.J., and Clements, J.A.: Control of lung surfactant by ventilation, adrenergic mediators, and prostaglandins in the rabbit. *Am. Rev. Resp. Dis.* **117**: 879, 1978.
37. Appenzeller, O.: *The Autonomic Nervous System.* New York, American Elsevier Publishing Co., Inc., 1976.
38. Stremel, R.W.: Role of vagal afferents and the carotid bodies in the hypopnea consequent to diminished pulmonary blood flow. *Chest* **73** (2) Suppl.: 270–272, 1978.
39. Carroll, J.E., Zwillich, C., Weil, J.V., and Brooke, M.H.: Depressed ventilatory response in oculo-craniosomatic neuromuscular disease. *Neurology* **26**: 140, 1976.
40. Riley, D.J.: Blunted respiratory drive in congenital myopathy. *Am. J. Med.* **63**: 459–466, 1977.
41. Cherniack, N.S.: Abnormal breathing patterns. *D. M.:* 1–45, July 1975.
42. Read, D.J.C.: A clinical method of assessing the ventilatory response to carbon dioxide. *Australian Ann. Med.* **16**: 20, 1967.
43. Baker, A.B., and Baker, L.H.: *Clinical Neurology,* Vols. 1, 2, and 3. Hagerstown, Md., Harper and Row, 1975.
44. Lesser, R.P., Hauser, W.A., et al.: Epidemiologic features of the Guillain-Barré Syndrome: Experience in Olmstead County, Minnesota, 1935–1968. *Neurology* **23**: 1269–1274, 1973.
45. Haymaker, W., and Kernohan, J.: The Landry-Guillain-Barré Syndrome, a clinicopathologic report of 50 cases and a critique of the literature. *Medicine* **28**: 59–141, 1949.
46. Appenzeller, O., Arnason, B.G., and Adams, R.D.: Experi-

mental autonomic neuropathology: an immunologically induced disorder of reflex vasomotor function. *J. Neurol. Neurosurg. Psychiat.* **28**: 510, 1965.

47. Arnason, B.G.W.: Inflammatory polyradiculopathies. In Dyck, P.J., Thomas, P.K., and Lambert, E.H. (eds.): *Peripheral Neuropathy,* Vol. II. Philadelphia, W.B. Saunders Co., 1975, pp. 1110–1148.
48. Asbury, A.K., and Arnason, B.G.: Experimental allergic neuritis; a radioautographic study. *J. Neuropath. Exp. Neurol.* **27**: 581-589, 1968.
49. Pollard, J.D., King, R.H.M., and Thomas, P.K.: Recurrent experimental allergic neuritis: an electron microscope study. *J. Neurol. Sci.* **24**: 365–370, 1975.
50. McFarland, H.R., and Heller, G.L.: Guillain-Barré disease complex: a statement of diagnostic criteria and analysis of 100 cases. *Arch. Neurol.* **14**: 196–201, 1966.
51. Hewer, R.L., Hilton, P.J., Crampton Smith, A., and Spalding, J.M.K.: Acute polyneuritis requiring artificial respiration. *Quart. J. Med.* **37**: 479, 1968.
52. Dyck, P.J., Lais, A., Michiya, O., Bastron, J., Okazaki, H., and Groover, R.: Chronic inflammatory polyradiculoneuropathy. *Mayo Clin. Proc.* **50**: 621–637, 1975.
53. Brody, I., and Wilkins, R.: Guillain-Barré-Strohl syndrome. *Arch. Neurol.* **18**: 449–452, 1968.
54. Marshall, J.: The Landry-Guillain-Barré syndrome. *Brain* **LXXXVI**: 55–66, 1963.
55. Asbury, A.K., Arnason, B.G.W., Kard, H.R., and McFarlin, D.E.: Criteria for diagnosis of Guillain-Barré syndrome. *Ann. Neurol.* **3**: 565, 1978.
56. Polk, B.V.: Cardiopulmonary complications of Guillain-Barré syndrome. *Heart Lung* **5**: 967–970, 1976.
57. Briskier, A.A.: Unusual rapid evolution of Guillain-Barré syndrome with bulbar palsy. *J. Nerv. Ment. Dis.* **100**: 462, 1944.
58. Forster, F.M., Brown, M., and Merritt, H.H.: Polyneuritis with facial diplegia, a clinical study. *N. Eng. J. Med.* **225**: 50–51, 1941.
59. Whitehouse, A.C., and Petty, T.L.: Recovery in Landry-Guillain-Barré syndrome after prolonged respiratory support. *Lancet* **1**: 1029–1030, 1969.
60. Castaigne, P., Brunet, P., and Novailhat, F.: Enquete clinique sur les polyradiculonèvrites inflammatoires en France. *Rev. Neurol. (Paris)* **115**: 849, 1966.

61. Margairaz, A., and Emile, J.: Syndromes polyradiculonèvritiques extensifs et techniques de réanimation neuro-respiratoires. *Rev. Neurol. (Paris)* **115**: 873, 1966.
62. Hall, W.J.: Respiratory failure as a complication of neuromuscular disease. In *Advances in Neurology,* Vol. 17. New York, Raven Press, 1977, pp. 317–324.
63. Osler, W.: *The Principles and Practice of Medicine.* New York, Appleton Press, 1892, pp. 777–778.
64. Birchfield, R.I., and Shaw, C.M.: Postural hypotension in the Guillain-Barré syndrome. *Arch. Neurol.* **10**: 149–157, 1964.
65. Appenzeller, O., and Marshall, J.: Vasomotor disturbance in Landry-Guillain-Barré syndrome. *Arch. Neurol.* **9**: 368, 1963.
66. Mitchell, P.L., and Meilman, E.: The mechanism of hypertension in the Gullain-Barré syndrome. *Am. J. Med.* **42**: 986–995, 1967.
67. Watson, W.E.: Some circulatory response to Valsalva's maneuver in patients with polyneuritis and spinal cord dysfunction. *J. Neurol. Neurosurg. Psychiat.* **25**: 19–23, 1962.
68. Hobday, J.D., and Baker, A.J.: Gullain-Barré syndrome complicated by hypertension and ileitis. *Med. J. Austr.* **2**: 536, 1968.
69. Davies, A.G., and Dingle, H.R.: Observations on cardiovascular and neuroendocrine disturbance in the Guillain-Barré syndrome. *J. Neurol. Neurosurg. Psychiat.* **35**: 176–179, 1972.
70. Clarke, E.S., Bayliss, R.S., and Cooper, R.: Cardiovascular manifestations of the Guillain-Barré syndrome. *Br. Med. J.* **2**: 1504, 1954.
71. Lichtenfeld, P.: Autonomic dysfunction in the Guillain-Barré syndrome. *Am. J. Med.* **50**: 772, 1971.
72. Chuttani, P.N., Chawla, L.S., Chugh, D.S., and Singh, H.: Landry-Guillain-Barré-Strohl syndrome in India. *J. Neurol. Sci.* **7**: 581, 1968.
73. Rolleston, J.D., and Ronaldson, G.W.: *Acute Infectious Diseases,* 3rd Ed. London, Heinemann, 1940.
74. Fisher, C.M., and Adams, R.D.: Diphtheritic polyneuropathy—a pathological study. *J. Neuropath. Exp. Neurol.* **15**: 243–268, 1956.
75. Alesen, L.A.: Post diphtheritic paralysis of the diaphragm. *J.A.M.A.* **84**: 730, 1925.
76. Scheid, W.: Diphtherial paralysis: An analysis of 229 cases of

diphtheria including more than 174 cases of polyneuritis. *J. Nerv. Ment. Dis.* **116**: 1095–1101, 1952.

77. McDonald, W., and Kocen, R.S.: Diphtheritic neuropathy. In Dyck, P.J., Thomas, P.K., and Lambert, E.H. (eds.): *Peripheral Neuropathy,* Vol. II. Philadelphia, W.B. Saunders Co., 1975, pp. 1281–1300.
78. Walshe, F.M.R.: On the pathogenesis of diphtheritic paralysis. II. Clinical observations on the paralysis of faucial and extrafaucial diphtheria, with an analysis of thirty cases following skin and wound infections. *Quart. J. Med.* **12**: 14–17, 1918–1919.
79. Emile, J., Bazin, C., and Truelle, J.L.: Extensive neuropathies caused by diphtheria. Apropos of the respiratory forms. *Rev. Neurol. (Paris)* **130** (1-2): 76–84, 1974.
80. Mustajoki, P., and Seppäläinen, A.M.: Neuropathy in latent hereditary hepatic porphyria. *Br. Med. J.* **2**: 310–131, 1975.
81. Sweeney, V.P., Patnak, M.H., and Asbury, A.K.: Acute intermittent porphyria: increased ALA synthetase activity during an acute attack. *Brain* **93**: 369–380, 1970.
82. Dean, G.: The porphyrias. *Br. Med. Bull.* **25**: 48–62, 1969.
83. Goldberg, A.: Acute intermittent porphyria: a study of 50 cases. *Quart. J. Med.* **28**: 183–209, 1959.
84. Baker, N.H., and Messert, B.: Acute intermittent porphyria with central neurogenic hyperventilation. *Neurology* **17**: 559–567, 1967.
85. Walton, J.N.: *Brain's Disease of the Nervous System,* 8th Ed. New York, Oxford University Press, 1977, p. 827.
86. Goldberg, A.: Diagnosis and treatment of the porphyrias *Proc. Roy. Soc. Med.* **61**: 193–198, 1968.
87. Welby, K., Street, J.P., and Watson, C.J.: Chlorpromazine in the treatment of porphyria. *J.A.M.A.* **162**: 174–176, 1956.
88. Atsmon, A., and Blum, I.: Treatment of acute porphyria variegata with propranolol. *Lancet* **1**: 196–197, 1970.
89. Riley, E.A.: Idiopathic diaphragmatic paralysis. *Am. J. Med.* **32**: 404, 1962.
90. Lieberman, A.: Spontaneous unilateral diaphragmatic paresis. *N.Y. State J. Med.* **54**: 2737, 1954.
91. Douglas, B.E., and Clagett, O.T.: The prognosis in idiopathic diaphragmatic paralysis. *Dis. Chest* **37**: 294, 1960.
92. Sandham, J.D.: Acute supine respiratory failure to bilateral diaphragmatic paralysis. *Chest* **72**: 96–98, 1977.

93. McCredie, M., Lovejoy, F.W., and Kaltreider, N.L.: Pulmonary function in diaphragmatic paralysis. *Thorax* **17**: 213–217, 1962.
94. Loeb, C.M., and Greenebaum, R.S.: Beriberi: secondary to hernia of mesentery. *J.A.M.A.* **112**: 1810–1814, 1939.
95. Novak, D.J., and Victor, M.: Affection of the vagus and sympathetic nerves in alcoholic polyneuropathy. *Arch. Neurol.* **30**: 273–284, 1974.
96. Brostoff, J.: Diaphragmatic paralysis after herpes zoster. *Br. Med. J.* **2**: 1571, 1966.
97. Logothesis, J., Silverstein, P., and Coe, S.: Neurologic aspects of Waldenström's macroglobulinemia. *Arch. Neurol.* **3**: 564, 1960.
98. Liske, E., Chou, S.M., and Thompson, H.G.: Peripheral and autonomic neuropathy in amyloidosis. *J.A.M.A.* **186**: 432, 1963.
99. Comroe, J.H., Wood, F.C., Kay, C.F., et al.: Motor neuritis after tetanus antitoxins with involvement of the muscles of respiration. *Am. J. Med.* **10**: 786–789, 1951.
100. Schott, B., Tommasi, N., et al.: Neuropathie périphérique demyelinisante au cours d'une intoxication par l'oxyde de carbone. *Rev. Neurol.* **116**: 429–437, 1967.
101. Asbury, A.K.: Hepatic neuropathy. In Dyck, P.J., Thomas, P.K., and Lambert, E.H. (eds.): *Peripheral Neuropathy,* Vol. II. Philadelphia, W.B. Saunders Co., 1975, pp. 993–998.
102. Isaacs, H.: Syndrome of continuous muscle fibre activity. *J. Neurol. Neurosurg. Psychiat.* **24**: 319–325, 1961.
103. Hughes, R.C., and Mathews, W.B.: Pseudo-myotonia and myokymia. *J. Neurol. Neurosurg. Psychiat.* **32**: 11–14, 1969.
104. Wallis, W.E., Poznak, A.V., and Pulm, I.: Generalized muscular stiffness, fasciculations and myokymia of peripheral nerve origin. *Arch. Neurol.* **22**: 430–439, 1970.
105. Jackson, D.L., Satya-Murti, S., Davis, L., and Drachman, D.B.: Isaacs syndrome with laryngeal involvement: An unusual presentation of myokymia. *Neurology* **29**: 1612–1615, 1979.
106. Isaacs, H.: Continuous muscle fibre activity in an Indian male with additional evidence of terminal motor fibre activity. *J. Neurol. Neurosurg. Psychiat.* **30**: 126–133, 1967.

6

Respiratory Complications of Neuromuscular Disease

Steven P. Ringel, M.D., and James E. Carroll, M.D.

As physicians who manage numerous patients with neuromuscular diseases, we are confronted with pulmonary complications almost daily. Respiratory failure or aspiration pneumonia may occur as an initial manifestation, particularly if the patient presents with acute muscle weakness, or the same symptoms may occur much later in a patient that already has chronic, debilitating weakness. The end stage neuromuscular patient can become a pulmonary cripple; he is unable to adequately ventilate the lungs, compromised not only by weakened muscles of respiration, but also by recurrent aspiration, insufficient cough reflex, and shrinking pulmonary reserve from progressive scoliosis. Less frequently, a patient with mild neuromuscular disease can suddenly deteriorate and have an acute respiratory crisis which is not associated with pneumonia or a sudden decline in strength. This event can be produced by relatively isolated diaphragmatic weakness or by an unresponsive chemoreceptor mechanism in association with weakening respiratory muscles. In spite of all these pulmonary complications, it is only the rare neuromuscular patient that has primary pulmonary pathology such as pulmonary fibrosis in association with an inflammatory myopathy.

This chapter is designed to illustrate the myriad pulmonary complications that can occur in patients with neuromuscular disease. The first section gives a classification of the neuromuscular diseases, along with a brief discussion of the common symptoms, signs and laboratory tests that aid in making a diagnosis. Our intent is to provide the physician with a useful framework of neuromuscular diseases rather than with a comprehensive review. For details of particular disorders, the reader is referred to several recent, comprehensive textbooks of neuromuscular disease.[1-7]

The second section discusses neuromuscular diseases in relation to pulmonary physiology and the tests that are most useful in assessing the patient's pulmonary capacity. Neurologists should find practical value in this section but may wish to read in greater detail from several excellent pulmonary reviews.[8-12]

The remainder of the chapter is organized around pulmonary complications the neurologist or pulmonary physician may encounter in managing a patient with neuromuscular disease. Since the same pulmonary complication can occur with a variety of neuromuscular diseases, each disorder will be discussed only as it relates to the complication under discussion.

CLASSIFICATION OF NEUROMUSCULAR DISEASES

A motor unit is a functional anatomical entity that is the basic unit of muscle movement. In the major limb muscles, a single motor unit consists of an anterior horn cell, its accompanying axon, and the 400 to 1,000 muscle fibers it innervates. These muscle fibers are not grouped together in independent fascicles; rather, they interdigitate with fibers of other motor units producing a checkerboard pattern. Two major physiologic types of motor units are present in man, each having a unique enzymatic staining reaction or histochemical profile.

Diseases are conveniently described depending on the part of the motor unit they affect (Table I). They can be categorized as: diseases of the anterior horn cell (neuronal disorders); diseases of nerve (neuropathies); diseases of the neuromuscular junction; and diseases of muscle (myopathies). In many cases, the physician will find these tradi-

TABLE I
Classification of Common Neuromuscular Diseases

I. *Anterior Horn Cell* (neuronal)
- Spinal muscular atrophies (Werdnig Hoffman; Kugelberg Welander)
- Motor neuron disease (ALS)
- Poliomyelitis

II. *Peripheral Nerve* (neuropathy)
- Metabolic (uremia, hepatic failure)
- Endocrine (diabetes, thyroid)
- Toxic (lead, arsenic, vincristine, Dilantin, etc.)
- Hereditary (Charcot-Marie-Tooth)
- Immunologic (Guillain Barré, lupus, rheumatoid arthritis)
- Vitamin deficiency

III. *Neuromuscular Junction*
- Myasthenia gravis
- Botulism

IV. *Muscle* (myopathy)
- Dystrophies (Duchenne, FSH, limb girdle, CPEO)
- Myotonic disorders
- Congenital myopathics (central core, rod, myotubular)
- Periodic paralysis
- Inflammatory myopathies (polymyositis, dermatomyositis)
- Metabolic myopathies (glycogen and lipid storage diseases)
- Endocrine myopathies (thyroid, adrenal)
- Toxic myopathies (alcohol, chloroquine, etc)

tional disease categories simple and convenient to use since they have certain features common both in the neurological examination and in special laboratory investigations including serum enzyme determinations, electrodiagnostic studies such as electromyography (EMG) and nerve conduction velocities (NCV), and muscle or nerve biopsy. In a small percentage of diseases, the classification scheme is less useful, particularly when the pathogenesis of the disease is poorly defined, or when more than one part of the motor unit is affected. For example, since a nerve has a trophic influence on muscle physiology, histochemistry and biochemistry, any primary disease of the anterior horn cell or peripheral nerve would be expected to produce both neuronal and muscular changes.

Neuronal Diseases

In diseases of the anterior horn cell, a patient may note cramps, symmetrical or asymmetrical weakness of the extremities, and bulbar dysfunction. Examination will reveal varying amounts of atrophy, hyporeflexia, and fasciculations. Classification of the anterior horn cell diseases is based on the age of onset, rate of progression, difference in inheritance if the disorder is familial, and the anatomical distribution of the weakness. EMG in these patients will usually show diffuse fibrillations, which represent individual muscle fibers firing spontaneously, positive sharp waves, and prolonged, high voltage polyphasic motor unit potentials. These giant polyphasic potentials probably represent enlarged motor unit territories produced as a result of sprouting of nerves with reinnervation of previously denervated muscle fibers. Nerve conduction velocities are usually normal. Muscle biopsy often shows a combination of atrophic, angular appearing fibers which stain darkly with the oxidative enzyme reactions, and a rearrangement of the histochemical fiber types with type grouping and group atrophy.

The most common anterior horn cell syndromes include infantile and juvenile spinal muscular atrophy, motor neuron disease and poliomyelitis. Infantile spinal muscular atrophy, or Werdnig Hoffman disease, is usually recognized before the age of three months and is fatal before the age of two. Some children may live for many years although they remain extremely incapacitated because of severe weakness and progressive scoliosis. This scoliosis can contribute significantly to abnormal respiratory function so that many patients eventually die of pulmonary complications if spinal collapse is not arrested. In juvenile spinal muscular atrophy, or the Kugelberg Welander syndrome, symptoms begin later in childhood or adolescence, and the proximal muscles are primarily affected. The earlier the onset of symptoms the more severe the disease is likely to become, but in most patients it is slowly progressive. Because of the proximal distribution of weakness many of these patients' symptoms are easily confused with primary muscle diseases. However, electrophysiological studies and muscle biopsy will confirm the neuronal nature of the disorder. The spinal muscular atrophies are usually autosomal recessively inherited but occasional autosomal dominant, sex-linked recessive, or sporadic cases have been described.

In motor neuron disease (amyotrophic lateral sclerosis) signs of spasticity and hyperreflexia (progressive lateral sclerosis) indicating damage to the upper motor neurons often accompany weakness and wasting of the extremities (progressive muscular atrophy). Weakness of bulbar musculature (progressive bulbar palsy) can cause great difficulty in speaking and swallowing. Confinement to a wheelchair can occur within one to two years, and death usually occurs from respiratory failure. The disease is typically sporadic but rarely can be inherited in an autosomal dominant pattern. The diagnosis is likely if weakness, wasting and fasciculations are found in three or more limbs associated with hyperreflexia.

Poliomyelitis is an acute infectious disease caused by a virus that has an affinity for the large motor cells in both the medulla and the ventral horn of the spinal cord. The end stage of the disease is characterized by flaccid paralysis of muscles innervated by affected anterior horn cells. The extent of muscle paralysis may range from minimal to widespread, involving extremities, truncal, and bulbar muscles. With worldwide immunization programs since the Salk vaccine was developed in 1955 and the Sabin vaccine in 1960, poliomyelitis is rarely seen today. Nevertheless, the principles of pulmonary care and the effects of respiratory muscle paralysis on breathing which were learned in the management of polio play an important role today in the management of other patients with neuromuscular disease.

Neuropathies

In peripheral neuropathies, early symptoms are usually related to a loss of strength in the small hand muscles or to a foot drop. In addition, there may be associated stocking-glove sensory loss since the distal afferent sensory fibers in the peripheral nerve may also be involved. Atrophy and hyporeflexia are usually early signs. The EMG and muscle biopsy are indistinguishable from diseases of the anterior horn cell, but motor or sensory nerve conduction velocities are often prolonged and may be slowed in some patients before the onset of clinical weakness. Terminal latency times may be impaired before the conduction velocities and are helpful in determining peripheral entrapment syndromes. Numerous classifications have been devised for peripheral neuropathies, since the causes are so numerous and diverse. Several excellent reviews are available for the reader who wishes to study these in greater detail.[2,5]

Diseases of the Neuromuscular Junction

The most common disorder of the neuromuscular junction is myasthenia gravis. In this disease, in which pathologic fatigue of bulbar and extremity muscles is a prominent manifestation, sudden respiratory compromise can occur with little warning. Recent studies have shown that the primary abnormality in this disorder is an immune reaction directed against the acetylcholine receptor site on the postsynaptic membrane of the neuromuscular junction.[13] During impulse conduction, acetylcholine is released normally from the presynaptic nerve ending but has an attenuated affect on the altered postsynaptic membrane. This produces the symptoms of pathologic fatigue.

Exposure to several chemicals and neurotoxins which have marked effects at the neuromuscular junction can result in acute weakness. Organophosphate insecticides, botulinum toxin, and succinylcholine administration to a patient without pseudocholinesterase can result in life-threatening weakness in a person otherwise normal.

Myopathies

Myopathies are disorders of muscles in which there is no evidence of neural abnormality. They include the genetic dystrophies, congenital myopathies, myotonic disorders, the periodic paralyses, glycogen and lipid storage diseases, the inflammatory myopathies, and several endocrine or toxic disorders. In these diseases, the fundamental defect may be either in the muscle membrane (myotonia) or in the contractile process (myophosphorylase deficiency), or the muscle may be the target of a generalized disorder such as an enzyme defect (acid maltase deficiency) or an endocrine disorder (thyroid myopathy). Similarly, in the inflammatory myopathies, a virus (influenza B), parasite (trichinosis), toxin (chloroquin), or collagen vascular disease (dermatomyositis) may produce widespread inflammation in muscle.

In a myopathy, weakness is usually symmetrical, involves all four limbs, and is more prominent proximally. Patients will have difficulty in raising arms over their heads, climbing stairs, and getting out of chairs. Unlike the neuropathies, deep tendon reflexes persist until late in the disorder, and the degree of atrophy is proportionally less than the amount of weakness.

The characteristic EMG abnormality in a myopathy is a motor unit that is polyphasic, shortened in duration and of low voltage. Features seen in denervation are uncommon in myopathies, but scattered fibrillatory activity can occur. Furthermore, motor units similar to those in myopathies can be seen in longstanding denervating diseases, so that the EMG, although helpful, may not always allow a specific diagnosis. The nerve conduction velocities are normal in a myopathy, as in anterior horn cell disease.

Serum enzymes, particularly creatine kinase (CK) are often elevated in myopathies, presumably as a result of the efflux of intramuscular enzymes from a damaged cell. In acute and subacute myopathies, CK is often markedly elevated, while in chronic myopathies it may be normal or only mildly elevated. In peripheral neuropathies, spinal muscular atrophies, and ALS a modest elevation of CK is occasionally seen so that CK may not distinguish myopathic from neuropathic disease.

In a myopathy, the muscle biopsy shows a variety of changes in individual fibers, rather than abnormalities of the entire motor unit. Fibers in various stages of degeneration or regeneration are seen, but an alteration of histochemical fiber types is not prominent. This distinction is useful in many of the diseases but is of less value in the study of congenital disorders associated with neuromuscular weakness. In these congenital myopathies, or perhaps more appropriately termed congenital neuromuscular diseases, children are often born weak and hypotonic or have delayed motor milestones. Unique structural alterations are seen in the muscle biopsy associated with a variety of histochemical fiber type changes. Alteration of the trophic influence of nerve on muscle has been hypothesized as partly responsible for these disorders.

The genetic dystrophies are characterized by progressive muscle weakness. Their classification has been, for the most part, on clinical grounds although recent morphological evidence has suggested that there may be altered neuronal influence as well as "dystrophic" muscle changes in several of them. The most common varieties include Duchenne dystrophy, myotonic dystrophy, limb girdle dystrophy, facioscapulohumeral dystrophy, and the progressive external ophthalmoplegias. Duchenne dystrophy is a sex-linked recessive disease which begins from ages three to five and is inexorably progressive with death in the second or third decade. A combination of proximal weakness, large gastrocnemii, tight heel cords, and markedly elevated serum CK is seen. In myotonic dystrophy, an autosomal dominantly inherited disease, varying amounts of diffuse facial and extremity weakness as well as delayed relaxation of muscles (myotonia) are characteristic along with cataracts, gonadal atrophy, ptosis and frontal balding. Limb girdle dystrophy is recessively inherited and is characterized by the slow development of proximal weakness of the shoulders and hips. It usually begins in the first two decades of life. In facioscapulohumeral dystrophy, slowly progressive weakness of the face, shoulders, and upper arms is seen. As with other autosomal dominant disorders, there is marked variability in the degree of impairment of the patients so that minimally affected family members often go undetected for years. The progressive external ophthalmoplegias are actually a group of diseases which have in common ptosis and ophthalmoparesis. In addition to these findings, a variety of disturbances of the neuraxis may be present.

PULMONARY PHYSIOLOGY

Under normal circumstances the diaphragm is the principal muscle of inspiration. During quiet breathing, intercostal muscles function primarily in stabilizing the chest wall during changes in intrathoracic pressure.[8-12] However, the intercostals and accessory muscles of respiration may become the primary inspiratory muscles and sustain ventilation without leading to respiratory failure in certain cases, such as bilateral diaphragmatic paralysis.[14]

Expiration is completely passive and does not require muscle contraction. Thus, expiratory flow limitation is important only in the neuromuscular disease patient having an obstructive component due to another disorder such as asthma or emphysema.

With neuromuscular disease the lack of tone in the chest musculature leaves the recoil pressures of the lung relatively unopposed, producing a smaller resting lung volume or functional residual capacity. The result of this underinflation of the lungs is both atelectasis and airway closure. This results in an abnormal distribution of inspired air, particularly in the region of the lower lung fields, producing decreased regional ventilation with continued perfusion. Therefore, blood is shunted from the right to the left side of the heart without benefit of oxygenation, and progressive hypoxemia results. Even though the lungs are structurally normal, the neuromuscular patient with continuing reduction in total alveolar ventilation will eventually experience CO_2 retention.[15-23]

As patients become weaker their inspiratory muscles become so ineffective that often use of accessory muscles of respiration such as the muscles of the neck, shoulder girdle, and abdomen are needed to maintain normal levels of ventilation. The patient is further compromised by this less efficient breathing which results in increased oxygen cost.

For an effective cough, a patient must forcibly contract the diaphragm, intercostals and accessory muscles against a closed glottis.[8,9,18] The high intrathoracic pressure gradient that is produced accelerates air flow when the glottis is suddenly opened so that clearance of tracheobronchial secretions can occur. If the patient's respiratory muscles are weakened, retention of secretions along with atelectasis leads to further impairment in ventilation-perfusion ratios. A depressed cough reflex is particularly troublesome in a patient who has recurrent aspiration from accompanying weakness of the palate and pharyngeal muscles.

Many patients with neuromuscular disease have weak abdominal muscles. Although these muscles play only a supportive role in normal respiratory effort, they can add significantly when additional respiratory effort is required. Paralysis of these muscles allows the abdominal contents to sag and lowers the level of the diaphragm decreasing its mechanical advantage and its effect on respiration. Similarly, if there is intercostal muscle dysfunction and the diaphragm is functioning normally, the chest will retract inward during inspiration, leading to less efficient parodoxical breathing.

In an office setting where complicated pulmonary respiratory apparatus is not available, it is still valuable to do clinical spirometry. A patient with neuromuscular disease will often show a characteristic diminution in the inspiratory flow rate, vital capacity (VC), and in maximum voluntary ventilation (MVV). In contrast, patients with chronic obstructive disease will demonstrate impaired expiratory flows measured as low forced expiratory volume in the first second (FEV_1) and decreased midexpiratory flow rate (MMEF).

Black and Hyatt[24] have emphasized the value of the maximal static expiratory and inspiratory pressures in detecting muscle weakness. This test, which is performed using a simple hand-held device, may give the most sensitive measure of early respiratory muscular weakness. They found that pressures exerted during dynamic maneuvers, such as the MVV, MMEF, or forced VC, were less impaired than maximal static expiratory and inspiratory pressures at every lung volume, making the dynamic maneuvers less sensitive than the maximal static pressures in detecting muscle weakness. Maximal static pressures are a direct measure of respiratory muscle strength, because no actual flow of air results. Since abnormalities in these pressures are not seen in intrinsic pulmonary disease, they are valuable in defining specific neuromuscular impairment.

Many patients with neuromuscular disease are able to compensate for respiratory muscle weakness so they do not develop any alteration in arterial blood gases. The first blood gas abnormality which usually develops with slowly progressive weakness is a reduction in arterial pO_2 which occurs because of abnormalities in the ventilation-perfusion ratio. This hypoxia often remains asymptomatic for prolonged periods. At times a mild hyperventilation ensues with a reduction in the arterial pCO_2. Decompensation is signaled by a progression to alveolar hypoventilation and CO_2 retention.

A patient who is developing chronic hypoxia may first begin to complain of abnormalities during sleep. These may consist of frequent awakening, daytime sleepiness, or perhaps nightmares. Later on, more evident signs such as increasing hematocrit, hypercapnia, and cor pulmonale may intervene. The latter findings are uncommon in neuromuscular disease patients in our experience.

Periodic assessment of pulmonary function in the patient with chronic neuromuscular disease is valuable in several respects. It assists the physician in determining the patient's prognosis as the disease progresses, and may alert him to inpending acute respiratory failure. It also helps the doctor determine the appropriate therapy when the patient requires surgery and general anesthesia or certain medications which might depress respiration. Furthermore, since patients with neuromuscular disease are not immune to coincidental chronic obstructive pulmonary disease, it helps differentiate the contribution of pulmonary dysfunction produced by the neuromuscular disease from that of intrinsic lung disease. In this way the patient can be adequately assessed for the efficacy of various forms of respiratory therapy, particularly for those aspects caused by primary pulmonary dysfunction.

PULMONARY COMPLICATIONS

Pulmonary complications have been divided into those associated with acute or chronic weakness. In patients who first come to the physician's attention because of respiratory failure secondary to acute muscle weakness, an intensive diagnostic evaluation must be undertaken immediately after the patient has received adequate respiratory support. Such an evaluation is performed promptly, since with some diseases early treatment can favorably affect the prognosis of the patient.

In the case of a patient with an established, progressive neuromuscular disease, the physician no longer relies on his neurodiagnostic skills, but must be constantly alert for an impending pulmonary complication. Respiratory infections caused by unrecognized recurrent aspiration can be fatal to a patient who already has chronic respiratory failure with a depressed cough reflex, atelectesis and marginal pulmonary reserve. All too familiar is the story of a patient that appeared only slightly dyspneic one minute and had a life-threatening respiratory arrest several minutes later.

These same patients with inadequate pulmonary reserve must be carefully managed at times of stress, such as a pregnancy, intercurrent illness, or at the time of emergency or elective surgery. It can be a difficult decision to balance the risk of major spinal surgery in patients with compromised pulmonary function against the inevitable respiratory failure they will undergo as the spine progressively collapses from increasing weakness.

Acute Muscle Weakness

Management

Diseases which produce acute paralysis are devastating to the patient and provide a major challenge for the physician. Many of these disorders are life-threatening because of accompanying respiratory muscle paralysis. As the physician hastens to determine the cause of the patient's sudden deterioration (Table II) it is critical to observe simultaneously the tempo and trend of the progressive weakness to anticipate acute respiratory dysfunction. Symptoms of respiratory distress can be very mild and nonspecific although confusion, restlessness, and a sensation of dyspnea are often present. The hypoxic patient may have associated bradycardia and hypotension because of decreased sympathetic response. Physicians cannot rely on cyanosis as an index of hypoxemia, nor can they be certain that the equally nonspecific symptoms of headache, drowziness, and hypertension are caused by CO_2 narcosis. The physician must, therefore, be acutely aware of the nonspecificity of these signs and symptoms and be extremely alert to potential ramifications. Arterial blood gases should be obtained if

TABLE II
Causes of Acute Muscle Weakness

I. Peripheral Nerve
- Guillain Barré syndrome
- Diphtheria
- Tic paralysis
- Porphyria

II. Neuromuscular Junction
- Myasthenia gravis
- Botulism
- Organophosphate poisoning
- Succinylcholine (pseudocholinesterase deficiency)

III. Muscle
- Periodic paralysis
- Rhabdomyolysis
- Metabolic–hypercalcemia
  - –hypophosphatemia
  - hypokalcmia

there is any suggestion of ventilatory failure. In cases where there is any uncertainty, the patient should be admitted to an intensive care unit where specialized medical and nursing needs can be provided including oxygen therapy, intubation, and mechanical ventilation. In some cases of hypoxemia it may not be necessary to intubate the patient, and oxygen by mask will suffice. Although oxygen administration in patients with severe obstructive pulmonary disease may be dangerous because of their dependency on hypoxic ventilatory drive, these considerations do not extend to the patient with neuromuscular disease. If the patient develops any elevation of arterial pCO_2, he usually has severe ventilatory impairment, and intubation is almost always necessary.[8,9,18] Preparation for tracheal intubation should be made in advance since emergent intubation often precipitates disaster. A physician experienced in intubation should be present.

In the neuromuscular patient on a ventilator, arterial blood gases should be monitored frequently, and the inspired air should be adequately humidified with warm water vaporizers to prevent drying of bronchial secretions. The patient's position should be changed at regular intervals to allow for gravity drainage of the various segments of the bronchial tree. Sterile catheters and sterile gloves should be used for aspiration of the tracheobronchial secretions, and Gram stains and cultures should be obtained. Compliant, low pressure cuffs should be used with the tracheostomy tube to avoid pressure necrosis of the tracheal mucosa. Bronchoscopic aspiration can be performed daily, if necessary, but with meticulous attention to postural drainage and careful suctioning through the tracheostomy, daily aspiration can usually be avoided.

It is important to emphasize that the prognosis of a patient with acute respiratory failure secondary to neuromuscular disease is not necessarily ominous. Even in those patients who require long periods in respiratory intensive care units, the survival rate is much higher than in patients with primary pulmonary disease.[25,26] The major complications that occur in these acutely ill patients are respiratory and urinary tract infections, decubitus ulcers, thrombophlebitis, pulmonary emboli, localized complications of tracheostomy and generalized debilitation from malnutrition.[18] Early feeding by nasogastric tube or gastrostomy may stave off this malnutrition. Many of the neuromuscular patients may also have associated cardiovascular disease and, therefore, are prone to autonomic instability with wide swings in blood pressure and cardiac arrhythmias.[27]

One often overlooked but important aspect of caring for the severely incapacitated patient is communication.[28] Since a mechanical airway prevents talking, it is important that the medical staff allow the patient to vent feelings of anxiety, frustration, hope, and depression. It is not hard to imagine how anxiety can develop in a fully alert and intelligent patient who finds himself immobilized from head to toe, dependent on a respirator for breathing, a tube for feeding, and on another individual for basic body needs and comforts. Reassurance by doctors and nurses at this time has major therapeutic value.

As a patient is recovering from acute weakness, physicians and nurses must be alert for the dangers of aspiration. Swallowing is often the last important function to return, yet the patient will be eager to take nourishment by mouth to get rid of the nasogastric tube. It is helpful to use small sips of water colored with food dye for initial evaluation. Aspiration is suggested if the patient coughs or if the dye is seen in endotracheal suctioning or around the tracheostomy tube. All too often a patient recovering from acute paralysis can have a life-threatening relapse caused by unrecognized, recurrent aspiration.

Causes of Acute Weakness

Several diseases of the motor unit, whether they involve the anterior horn cell, peripheral nerve, neuromuscular junction, or muscle, can produce acute weakness (Table II). Although there are clinical features which are useful to the physician in localizing the disturbance, the abrupt onset of weakness may mask these distinctions. Peripheral nerve diseases that can be associated with acute weakness include the Guillain-Barré syndrome, diphtheritic neuropathy, and tic paralysis. In the Guillain-Barré syndrome, or acute idiopathic polyradiculopathy, weakness usually begins about one to three weeks after an upper respiratory infection or other viral illness. The patient may initially note numbness or a tingling sensation in the arms or legs although there are rarely accompanying sensory findings on examination. Shortly thereafter, progressive weakness often begins in the lower limbs and ascends to include the upper extremities. Later, respiratory and bulbar muscles may become affected. The most helpful laboratory investigation is examination of the cerebrospinal fluid, which at some stage of the disease demonstrates an elevated protein with a normal cell count (albumino-cytologic dissociation). Peripheral nerve conduction velocities will often show slowing, particularly in the proximal segment.

In diphtheritic neuropathy, a disease rarely seen today, the patient will have a characteristic pharyngeal membrane with a mousey odor. Paralysis of bulbar muscles and loss of ocular accommodation occur early in the disease. A distal sensorimotor polyneuropathy does not occur until four to eight weeks after the acute illness. Associated myocardial and renal involvement can provide a clue to the etiology of this neuropathy.

Another neurotoxin which results in a progressive, symmetrical paralysis is produced by the female Dermacentor andersoni or North American tic. Most cases of tic paralysis occur in children after the tic has been embedded for five to six days. Often the tic is embedded near the hairline and goes unnoticed. Symptoms include difficulty with speaking and swallowing, facial weakness, blurred vision, and paralysis of arms and legs with associated arreflexia. Occasional sensory symptoms including numbness and tingling of the extremities and face are also described. If an engorged tic is found, it should be removed immediately, and the patient will generally improve within hours. Electrophysiological studies show both slowing of motor conduction and reduced amplitude of the evoked muscle action potential suggesting that the toxin acts both at the nerve terminals and on large myelinated axons.

Disorders of the neuromuscular junction are much more commonly associated with acute muscle weakness. In botulism, acute weakness occurs within 12 to 36 hours after ingestion of the toxin produced by the bacteria *clostridium botulinum.* This toxin is estimated to cause death in man in doses as small as 0.1 to 1.0 micrograms. Although the toxin is heat-labile and destroyed by the cooking process, spores of botulinum are heat-resistant and continue to produce toxin at room temperature under anaerobic conditions.

The signs and symptoms begin in the cranial nerves and include blurred vision, dysarthria, and dysphagia and then rapidly descend. Respiratory paralysis can follow quickly and without treatment is often fatal. Alertness, mentation, and the sensory system remain normal. The pupils are usually spared, but marked extraocular muscle weakness and ptosis are common. Weakness of the face, tongue, pharynx, neck, and extremities may progress for the first four to five days and is usually bilateral although occasionally asymmetrical. Laboratory confirmation usually requires the detection of the toxin in the patient's serum, stool, or in the contaminated food. Specimens that should be examined include serum, gastric contents, feces, exudates from wounds, and contents of suspected jars or cans. Electrodiagnostic studies are often helpful in the diagnosis after the patient's respiratory needs have been adequately treated. Often the amplitude of the evoked muscle action potential with supramaximal nerve stimulation is reduced. Repetitive studies at rapid rates of nerve stimulation can show potentiation in some but not all cases. Needle electromyography will show small motor unit potentials of short duration in affected muscles. Botulinum toxin causes paralysis by blocking the release of acetylcholine from nerve terminals. It does not impair impulse conduction in nerve or muscle.

Botulism has now also been reported to occur in infants with intestinal production of toxin occurring after ingestion of the bacteria. With constipation as the first sign, these infants later develop cranial nerve palsies and generalized muscle weakness. Diagnosis is best made by recovery of the organism from the feces.[29,30]

The major treatment of botulism is medical care which consists of providing artificial ventilation for patients with respiratory paralysis. Artificial ventilation may be necessary for as long as weeks or months since recovery, if it occurs, is prolonged and is probably a reflection of the delayed sprouting of nerve terminals which eventually reinnervate the muscle fibers. Other adjuncts of therapy which have been tried include early administration of antitoxin particularly in cases of Type B botulism and guanidine hydrochloride, which has been shown to reverse the neuromuscular block of botulism in animals.

Similar acute muscle weakness due to disorder of the neuromuscular junction occurs if an individual is exposed to insecticides containing organophosphates or after succinylcholine administration in patients with cholinesterase deficiency. Succinylcholine is commonly used in surgery to produce muscle relaxation. The paralysis is short-lived, usually lasting only three minutes, due to the rapid hydrolysis of the succinylcholine by cholinesterase to succinic acid and choline. In patients with low plasma pseudocholinesterase activity, prolonged paralysis and apnea may follow administration of succinylcholine. The causes of low cholinesterase activity include genetic disorders, liver disease, malnutrition, uremia, hyperpyrexia, poisoning by organophosphates and pregnancy. Most patients will recover in four to six hours if artificial ventilation is maintained. A purified and concentrated preparation of serum cholinesterase may terminate the paralysis and apnea when administered intravenously.

In myasthenia gravis, another disorder of the neuromuscular junction, clinical signs and symptoms consist of pathological fatigue. Often the onset is insidious but occasionally a patient may present with acute respiratory depression. If the eyes are predominantly involved, the patient will experience diplopia and ptosis. With bulbar involvement, there is difficulty in speaking, swallowing, and chewing; and recurrent aspiration can be a severe problem. The symptoms produced by the involvement of the limb and trunk differ from chronic neuromuscular diseases in that the prominent manifestation is fatigue rather than fixed weakness. Electrical testing often confirms the defect in neuromuscular transmission. With repetitive stimulation, the amplitude of the evoked potential becomes progressively smaller. Edrophonium (Tensilon), an anticholinesterase medication, will reverse this decrement in the compound muscle action-potential as well as improve the patient's strength. Antireceptor antibody titers are usually elevated as well.[13]

Because of the marked fluctuation in strength in these patients, acute respiratory depression can occur suddenly in a patient who appeared relatively normal only minutes before. Occasionally this weakness can be attributed to the patient's medication. With anticholinesterase compounds, overdosing can easily occur and will produce weakness. Often it can be difficult to distinguish if weakness is due to myasthenia or to over-medication, although the latter is frequently associated with other cholinergic side effects such as abdominal pain, diarrhea, and widespread fasciculations. The absence of side effects does not necessarily mean that the patient is experiencing an exacerbation of myasthenia, however. For any patient with myasthenia gravis who is getting weaker either from myasthenic crisis or a cholinergic crisis, an edrophonium test should be performed. An advantage of edrophonium is that its action is short-lived, lasting only two to three minutes. If the patient is, in fact, in cholinergic crisis, any worsening can be rapidly reversed. If there is clear improvement with edrophonium, the patient's medication can be increased accordingly.

In many patients during an acute exacerbation, it may be difficult to tell if there has been any improvement with edrophonium. In such a situation it is worthwhile to discontinue all medications and to assist respiration. The patient should be admitted to an intensive care unit and intubated or a tracheotomy should be performed with an endotracheal tube in place, followed carefully for one to two weeks, and then anticholinesterase medications can be reinstated in small doses. Several authors have commented that after this period of withdrawal, the patient becomes sensitive once again to the cholinergic medication, and management can be undertaken as an out-patient.

A word of warning should be given concerning the edrophonium (Tensilon) test since an occasional patient will suddenly collapse immediately after injection of the medication intravenously. An ambu bag and oral airway should be readily accessible whenever the test is performed.

Corticosteroids are now commonly used in myasthenia gravis because of their immunosuppressive effects. After starting the medication the patient may become weaker in the first week to ten days and will then gradually improve. At the onset of treatment, caution must be taken to avoid aspiration or respiratory depression. It is often helpful to admit the patient to the hospital and monitor the vital capacity. Temporary respiratory assistance may be necessary but usually can be avoided. If possible, any anticholinesterase medication should be stopped since it can be difficult to determine if this medication is contributing to the patient's weakness. If it is not practical to bring the patient into the hospital, an alternative approach is to use gradually increasing alternate day prednisone. Seybold et al.[31] have recommended treatment with 25 mg every other day and gradually increasing the dosage to 100 mg by 12.5 mg steps at each third dose. Using this protocol, patients experienced less weakness as the steroids were instituted.

In recording pulmonary function in myasthenic patients on alternate day prednisone, one group[28] found monitoring a patient's vital capacity at the bedside during periods of marginal ventilatory reserve provided the most useful information. A decrease in vital capacity to 25 percent of the predicted value, that is about 1 to 1.2 liters, was an indication that ventilatory failure was immanent. The authors emphasized that classical signs of respiratory difficulty, including intercostal and suprasternal retraction and flaring of the nasal alae, were not seen because of the patient's weakness. They cautioned the physician to be alert for loss of ability to speak for more than a few seconds, dysphonia, headaches, rising blood pressure because of CO_2 retention, rising pulse rate, choking, aspiration and restlessness. The patient generally showed improvement in vital capacity during the prednisone on-day and relative decline on the off-day. Arterial blood gases are also a useful way of following patients during an acute illness.

Thymectomy is commonly used as another form of therapy in myasthenia gravis since either thymic hyperplasia or thymoma occurs in this disease, and patients often improve when the thymus is removed. If this procedure is undertaken, it is important to assess carefully the preoperative pulmonary function of the patient. The anesthesiologist should be encouraged to avoid neuromuscular blocking agents or other medications that have adverse effects on neuromuscular transmission, such as quinine, diphenylhydantoin, quinidine, procaine, propranolol, or other beta-adrenergic blockers and antibiotics such as neomycin and streptomycin. Several authors have recommended that in severe myasthenia gravis, in which a thorocotomy may be contraindicated, a suprasternal removal of the thymus may be more advisable.[32]

When a myasthenic is to have surgery of any kind, anticholinesterase drugs are often withdrawn for at least 24 hours preoperatively and no preoperative sedation is used. Muscle relaxants should also be avoided either for intubation or during maintenance of anesthesia. The wary physician should not be misled when patients ventilate well immediately following surgery since they may deteriorate in muscle power within the next 24 hours due to fatigue. Anticholinesterase drugs will improve muscle power but, unfortunately, will simultaneously increase bronchial secretions. If narcotics are administered for control of pain, the physician should be aware that these may potentiate the neuromuscular blockade. However, the doctor will want to take advantage of this relatively pain-free period to encourage the patient to cough and perform better chest physiotherapy. The anesthesiologist must be aware of the potential for long-term ventilatory support.

It cannot be emphasized too strongly that intensive care nursing and continuous medical supervision is mandatory. Adequacy of ventilation must be evaluated repeatedly bearing in mind that excessive manipulation and measurements will fatigue the patient unduly. A low vital capacity in the postoperative period may not indicate just increased muscle weakness but also could be caused by a mucous plug in a bronchus, the onset of a pulmonary infection, restriction of chest movement because of pain, or weak facial and lip muscles allowing air to escape as the patient expires into the respirometer. Although edrophonium tests in the postoperative period are a good guide to therapy, it is often more advantageous to maintain endotracheal intubation and not use the cholinesterase inhibitors until later as the patient recovers.[28] Because patients are frequently so improved on prednisone before thymectomy, operative morbidity and mortality has sharply declined in the last several years.

Similar precautions should be taken in the patient with myasthenia gravis during labor, delivery, and the puerperium. Numerous circumstances can precipitate weakness such as emotional stress, exertion and infection, particularly of the upper respiratory or urinary tract. Since the myasthenic is sensitive to drugs, sedatives, analgesics, tranquilizers, and narcotics, these medications should be used cautiously during labor. Local anesthesia in the form of pudendal block or regional anesthesia is preferable. If general anesthesia is used, muscle relaxants should be avoided. The puerperium in the patient with myasthenia gravis is particularly dangerous since severe exacerbations can occur at that time. Careful observation of the patient for signs of respiratory failure is mandatory.

If the baby of a mother with myasthenia gravis is born with generalized weakness, a mask-like face, poor sucking and swallowing, and respiratory distress, neonatal myasthenia gravis should be considered. This disease can be confirmed by testing the infant's response to edrophonium. If the child improves, he can usually be treated with intramuscular neostigmine, and the majority of symptoms will disappear within the first two weeks.

Primary disorders of the muscle are an uncommon cause of severe, acute muscle weakness and respiratory failure. Occasionally a patient may develop acute rhabdomyolysis with associated myoglobinuria. The patient notices muscle pain, swelling and weakness. Often there is a risk of acute renal failure with associated hyperkalemia, and serum enzymes will be markedly elevated. The urine may be red and turn brown on standing due to myoglobinuria. The etiology can include primary metabolic disease of muscle, an inflammatory myopathy, vigorous and unaccustomed exercise, potassium depletion or other metabolic imbalance, or exposure to a variety of toxic substances. In all cases the treatment includes forced diuresis and alkalinization of the urine. Renal dialysis may be necessary.

A reversible loss of membrane excitability may result in primary muscle weakness. Such a loss is common with either acute hypo- or hyperkalemia. Hyperkalemia may be a manifestation of a periodic paralysis but is usually seen in response to intravenous replacement of potassium, renal insufficiency, Addison's disease, or treatment with spironolactone. It also may be produced with sudden damage to large tissue mass such as with acute rhabdomyolysis. The treatment in all cases is to reduce the serum potassium. Acute respiratory failure is uncommon in these disorders but has been occasionally reported.

Chronic Neuromuscular Weakness

The physician who follows patients for many years with chronic neuromuscular weakness is often confronted with a series of pulmonary complications. The most important of these are: progressive dysphagia with recurrent aspiration; progressive scoliosis, which produces decreased pulmonary reserve; sudden respiratory failure from superimposed primary alveolar hypoventilation or diaphragmatic paralysis; and, end-stage respiratory failure which usually results from weakness of the muscles of respiration in addition to the complications listed above. If each of these complications is anticipated by the examining physician as it first develops, a fatal pulmonary event can often be avoided. In the long run, some of the same patients will succumb to pulmonary disease, but at least their lives can be prolonged, often for years, so that they do not die prematurely from a potentially reversible complication.

Progressive Dysphagia

Progressive dysphagia with recurrent aspiration can occur with involvement of any part of the motor unit. It is particularly prominent in amyotrophic lateral sclerosis,[33] X-linked spinal muscular atrophy,[34] myasthenia gravis,[28] and oculopharyngeal dystrophy[35] but can also occur in a variety of other neuromuscular diseases as diverse as myotonic dystrophy[36] and the inflammatory myopathies.[37] Early difficulty frequently goes unrecognized; the physician, therefore, must be alert to this possibility in any patient with recurrent pneumonia. A barium swallow with cine radiography will often demonstrate aspiration (Fig. 1). As dysphagia pro-

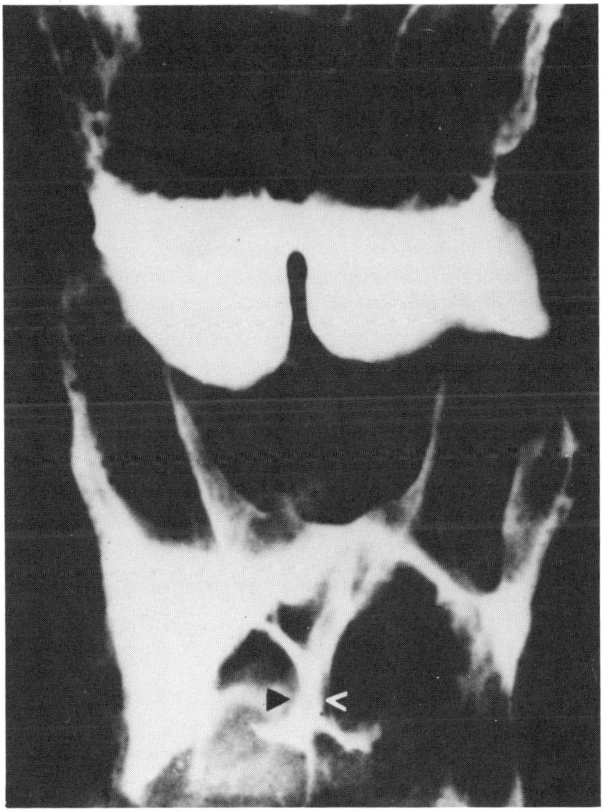

A

Figure 1. Anterior (*A*) and lateral (*B*) views of esophagram in a patient with X-linked spinal muscular atrophy. The hypopharynx is dilated, with pooling of barium in the epiglottal recesses. With swallowing, contrast material spills into the larynx (*arrows*). (Reprinted with permission from Ringel. S.P., et al.: *Muscle Nerve* **1**:297–301, 1978.)

B

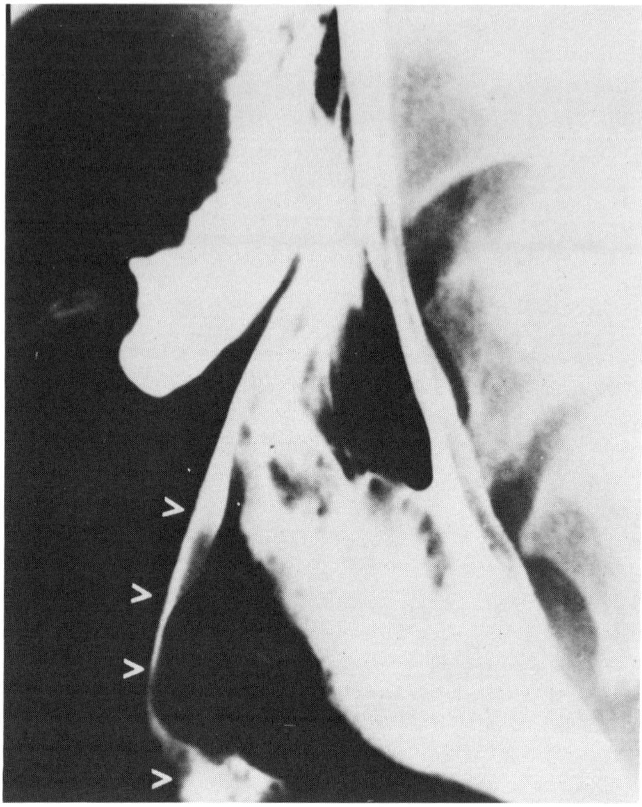

Figure 1. (Continued)

gresses, the patient initially has difficulty with hard solids, and later liquids may become more difficult to swallow. Soft, ground materials are easier to get down, and a dietician may be helpful in instructing the patient in food preparation. Patients will often throw the head back in order to get liquids past the tongue and are more successful drinking from a straw. Maneuvering solids into the oral pharynx can be quite difficult if there is associated weakness of the facial and tongue muscles. Patients may lose fluids through the lips and into the air passages or may regurgitate through the nose.

Several forms of therapy have been attempted in people with functional disorders of swallowing with only limited success. Therapists teach patients to keep their heads erect or their chins tilted somewhat forward during swallowing and to position their posterior tongue down and back while making the "K" sound.[38] Mouths are kept open while doing so, and patients are instructed to swallow quickly and to say "gah" at the very end of the swallow. Another method that has been tried is Teflon injection of the vocal cords for the prevention of chronic aspiration.[39] By making the glottis more competent, subglottic pressure can build, restoring the coughing reflex and preventing reaspiration when foreign material has been expelled. Glottic competence can be evaluated by testing not only the patient's ability to cough but also his ability to sustain a note, to hold his breath and to laugh. A crycopharyngeal sphincterotomy or myotomy has proved highly effective[35,40] for both relief of dysphagia and the control of aspiration in several neuromuscular diseases including oculopharyngeal dystrophy, amyotrophic lateral sclerosis, and polymyositis. If patients are noted by cineradiography to have an appreciable amount of food and fluid trapped in the hypopharynx after the supposed completion of the swallow, they may benefit from this procedure. The best results are obtained in those cases in which there is a moderate degree of tongue movement. If the tongue can be protruded as far as the lower lip, there is enough propulsion to initiate deglutition.

Lesser degrees of obstruction accompanied by stridor and produced by aspiration of saliva or food can be quite alarming to the patient and should be dealt with as calmly as possible. Supplemental oxygen often gives reassurance to the patient and may help facilitate breathing. Pharyngeal suction is beneficial, and family members can be instructed in the use of a suction machine at home.

Feeding via a nasogastric tube is not satisfactory for long-term management because of irritation and ulceration of the nasal mucosa and pharynx. If the patient is unable to take any food by mouth, alternative procedures include gastrostomy or cervical esophagostomy,[41] which avoids the risk of peritonitis. In the latter procedure, a tube is passed through a neck incision into the piriform recess, through the esophagus, and into the stomach. This tube is changed every three to four weeks, and the esophagostomy can remain in place for at least a year.

Above all, the physician must be sensitive to the patient's wishes. Some will understandably choose not to have any of these procedures since life has lost meaning under these circumstances. A doctor's emotional support at this difficult time can be more valuable to the patient than the prolongation of his life.

All families should be instructed how to manage their patient should he suddenly develop obstruction of the respiratory pathway. The Heimlich maneuver, or abdominal hug of life, can be life-saving. The patient is bent forward over a chair or the rescuer's arm so that his head is lower than his chest. The rescuer stands behind the patient, encircling him with his arms, hands interlocked, and presses forcefully upward on the upper abdomen. This sudden pressure forces the diaphragm up, expelling residual air from the chest cavity and dislodges the foreign body.[33]

Progressive Scoliosis

In chronic neuromuscular disease, deformities of the axial skeleton from weakness of the muscles balancing the spine can further affect pulmonary function (Fig. 2). As the spine collapses, vital capacity and total lung capacity decrease and an unequal matching of ventilation to lung perfusion with an increased physiological deadspace is produced. The amount of abnormality is directly proportional to the degree of scoliosis although changes have already been demonstrated in cases in which the spinal deformity was quite slight.[42] As a result, patients with spinal collapse from neuromuscular disease will have a high morbidity if progressive deformity is not prevented.

For many patients who are wheelchair-bound, the use of polypropylene thoracic body jackets as external support for the spine is recommended (Fig. 2*C*). Forced vital capacity and maximum voluntary ventilations are often mildly reduced when the patient is wearing the jacket. However, it is our impression that these jackets maintain better pulmonary function in the long run. It is useful to remember that with an acute infection, even a mild one, the body jacket must be removed to allow the patient to take advantage of his full pulmonary reserve.

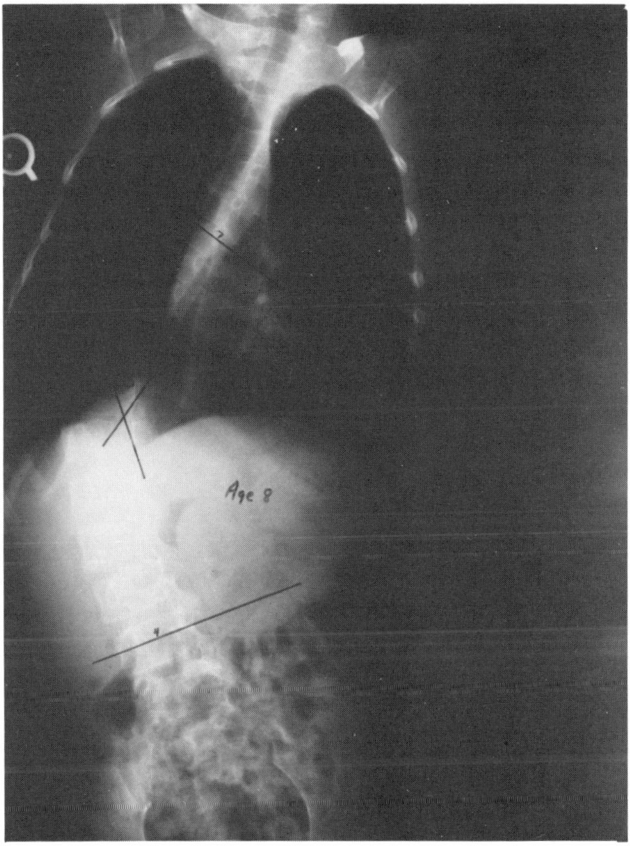

A

Figure 2. Sequential treatment of spinal collapse in a patient with spinal muscular atrophy. The patient progressed from a 55° curve at age 8 (*A*) to 75° at age 9 (*B*). With the use of a polypropylene body jacket, the curve could be reduced to 57° (*C*) but did not significantly slow down progression. At age 10 (*D*) spinal stability was achieved in two stages. An anterior fusion along with Dwyer instrumentation was performed initially. Three weeks later posterior fusion and two Harrington distraction rods were used to distribute the force over a larger area.

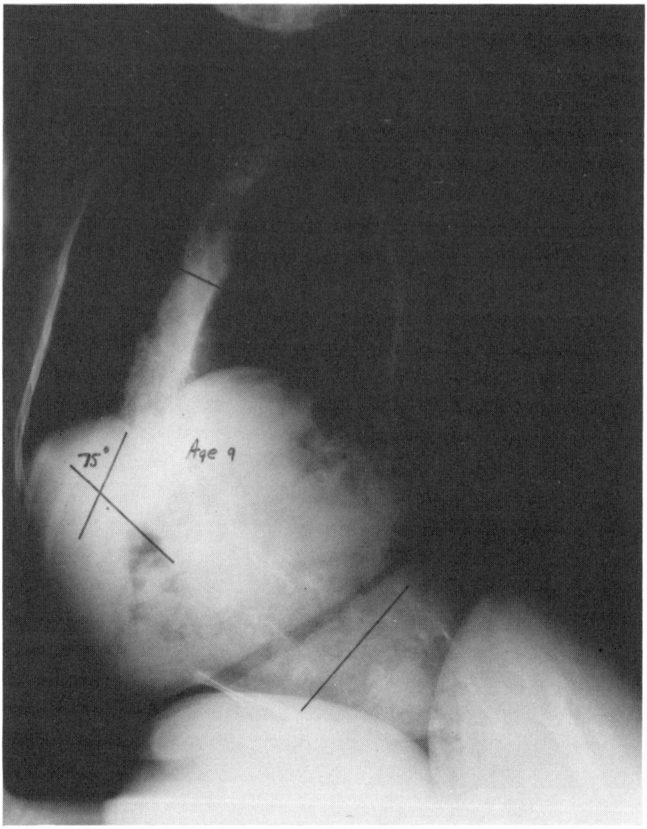

B

Figure 2. (Continued)

One author has proposed that severe scoliosis can be prevented if the spine is maintained hyperextended,[43] locking the posterior facet joints and preventing lateral collapse. Such hyperextension can be maintained with a brace or body jacket, or with a modified wheelchair that accentuates hyperextension. The chair should not be too wide, so that the patient does not have to lean to the side to gain arm support.

An early, aggressive surgical approach has been advocated by some in the treatment of scoliosis since the risk of further pulmonary decompensation increases when surgery is postponed.[44] In a patient with chronic neuromuscular dis-

C

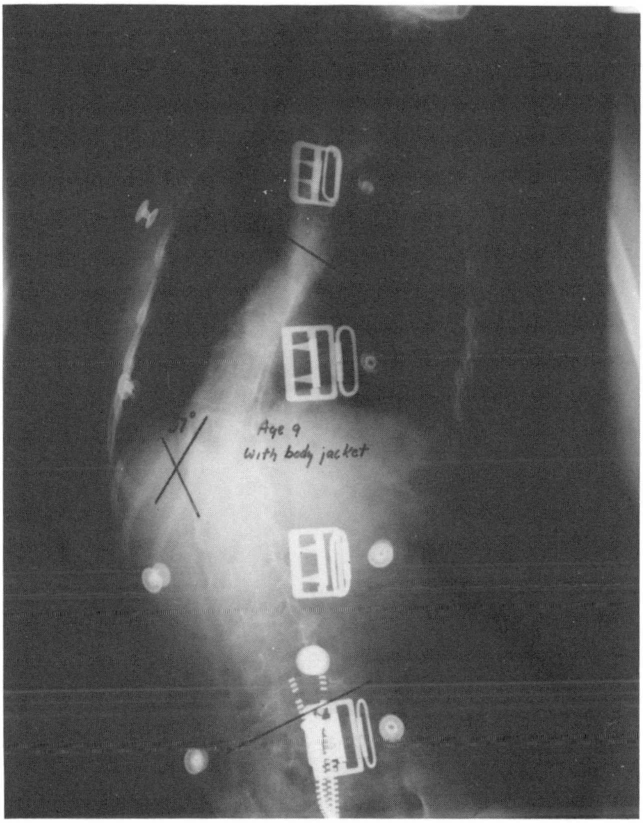

Figure 2. (Continued)

ease who has decreased pulmonary reserve because of both spinal deformity and weakened respiratory muscles, pulmonary reserve may be markedly decreased. These patients may experience almost no difficulty at rest, but little movement such as transferring from a wheelchair to a bed or an emotional stress may cause the patient to have increasing respiratory difficulty. Furthermore, these patients may develop respiratory failure so slowly that the only manifestation will be a secondary problem such as polycythemia or edema.

The physician must take into account the natural history of the disease as well as the patient's level of disability

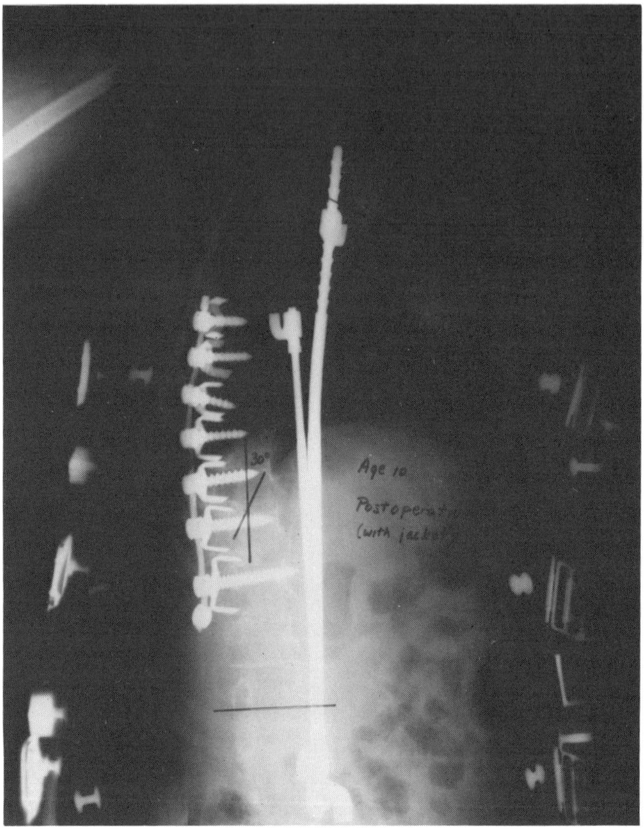

D

Figure 2. (Continued)

before surgery can be considered. Few recommend surgery in Duchenne dystrophy since the prognosis is uniformly fatal. On the other hand, the patient with a fixed deficit, such as polio, or with slow progression, such as in spinal muscular atrophy, is better suited for such a procedure.

If a patient with neuromuscular disease is to have surgery, extensive preoperative evaluation should be performed by a team of physicians including the orthopedist, anesthesiologist, neurologist, and pulmonary specialist. In general, patients whose vital capacity is more than 70 percent of normal tolerate surgery well. However, the majority of patients with neuromuscular disorders and a spinal deformity have a vital capacity between 30 and 70 percent. In patients whose vital capacity is under 30 percent of predicted normal, a period of postoperative mechanical ventilation is almost mandatory.[44]

Arterial blood gases should be obtained prior to surgery to obtain a baseline for evaluation both during surgery and in the postoperative management. Surgery should be delayed if there is a history of recent chest infection. Preoperative sputum culture has been advocated by some physicians in all patients with decreased respiratory function but is probably not of much value. Preoperative medication should be kept to a minimum to prevent undue respiratory depression or oversedation. Often, it is advantageous to have a pulmonary physiotherapist visit the patient and start treatment several days before surgery is planned. Using and strengthening accessory muscles of respiration preoperatively may make a considerable difference in the pulmonary function after surgery. The patient can also be taught to cough adequately, particularly if the abdominal muscles are weak. Postural drainage should be taught and can be valuable in the postoperative period if respiratory muscle function is decreased. Intermittent positive pressure breathing several days before the operation has also been suggested to help the patient expand the lungs but its major value is probably in familiarizing the patient to the apparatus that may be required in the postoperative period. Bronchial dilators are usually not necessary unless an obstructive element is present. The patient should be made fully aware that he might require an endotracheal tube postoperatively so that he is not alarmed when he awakens from general anesthesia and is unable to talk.

An anesthetic agent should be selected that is not irritative to the respiratory tract and is free of pulmonary vasoconstrictive activity. It should be stressed that careful blood gas monitoring in these patients may be necessary during surgery to provide a safe arterial pO_2. A large right-to-left shunt may be present before anesthesia and may increase intraoperatively. This shunt can be demonstrated by low arterial oxygenation even when the patient is receiving a high oxygen fraction. The physiotherapist can visit the patient in the recovery room and start intensive chest physiotherapy. Weaning from ventilatory support can be undertaken when the patient is stabilized.

Respiratory Failure

Sudden respiratory failure has been reported in patients with a variety of neuromuscular diseases in which sufficient weakness is not present to account for the respiratory embarrassment. This situation has been described in myotonic dystrophy,[45-52] polio,[53] acid maltase deficiency,[54,55] progressive external ophthalmoplegia,[56] and in several congenital or nonspecific myopathies.[57-79] The phenomenon of abnormal ventilatory control or primary alveolar hypoventilation probably plays a role in respiratory failure in many of these patients. This phenomenon has been investigated by many workers, who have noted a diminished response to decreases in oxygen tensions (Fig. 3) or increases in CO_2 tensions. Hypoxic response is mediated by the carotid body through the ninth cranial nerve to the brain stem. Hypercapnic response is mediated by the carotid body and also by the brain stem directly. Decrements in ventilatory response have been documented in these patients and exhibit more reduction than routine pulmonary functions would indicate, suggesting that these patients have the muscular power to ventilate but not the reflex stimulation to do so. These reductions suggest that in addition to an underlying myopathic involvement of the respiratory muscles, a central chemoreceptor hyporesponsiveness may be present. This hyporesponsiveness either to hypoxemia or increased carbon dioxide may be important to evaluate since it might identify a group of patients prone to develop respiratory failure following general anesthesia, exposure to depressant drugs, or perhaps with respiratory infection or high altitude.

Occasionally a patient with only a mild weakness of accessory muscles of respiration may develop acute respiratory failure from isolated or dominant diaphragmatic weakness. This respiratory failure has been noted with polio,[60] brachial plexus neuropathy,[61-64] the Guillain-Barré syndrome,[65] and in several unclassified neuropathies.[14,66] It has been reported as an early manifestation of motor neuron disease (ALS)[67,68] and also rarely in newborns with infantile spinal muscular atrophy,[69] infantile myotonic dystrophy,[70] or with an isolated myopathy of the diaphragm.[71]

With paralysis of the diaphragm, abdominal muscles can assist in respiratory function but only when the patient

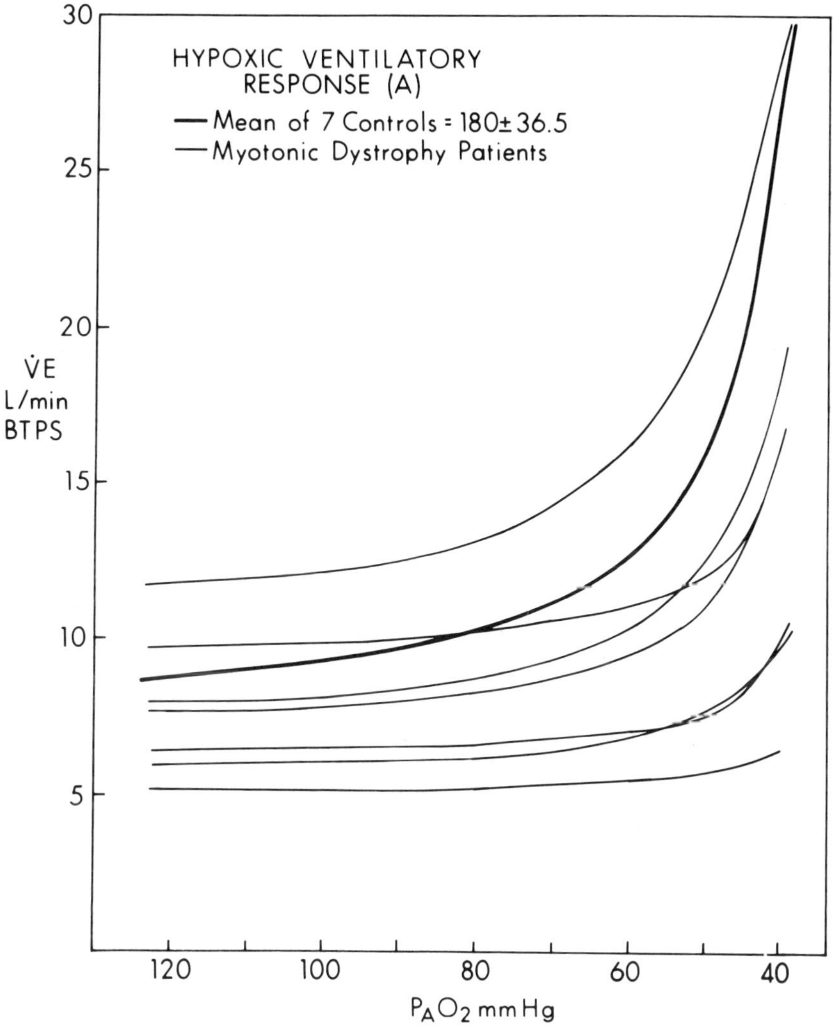

Figure 3. Hypoxic response is normally a hyperbolic function when plotted against P_AO_2. Seven patients with myotonic dystrophy had significantly reduced hypoxic response (74 ± 24.4) when compared to seven height-matched controls (Reprinted with permission from Carroll, J.E., et al.: Ventilatory response in myotonic dystrophy. *Neurology* **27**: 1125–1128, 1977.)

is erect. When abdominal muscles contract, there is an increase in intraabdominal pressure raising the diaphragm and assisting expiration. Similarly, with relaxation of the muscles and lowering of the intraabdominal pressure, gravity will cause the diaphragm to descend, producing a passive inspiratory phase. If the patient is supine, the force of gravity is lost and alternating inspiration-expiration can no longer be accomplished, which is particularly difficult for the patient during sleep. Furthermore, the neck and shoulder girdle muscles, although they allow greater chest expansion and may substitute for other paralyzed respiratory muscles, lack rhythmical control and endurance during sleep so that it may be necessary for the patient to have assisted respiration at night. It is important when diaphragmatic weakness is suspected to check vital capacity in both upright and recumbent positions since the vital capacity may be normal in the upright position but decreased by one-half when tested in the patient in the supine position.[72] In addition, the ineptness of trying to assess diaphragmatic function with fluoroscopy has been frequently demonstrated.[72] The measurement of transdiaphragmatic pressure is a sensitive indicator of diaphragmatic weakness but is infrequently used.[73] Phrenic nerve pacing has been used successfully in several patients with diaphragmatic weakness[74] but has not gained wide acceptance. A currass ventilator or a rocking-chair device may also be useful.

Respiratory Therapy

The efficacy of respiratory therapy in neuromuscular disease without accompanying pulmonary disease is not clearly established. Several groups have advocated positive pressure breathing in children with Duchenne dystrophy[15] and have suggested a modest increase in lung volume over a three-month period,[22] but there is no evidence that this increase alters overall prognosis.[16,17,19-21] In a review of 38 patients with Duchenne dystrophy[23] the total lung volumes were almost normal before the children were wheelchair-bound, although there were mild changes in the inspiratory and expiratory pressures and in the residual lung volume. No changes were noted in going from a supine to a standing position, suggesting that the diaphragm was well maintained. Blood gases were normal in these children. Respiratory infections were frequently managed successfully in an ambulatory setting until the pulmonary function began to deteriorate, usually concomitant with the child going into a wheelchair. No child died of a pulmonary complication before he had advanced disease and was confined to a wheelchair. These authors suggest that physicians should use energetic pulmonary therapy in all patients who are not severely affected since the prognosis is so good. They urge that the family be instructed in techniques of postural drainage, pharyngeal suctioning and percussion of the chest, although the latter is usually best done by a trained pulmonary therapist. They also emphasize that the two major errors in management of Duchenne patients are the failure to recognize the emergent nature of pulmonary infections and the failure to hospitalize the patient promptly for comprehensive pulmonary treatment. They stress that a respiratory infection causing difficulty in breathing is a medical emergency in a child with compromised strength. The diagnosis of pneumonia can be missed early in Duchenne dystrophy so that a chest x-ray is mandatory in all seriously ill dystrophics with respiratory secretion problems. The most frequent bacterial organisms are Hemophilus influenza and pneumococcus.

Pulmonary Interstitial Fibrosis

Although underlying primary pulmonary disease is not usually associated with neuromuscular disease, pulmonary interstitial fibrosis has been reported in association with the inflammatory myopathies (Fig. 4).[37,75-82] In patients receiving methotrexate it can be difficult to determine if the chest x-ray changes are secondary to medication[83,84] or are a primary manifestation of the disease. If there is any doubt, the methotrexate should be discontinued.

Hypotonia

In newborns, severe hypotonia and weakness can be the presenting manifestations of neuromuscular disease. Premature infants and children with central nervous system dysfunction may also have prominent hypotonia since mo-

A

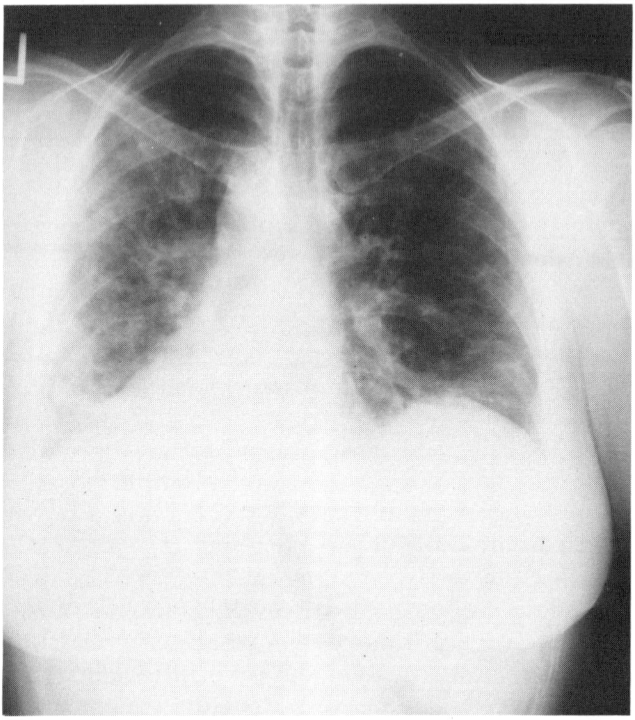

Figure 4. Serial chest x-rays from a 54-year-old female with an inflammatory myopathy of recent onset. The patient was hospitalized with acute respiratory failure. Although initial films revealed bilateral patchy infiltrates (*A*) which subsequently cleared, bibasilar interstitial changes have persisted (*B*). The patient has never received methotrexate to account for the pulmonary interstitial fibrosis.

tor control develops in an orderly manner during gestation and is incomplete even in the normal term newborn. No matter what the cause of the hypotonia, the complications that occur are rather uniform. Therefore, as the infant undergoes further laboratory evaluation to determine the etiology of this disorder, care must be exercised to avoid these complications. In some infants feeding difficulties are the earliest problem and can be particularly prominent in diseases in which the facial and bulbar muscles are weakened.

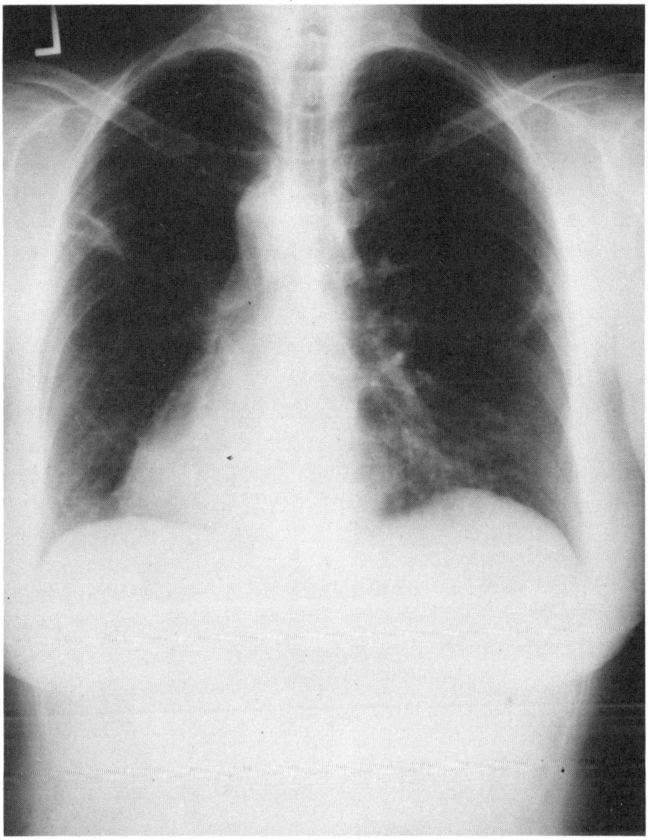

B

Figure 4. (Continued)

To prevent aspiration it may be necessary to gavage-feed the infant. A depressed cough reflex may also be present making clearance of secretions difficult and any respiratory infection potentially serious. Any accompanying scoliosis will only further compromise pulmonary reserve. When the hypotonia impairs pulmonary reserve or reduces the cough reflex, it is important to provide postural drainage, suctioning, and vigorous treatment of respiratory illness. Constipation or abdominal distention can further impair pulmonary reserve so that dietary control, stool softeners, or laxatives may be needed to prevent this.

SUMMARY

In this chapter we have illustrated the numerous respiratory complications that occur in patients with weakness of skeletal muscle. In the patient with acute onset of muscle weakness, early diagnosis is essential since accurate therapy can favorably affect the patient's outcome. With chronic progressive weakness, careful management of the patient will often prevent or forestall for many years a fatal respiratory disturbance.

Acknowledgments

This work was supported in part by a grant from the Muscular Dystrophy Association to Dr. Steven P. Ringel.

Special thanks to Clifford Zwillich, M.D. for careful editing, to Candy DeLapp for typing the chapter, and to Joan Ringel who continually transforms scientific jargon into simple, understandable language.

REFERENCES

1. Adams, R.D.: *Diseases of Muscle. A Study in Pathology.* New York, Harper and Row, 1975.
2. Bradley, W.G.: *Disorders of Peripheral Nerves.* Oxford, Blackwell Publishing, 1974.
3. Brooke, M.H.: *A Clinician's View of Neuromuscular Diseases.* Baltimore, Williams and Wilkins Co., 1977.
4. Dubowitz, V.: *Muscle Disorders in Childhood.* London, W.B. Saunders Co., 1978.
5. Dyck, P.J., Thomas, P.K., and Lambert, E.H. (eds.): *Peripheral Neuropathy.* Philadelphia, W.B. Saunders Co., 1975.
6. Vinken, P.J., and Bruyn, G.W.: Diseases of muscle. In *Handbook of Clinical Neurology,* Vol. 40–41. Amsterdam, North Holland Publishing Co., 1979.
7. Walton, J.N.: *Disorders of Voluntary Muscle,* 3rd Ed. London, Churchill Livingston, 1974.
8. Cherniak, R.M., Cherniak, L., and Naimark, A.: Diseases of the chest wall and diaphragm. In *Respiration in Health and Disease.* Philadelphia, W.B. Saunders Co., 1972.

9. Harrison, B.D.W., Collins, J.V., and Brown, K.G.E.: Respiratory failure in neuromuscular diseases. *Thorax* **26**:579–584, 1971.
10. Hirshman, C.A., McCullough, R.E., Weil, J.V.: Normal values for hypoxic and hypercapnic ventilatory drives in man. *J. Appl. Physiol.* **38**:1095–1098, 1975.
11. Kory, R.C., Cullahan, R., and Boren, H.G.: Clinical spirometry in normal man. *Am. J. Med.* **30**:243–258, 1961.
12. Laurence, R.V. (ed.): Clinical methods for the study of regulation of ventilation. Symposium. *Chest* **70** (Suppl.):109–186, 1976.
13. Drachman, D.B.: Myasthenia gravis. *N. Eng. J. Med.* **298**: 136–142; 186–193, 1978.
14. Blythe, J.A., Griffin, J.P., and Gonyea, E.F.: Bilateral diaphragmatic paralysis in association with neurogenic disease. *Arch. Int. Med.* **137**:1455–1457, 1977.
15. Adams, M.A., and Chander, L.S.: Effects of physical therapy program on vital capacity of patients with muscular dystrophy. *Phys. Ther.* **54**:494–496, 1974.
16. Arce-Gomez, E., Palma-Garcia, S., Yanez, J.L., Lopez-Portillo, M., Lombardo, L., Brandt, H., and Marquez, M.H.: Study of the cardiorespiratory function in patients with progressive muscular dystrophy. *Angiology* **15**:407, 1964.
17. Burke, S.S., Grove, N.M., Hauser, C.R., and Hohn, D.M.: Respiratory aspects of pseudohypertrophic muscular dystrophy. *Am. J. Dis. Child.* **121**:230, 1971.
18. Hall, W.J.: Respiratory failure as a complication of neuromuscular disease. In Griggs, R.L., and Moxley, R.T. (eds.): *Advances in Neurology,* Vol. 17. New York, Raven Press, 1977, pp. 317–324.
19. Hapke, E.J., Meek, J.C., and Jacobs, J.: Pulmonary function in progressive muscular dystrophy. *Chest* **61**:41, 1972.
20. Inkley, S.R., Oldenburg, F.C., and Vignos, P.J., Jr.: Pulmonary function in Duchenne muscular dystrophy related to stage of disease. *Am. J. Med.* **56**:297, 1974.
21. Gilroy, J., Cahalan, J.L., Berman, R., and Newman, M.: Cardiac and pulmonary complications in Duchenne's progressive muscular dystrophy. *Circulation* **27**:484, 1963.
22. Siegel, I.M.: Pulmonary problems in Duchenne muscular dystrophy. Diagnosis, prophylaxis and treatment. *Phys. Ther.* **55**:160–162, 1975.

23. Vignos, P.J.: Respiratory function and pulmonary infection in Duchenne muscular dystrophy. *Israel J. Med. Sci.* **13**:207–214, 1977.

24. Black, L.F., and Hyatt, R.E.: Maximal static respiratory pressures in generalized neuromuscular disease. *Am. Rev. Resp. Dis.* **103**:641, 1971.

25. Petty, T.L., Laksminarayan, S., Salin, S.A., Zwillich, C.W., and Nett, L.M.: Intensive respiratory care unit—a review of ten years' experience. *J.A.M.A.* **233**:34–37, 1975.

26. Pontoppidan, H., Griffin, B., and Lowenstein, E.: *Acute Respiratory Failure in the Adult.* Boston, Little, Brown and Co., 1972.

27. O'Donohue, W.J., Baker, J.P., Bell, G.M., Muren, O., Parker, C.L., and Patterson, J.L.: Respiratory failure in neuromuscular disease. *J.A.M.A.* **235**:733–735, 1976.

28. Engel, W.K., Festoff, B.W., Patten, B.M., Swerdlow, M., Newball, H.H., and Thompson, M.D.: Myasthenia gravis. *Ann. Int. Med.* **81**:225–246, 1974.

29. Arnon, S.S., Midura, T.F., Clay, S.A., Wood, R.M., and Chin, J.: Infant botulism. Epidemiological, clinical, and laboratory aspects. *J.A.M.A.* **237**:1946–1951, 1977.

30. Pickett, J., Berg, B., Chaplin, E., et al.: Syndrome of botulism in infancy: Clinical and electrophysiologic study. *N. Eng. J. Med.* **295**:770–772, 1976.

31. Seybold, M.E., and Drachman, D.B.: Gradually increasing doses of prednisone in myasthenia gravis. *N. Eng. J. Med.* **290**:81–84, 1974.

32. Papatestas, A.E., Genkins, G., Kornfeld, P., Horowitz, S., and Kark, A.E.: Transcervical thymectomy in myasthenia gravis. *Surg. Gynec. Obst.* **140**:535–540, 1975.

33. Goldblatt, D.: Treatment of amyotrophic lateral sclerosis. In Griggs, R.C., and Moxley, R.T. (eds.): *Advances in Neurology,* Vol. 17. New York, Raven Press, 1977, pp. 265–283.

34. Ringel, S.P., Lava, N.S., Treihaft, M.M., Lubs, M.L., and Lubs, H.A.: Late onset X-linked recessive spinal and bulbar muscular atrophy. *Muscle Nerve* **1**:297–307, 1978.

35. Montgomery, W.W., and Lynch, J.P.: Oculopharyngeal muscular dystrophy treated by inferior constrictor myotomy. *Trans. Am. Acad. Ophthal. Otolaryn.* **75**:986–993, 1971.

36. Pruzanski, W., and Profis, A.: Pulmonary disease in myotonic dystrophy. *Am. Rev. Resp. Dis.* **91**:874–879, 1965.

37. Medsger, T.A., Robinson, H., and Masi, A.T.: Factors affect-

ing survivorship in polymyositis. *Arth. Rheum.* **14**:249–258, 1971.

38. Barrett, R.H., and Hanson, M.L.: Oral myofunctional disorders. St. Louis, C.V. Mosby Co., 1974.
39. Rontal, E., Rontal, M., Morse, G., and Braun, E.M.: Vocal cord injection in the treatment of acute and chronic aspiration. *Laryngoscope* **86**:625–634, 1976.
40. Mills, C.P.: Dysphagia in pharyngeal paralysis treated by cricopharyngeal sphincterotomy. *Lancet* **1**:455–457, 1973.
41. Graham, W.P., and Royster, H.P.: Simplified cervical esophagostomy for long-term extra oral feeding. *Surg. Gynec. Obst.* **125**:127–128, 1967.
42. Shannon, D.C., Riseborough, E.J., and Kazemi, H.: Ventilation perfusion relationships following correction of kyphoscoliosis. *J.A.M.A.* **217**:579, 1971.
43. Gibson, D.A., and Wilkins, K.E.: The management of spinal deformities in Duchenne muscular dystrophy. *Clin. Orthop.* **108**:41–51, 1975.
44. Hardy, J.H.: *Spinal Deformity in Neurological and Muscular Disorders.* St. Louis, C.V. Mosby Co., 1974.
45. Benaim, S., and Worster-Drought, C.: Dystrophia myotonica with myotonia of the diaphragm causing pulmonary hypoventilation with anoxia and secondary polycythemia. *Med. Biol. Illus. (London)* **8**:221, 1954.
46. Cannon, P.J.: The heart and lungs in myotonic muscular dystrophy. *Am. J. Med.* **32**:765, 1965.
47. Gillam, P.M.S., Heaf, P.J.D., and Kaufman, L.: Respiration in dystrophia myotonica. *Thorax* **19**:142, 1964.
48. Kilburn, K.H., Eagen, J.T., and Heyman, A.: Cardiopulmonary insufficiency associated with myotonic dystrophy. *Am. J. Med.* **26**:929, 1959.
49. Kilburn, K.H., Eagen, J.T., Sielser, H.O., et al.: Cardiopulmonary insufficiency in myotonic and progressive muscular dystrophy. *N. Eng. J. Med.* **261**:1089–1096, 1959.
50. Carroll, J.E., Zwillich, C.W., and Weil, J.V.: Ventilatory response in myotonic dystrophy. *Neurology* **27**:1125–1128, 1977.
51. Coccagna, G., Mantovani, M., Parchi, C.: Alveolar hypoventilation and hypersonemia in myotonic dystrophy. *J. Neurol. Neurosurg. Psychiat.* **58**:977–984, 1976.
52. Bashour, F., Winchell, P., and Reddington, J.: Myotonia atrophica and cyanosis. *N. Eng. J. Med.* **252**:768, 1955.
53. Solliday, N.H., Gaensler, E.A., and Schwaber, J.R.: Impaired

central chemoreceptor function and chronic hypoventilation many years following poliomyelitis. Case Report. *Respiration* **31**:177, 1974.

54. Bellamy, D., Newsom Davis, J.M., and Hickey, B.P.: A case of primary alveolar hypoventilation associated with mild proximal myopathy. *Am. Rev. Resp. Dis.* **112**:867, 1975.
55. Rosenaw, E.C., and Engel, A.G.: Acid maltase deficiency in adults presenting as respiratory failure. *Am. J. Med.* **64**:485–491, 1978.
56. Carroll, J.E., Zwillich, C.W., Weil, J.V., and Brooke, M.H.: Depressed ventilatory response in oculocraniosomatic neuromuscular disease. *Neurology* **26**:140–146, 1976.
57. Buchsbaum, H.W., Martin, W.A., and Turino, G.M.: Chronic alveolar hypoventilation due to musuclar dystrophy. *Neurology* **18**:319, 1968.
58. Riley, D.J., Santiago, T.V., Daniels, R.P., Schall, B., and Edelman, N.H.: Blunted respiratory drive in congenital myopathy. *Am. J. Med.* **63**:459–466, 1977.
59. Tseuda, K., Shibutani, K., and Lefkowitz, M.: Postoperative ventilatory failure in an obese, myopathic woman with periodic somnolence. A case report. *Anesth. Analg.* **54**:523–526, 1975.
60. Smith, E., Harris, I.L., and Rosenblatt, P.: Acute poliomyelitis, a clinical and statistical study of 263 cases. *J. Ped.* **43**:9–20, 1953.
61. Comroe, J.H., Jr., Wood, F.C., and Kay, C.F.: Motor neuritis after tetanus antitoxin with involvement of the muscles of respiration. *Am. J. Med.* **10**:786–789, 1951.
62. Cape, C.A., Fincham, R.W.: Paralytic brachial neuritis with diaphragmatic paralysis. *Neurol.* **14**:191–193, 1965.
63. Tsairis, P., Dyck, P.J., and Mulder, D.W.: Natural history of brachial plexus neuropathy. *Arch. Neurol.* **27**:109–117, 1972.
64. Spitzer, S.A., Korczyn, A.D., and Kalaci, J.: Transient bilateral diaphragmatic paralysis. *Chest* **64**:355–357, 1973.
65. Goldstein, R.L., Hyde, R.W., and Lasham, L.W.: Peripheral neuropathy presenting with respiratory insufficiency as the primary complaint. *Am. J. Med.* **56**:443–449, 1974.
66. Schmalstieg, E.J., Peters, B.H., Schochet, S.S., and Findlay, S.R.: Neuropathy presenting as prolonged dyspnea. *Arch. Neurol.* **34**:473–476, 1977.
67. Miller, R.D., Mulder, D.W., and Fowler, W.S.: Exertional dyspnea: a primary complaint in unusual cases of progressive

muscular atrophy and amyotrophic lateral sclerosis. *Ann. Int. Med.* **46**:119–125, 1957.

68. Parhad, I.M., Clark, A.W., Barron, K.D., and Staunton, S.B.: Diaphragmatic paralysis in motor neuron disease. *Neurol.* **28**:18–22, 1978.
69. Mellins, R.B., Hays, A.P., Gold, A.P., et al.: Respiratory distress as the initial manifestation of Werdnig Hoffman's disease. *Pediatrics* **53**:33–41, 1974.
70. Bossen, E.H., Shelburne, J.D., and Verkauf, B.S.: Respiratory muscle involvement in infantile myotonic dystrophy. *Arch. Pathol.* **97**:250–252, 1974.
71. Bergen, B.J., Sangalang, V.E., and Aterman, K.: Isolated myopathic involvement of the diaphragmatic musculature in a neonate. *Ann. Neurol.* **1**:403–407, 1977.
72. Newsom, D.J., Goldman, M., and Loh, L.: Diaphragm function and alveolar hypoventilation. *Quart. J. Med.* **45**:87, 1976.
73. Newsom, D.J.: Phrenic nerve conduction in man. *J. Neurol. Neurosurg. Psychiat.* **30**:420–426, 1967.
74. Glenn, W.W., Holcomb, W.G., and Hogan, J.: Diaphragm pacing by radiofrequency transmission in the treatment of chronic ventilatory insufficiency: Present studies. *J. Thorac. Cardiovasc. Surg.* **66**:505–520, 1973.
75. Brundin, A.: Pulmonary fibrosis in scleroderma and dermatomyositis. *Scand. J. Resp. Dis.* **41**:160–170, 1970.
76. Camp, A.V., Lane, D.J., and Mawat, A.G.: Dermatomyositis with parenchymal lung involvement. *Br. Med. J.* **1**:155–156, 1972.
77. Duncan, P.E., Griffin, J.P., Garcia, A., and Kaplan, S.B.: Fibrosing alveolitis in polymyositis. A review of histologically confirmed cases. *Am. J. Med.* **57**:621–626, 1974.
78. Olson, G.N., and Sevenson, E.W.: Polymyositis and interstitial lung disease. *Am. Rev. Resp. Dis.* **105**:611–617, 1972.
79. Park, S., and Nyhan, W.L.: Fatal pulmonary involvement in dermatomyositis. *Am. J. Dis. Child.* **129**:723–726, 1975.
80. Schwarz, M.I., Matthay, R.A., Sahn, S.A., Stanford, R.E., Marmorstein, B.L., and Scheinhorn, D.S.: Interstitial lung disease in polymyositis and dermatomyositis. Analysis of six cases and review of the literature. *Medicine* **55**:89–104, 1976.
81. Webb, R.D., Gordon, C.D.: Pulmonary fibrosis masking polymyositis. Remission with corticosteroid therapy. *J.A.M.A.* **222**:1146–1149, 1972.
82. Weaver, A.L., Brundage, B.H., Nelson, R.A., et al.: Pulmo-

nary involvement in polymyositis. Report of a case with response to corticosteroid therapy. *Arth. Rheum.* **11**:765–773, 1968.

83. Arnett, F.C., Whelton, J.C., Zizac, T.M., and Stevens, M.B.: Methotrexate therapy in polymyositis. *Ann. Rheum. Dis.* **32**:536–546, 1973.
84. Everts, C.S., Westcott, J.L., and Bragg, D.G.: Methotrexate therapy and pulmonary disease. *Radiology* **107**:539–543, 1973.

7

RESPIRATORY DYSFUNCTION IN CEREBRAL VASCULAR DISEASE

Jeffrey Kramer, M.D.

Cerebrovascular disease, which often produces focal neurological deficits, has provided neurologists the opportunity to localize specific neurologic functions. Anatomic localization plays an integral role in delineation of diagnostic problems. It is within this framework that knowledge of abnormal respiratory patterns has gained clinical significance. Pathoanatomic localization of lesions resulting from cerebral vascular disease within the neuroaxis will be discussed in terms of altered patterns of respiratory rates and rhythms in the initial section of this chapter. Although some controversy exists pertaining to these various respiratory patterns and their associated neuroanatomical level of dysfunction, only the more widely accepted theories will be presented. A significant deficiency of recent reports regarding respiratory dysfunction in cerebral vascular disease presently exists in the medical literature. It has been suggested that this most likely reflects the frequent, early intubation of affected patients in an emergency room prior to delineation of a known or characteristic respiratory pattern. Klassen (personal communication) emphasizes that intubation of patients with acute strokes in his Intensive Care Unit is the exception rather than the rule.

Since this chapter is devoted to respiratory disturbances and their metabolic influences in cerebral vascular disease, it is beyond its scope to discuss specific pathology and pathogenesis and many of the clinical nonrespiratory neuroanatomic aspects of this disease. For more complete details of the prevalent clinical entity of cerebral vascular disease, the reader is referred to the monograph by E.C. Hutchinson and E.J. Acheson entitled *Strokes: Natural History, Pathology and Surgical Treatment* or other pertinent sources.[1-5]

LOCALIZATION BASED ON RESPIRATORY PATTERNS

In conjunction with motor and ophthalmic signs, localization of vascular lesions within the central nervous system may often be aided by observation of the patient's respiratory pattern.[6] This is especially true in cerebral vascular disease. The following discussion will consider the neuroanatomic basis of the abnormal respiratory patterns seen in vascular disease of the central nervous system following a descending or caudal pattern from cerebral hemispheral pathology to abnormalities within the medulla oblongata.

Posthyperventilation Apnea (PHVA)

Posthyperventilation apnea (although not always indicative of an abnormal respiratory state) is the most frequent pattern of altered breathing due to faulty neurologic control of the process or respiration.[7] PHVA is characterized by diminished or absent respirations following a period of deep breathing (hyperventilation). Rhythmic respirations resume again as the arterial carbon dioxide tension pCO_2 increases to a normal level. PHVA is seen in conscious patients whose underlying dysfunction is most often metabolic but has also been observed in patients with bilateral structural lesions within the cerebral hemispheres such as that seen in bilateral cerebral infarctions.[7,8] Klassen (personal communication) believes PHVA has been an overated clinically useful sign and PHVA may merely represent decreased inhibition of brainstem responses to alterations in arterial pCO_2.

To demonstrate the presence of PHVA, the patient must be asked to voluntarily hyperventilate. At least five to seven deep breaths are required to lower the arterial pCO_2 sufficiently to demonstrate this abnormal pattern. The apnea in PHVA lasts from 15 to 30 seconds, thus suggesting an abnormal respiratory response to hyperventilation since in normal subjects there is usually no delay in resumption of normal respiratory rhythm. Focal neurologic deficits or a prior history of multiple cerebral vascular accidents suggest that the underlying etiology is that of bilateral structural lesions in the cerebral hemispheres due to infarction. In one study, however, seventeen patients had unilateral pathology at the cerebral level, many of these due to vascular disease.[7] Plum and co-workers have suggested that the neural deficit responsible for PHVA is bilateral dysfunction of forebrain structures.[7]

Pathogenesis

As is the case with much of the material related to cerebral vascular disease and respiratory dysfunction, the pathophysiology of PHVA is debatable. The most widely accepted theory for this type of periodicity in respiration is that bilateral cortical infarctions in forebrain structures or their related tracts interrupt the normal neural influence which activates rhythmicity of breathing when carbon dioxide tension is reduced.[7-9] Most importantly, recognition of PHVA as an abnormal respiratory pattern can alert the physician to the possibility of underlying cerebral dysfunction, including subclinical cerebral vascular disease. In addition, PHVA lends credence to the contention that higher cortical centers play an integral role in the control of respiration.

Cheyne-Stokes Respiration (CSR)

CSR is a normal respiratory pattern during sleep in the infant and elderly populations. This pattern of respiration is characterized by a series of breaths initially of small tidal volume, increasing in size, and subsequently diminishing until a period of apnea ensues. CSR is a periodic pattern of breathing in which cycles are repeated at varying intervals, and is often accompanied by a periodicity in blood pressure and pulse.[10] The period of hyperpnea in this pattern is characteristically longer than the duration of apnea (Fig. 1).

In 1818, John Cheyne first described the periodic respiratory pattern which subsequently has come to bear his name.[11] Although necropsy showed both cardiac and cerebral pathology in Cheyne's original case, it is now generally recognized that CSR is due to structural lesions at or above the level of the diencephalon.[9] CSR may also be seen in patients with sleep disorders, head trauma, hypertensive heart disease and congestive heart failure, uremia, and narcotic overdose. However, the most common cause of this type of periodic respiration is cerebral infarction, either unilateral with secondary depression of the opposite hemisphere or bilateral as seen in embolic disease. The associated vascular lesions are often located deep in the cerebral hemispheres, within the basal ganglia and internal capsule. Although mainly associated with hemisphere pathology, CSR has been observed more frequently than originally thought in patients suffering brainstem infarction.[6,14,15]

Associated acute neurologic signs in patients with CSR due to cerebral vascular disease are altered levels of consciousness (lethargy, stupor, or coma), hemiparesis, hemianesthesia, and conjugate gaze palsy. Brown and Plum described more chronically afflicted patients with CSR who had pseudobulbar palsy, dementia, and pyramidal tract signs such as spasticity and Babinski signs.[12] In most patients with CSR, pupils dilate in the hyperpneic phase and

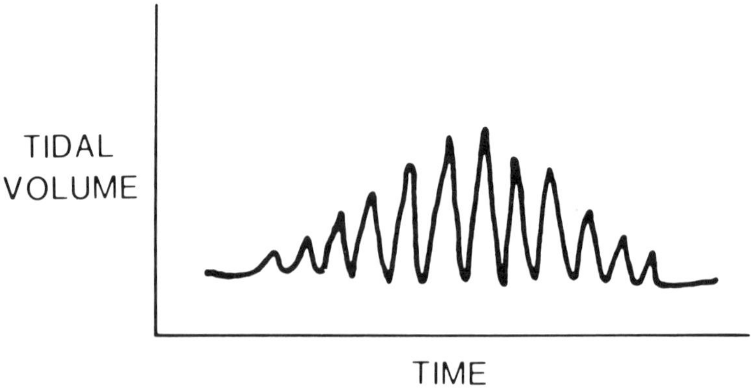

Figure 1.

constrict during the apneic phase. During the hyperpnea of CSR, the patient may become arousable and responsive, whereas during the apneic phase, decreasing levels of consciousness ensue. During this apneic period Babinski signs may appear and deep tendon reflexes may diminish. Just the opposite has been observed during the hyperpneic phase of CSR. Before discussing the pathogenesis of CSR, it should be emphasized that this pattern localizes the level of the vascular lesion (in almost all patients) at or above the level of the upper midbrain. In addition, when patients proceed from a normal respiratory pattern to one of CSR, this most often represents neurologic deterioration and close observation is warranted.

There have been multiple theories which have been proposed to explain Cheyne-Stokes respiration. The first and original proposition is that CSR is due to prolonged cerebral circulation time which most often is a result of heart failure.[14] The second theory suggests that CSR occurs because of cyclic depression of the respiratory centers in the medulla oblongata. A third proposal is that CSR is a result of medullary irritability and lastly, that periodicity of respiration as seen in CSR is a result of alterations in the descending influences on the respiratory centers located within the medulla oblongata.[13]

It has been demonstrated that patients with bilateral cerebral infarctions have an altered response to carbon dioxide stimulation.[9] Abnormally increased ventilatory response to carbon dioxide stimulation leads to hyperpnea. Structural cortical lesions of the forebrain (often bilaterally) is known to result in posthyperventilation apnea. The resultant combination of the two, increased ventilatory response to carbon dioxide stimulation and decreased forebrain stimuli on the lower respiratory centers located within the brain stem, results in the pattern of Cheyne-Stokes respiration. Although CSR is known to occur in pure neurologic lesions, the periodicity may be altered with oxygen therapy. Prevention of the apneic period can be accomplished by the administration of carbon dioxide.[16] This may indicate the peripheral receptors still maintain their influence of central neuroregulatory processes in most patients with CSR. However, the effect of carbon dioxide may more likely represent functional integrity of central chemoreceptors.

Prognosis

Blood gases obtained in patients with CSR usually reveal a pattern of respiratory alkalosis which is most likely due to the longer duration of the hyperpneic phase over the apneic period.[17,18] Rout and colleagues, in assessing prognosis of patients with cerebral vascular accidents in relation to respiratory patterns and blood gas tensions, determined that CSR carried a fair to good prognosis as long as no progression to rhythmic hyperventilation occurred. An arterial pCO_2 of less than 35 mmHg and an arterial pH greater than 7.46 are reported to be associated with a poor prognosis.[19]

Central Neurogenic Hyperventilation (CNH)

Central neurogenic hyperventilation is an abnormal respiratory pattern characterized by rapid, regular relatively deep hyperpnea which may continue for days at a time.[67] It is usually associated with a poor prognosis when it occurs as a result of a cerebral vascular accident and is often confused with the breathing seen in patients with acute metabolic acidosis. CNH is a regular hyperpnea at a rate of 24 to 38 breaths per minute (Fig. 2). Once acute metabolic disease and infection have been ruled out as the cause of a patient's hyperventilation, CNH suggests acute brain stem infarction or hemorrhage with subsequent dysfunction of the brain stem tegmentum (medially and paramedially).

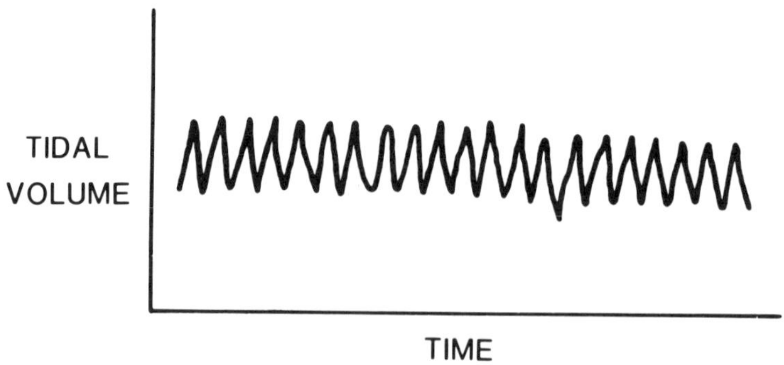

Figure 2.

Anatomically, the lesion may involve the midpons up to the midbrain.[16] Brain stem hemorrhage may be primary or may result from transtentorial herniation which is also known to cause secondary brain stem dysfunction.

Arterial blood gases reveal a pattern of respiratory alkalosis with diminished arterial carbon dioxide tensions, depressed arterial oxygen saturation, and an elevated arterial pH level.[16] Administration of oxygen therapy is of no value and does not modify the pattern of CNH, whereas in the periodic breathing of CSR, administration of O_2 has been demonstrated to suppress the periodicity. Administration of carbon dioxide to patients with CNH will tend to increase the depth but not the rate of the respiratory pattern. Associated neurologic signs in patients with CNH depend upon the distribution of lesions at the level of infarction. In midbrain lesions, contralateral hemiplegia, rubral tremor and ipsilateral pupillary dilatation may be present. In pontine lesions, various ophthalmologic signs (nystagmus and gaze palsies), hemiplegia, quadriplegia, and the "locked-in" syndrome, may be demonstrated upon examination.

Although CNH is the most accepted abnormal respiratory pattern with rostral median pontine or caudal midbrain infarction, Lee and colleagues have recently suggested that periodic breathing such as Cheyne-Stokes respiration and Cheyne-Stokes variant breathing are at least as frequent. Depending on the time the patient is observed and underlying metabolic conditions, variations in the abovementioned respiratory patterns are frequent and often mixed.[15] It is, therefore, more common to observe combinations of periodic breathing and rhythmic hyperventilation in patients with vascular lesions in these brain stem territories.

Experimental production of CNH has not provided an adequate understanding of the pathogenesis of this abnormal respiratory pattern. However, two hypotheses have been put forward: (1) medial pontine tegmental damage disinhibits descending cortical neuronal and lateral pontine reticular influences on the control of breathing, resulting in facilitation of the respiratory centers within the medulla (both inspiratory and expiratory), and (2) the incoming ascending afferent impulses from pulmonary stretch receptors are disinhibited because of dysfunction of the medial pons and thus result in hyperpnea.[16] Most of the original cases of CNH had coexistent pulmonary pathology at postmortem, although one patient clearly had only brain stem pathology.[16] Although the pathophysiology of CNH remains controversial, little doubt exists that isolated basilar artery thrombosis with subsequent necrosis in the upper one half of the medial pons can produce CNH in the absence of pulmonary pathology.

Apneustic Breathing

From the available literature concerning abnormal respiratory patterns in cerebral vascular disease, it is apparent that more has been described in relation to brain stem infarction or hemorrhage than for vascular lesions of the cerebral hemispheres. This is most likely the result of the earlier concept that the only neurologic control over the respiratory system existed from midpons to medulla.[20] However, various respiratory patterns can result from cerebral vascular disease which produces either cerebral hemispheral or brain stem dysfunction.[6] One of the least understood of the abnormal patterns in brain stem lesions is apneustic breathing.

First described in 1888 and subsequently named by Lumsden in 1923, apneusis is characterized by sustained inspiratory cramps and an abnormal duration of expiration.[8,21] Apneustic breathing is rare in man and in one recent series of twenty-three patients with acute brain stem infarction, this pattern was not even observed.[15] Apneusis presumably results from infarction or hemorrhage in the mid to caudal pons, just below the exit of the fifth cranial nerve. As with CNH, the site of the lesion associated with apneusis is the brain stem tegmentum, especially dorsolaterally.[6,21] However, with apneustic breathing the lower third of the pons is most affected and the implicated vessels are the basilar artery and its pontine perforating branches. Bilateral involvement of the pons is necessary to produce apneustic breathing.[22] Therefore, bilateral vertebral artery occlusion, basilar artery thrombosis, or pontine hemorrhage is required to produce the pathologic pontine lesion resulting in apneusis. The area of pontine infarction in man correlates with the area in animals known as the pneumotaxic center.[8] Associated neurologic signs seen with apneusia may involve the fifth, sixth, and seventh cranial nerves. Horizontal or vertical gaze palsies, severe vomiting, wild nystagmus, ocular bobbing, altered level of consciousness, and hemi- or quadriplegia may also frequently accompany apneustic respiration. Occasionally, apneustic breathing has been seen in severe basilar meningitis, anoxia, and hypoglycemia.[8] Transtentorial herniation, which may cause Cheyne-Stokes and central neurogenic hyperventilation respiratory patterns, does not cause the pattern of apneustic breathing. Apneustic respirations may rarely be observed in infarction of the medulla oblongata. In the occasional patient with brain stem compression secondary to cerebellar hematoma or infarction, early recognition of apneusis may be life-saving. In the experience of Klassen (personal communication), pure apneusis resulting from acute infarction has not been observed.

Pathogenesis

Apneustic breathing is believed to result from interference of the reciprocal inhibition that normally occurs between the inspiratory and the expiratory neuronal pools located within the brain stem.[22] This would then produce prolonged and uninhibited firing of the inspiratory neurons resulting in the inspiratory cramp seen in apneustic breathing. Similarly, uninhibited discharge of the expiratory neuronal pool would lead to the prolonged expiratory time also observed in this breathing pattern. A second explanation is that apneusis is merely the result of an extramedullary stimulus to inspiration superimposed on the basic rhythmic medullary respiratory center.[23]

Prognosis

Apneustic breathing is rarely seen as the only respiratory pattern in affected patients. Periodic respirations and more often cluster breathing is intermixed with apneusis.[21] Thus, the hyperpnea, respiratory alkalosis, and lowered pCO_2 seen in other tachypneic patients are associated with the poor prognosis described by Rout and colleagues.[19]

Ataxic Breathing

Ataxic breathing is an abnormal pattern of respiration which is completely irregular in both rate and rhythm. Random shallow and deep breaths alternate with short and long apneic pauses. There is little difficulty in distinguishing this pattern from Cheyne-Stokes respiration. Plum and Swanson have stated that ataxic breathing is due to decreased sensitivity to circulatory chemical stimuli. Ataxic respirations are reportedly sensitive to respiratory depressant drugs, seemingly more so than breathing patterns associated with more rostral brain stem dysfunction.[24] Ataxic breathing is rare in cerebral vascular disease of the brain stem. However, in conjunction with cluster or Cheyne-Stokes variant breathing, ataxic respirations are occasionally seen in patients with cerebellar hemorrhage and secondary compression of the medulla.[25] These patients with ataxic breathing may cease breathing without warning and immediate intubation is required as surgical decompression of the lower brain stem has been successful and life-saving in these instances.[25-27]

Ataxic breathing may result from vascular lesions within the lower pons and throughout much of the medulla oblongata. Except for low brain stem infarcts, cerebellar infarction or hemorrhage may cause ataxic breathing, usually as a result of compression of the medulla oblongata.[26,27] One must exclude severe neuronal depression from such clinical entities as narcosis, either drug-induced or due to elevated pCO_2, severe anoxia and primary lesions of the medulla such as compression from meningitis, neoplasm, and demyelinating disease.[2] Ataxic respirations carry a grave prognosis. Arterial blood gases usually reveal elevated arterial carbon dioxide tensions and usually a lowered arterial oxygen tension.[17]

The pathophysiologic basis for ataxic breathing has been postulated to result from disruption of the reciprocal interplay between expiratory neuronal population and medullary inspiratory neurons. This irregular pattern of breathing is also associated with hypersensitivity of the respiratory centers to endogenous chemicals as well as depressant drugs.

Ataxic breathing resulting from vascular disease is rare in pure medullary disease because of the bilateral vertebral arterial supply to this area. In order to produce ataxic breathing on the basis of central medullary disease, both vertebral arteries would have to be implicated in the pathogenesis.[8] Levin and Margolis recently reported acute failure of automatic respirations (Ondine's curse) due to a unilateral infarction of the medulla oblongata.[28] Ondine's curse has been reported more often in bulbar poliomyelitis and bilateral cervical cordotomy than in vascular lesions of the medulla.[29] However, these authors reported an unusual case of a fifty-two year old man with symptoms of brain stem infarction. This patient subsequently died due to hypertensive vascular disease with an infarction of the left pontomedullary lateral tegmentum. Although his respirations were described as erratic, he was never dyspneic. Depressants apparently led to a respiratory arrest. This case report with autopsy confirmation suggests that Ondine's curse can be caused by unilateral pontomedullary infarction. Devereaux, Keane, and Davis reported two cases of automatic respiratory failure due to bilateral infarctions of the medulla oblongata. Pathologic study of one case revealed an old infarct in the right tegmentum and a recent infarct on the left at the level of the midmedulla.[29]

Respiratory Dysfunction in Unilateral Cerebral Vascular Disease

Unilateral cerebrovascular accidents are often characterized by the abrupt onset of focal neurologic deficits on the side of the body contralateral to the vascular cerebral hemisphere lesion. Since Jackson's description in 1895,[30] diminished voluntary movement of the chest contralateral to the hemispheral pathology has been recognized. Others have also emphasized this point.[8,31] These clinical observations suggest that, at least in part, some of the fibers involved in cerebral control over the respiratory mechanisms travel amidst the corticospinal fibers to at least the pontine level. The exact location of the forebrain structures involved in voluntary respiration is not fully known in man. Orbitofrontal cortex and anterior cingulum have been implicated as higher cortical centers involved in the neurologic integration controlling the act of respiration.[33] These areas are supplied by branches of both the anterior and middle cerebral arteries and infarction in the distribution of these arteries may theoretically result in loss of voluntary deep breathing. Plum has described a unique abnormality of voluntary breathing which has been called respiratory apraxia.[8]

It is not infrequent to hear an examiner yelling at a patient with an acute cerebrovascular accident to "take a deep breath." If one understands that voluntary deep breathing may be absent unilaterally or bilaterally (if a second lesion exists or if there is secondary involvement of the uninvolved hemisphere which may be seen in large unilateral CVA's), the examiner may spare his vocal cords and the patient's stapedius.

Although the pathoanatomic correlate has not yet been demonstrated, bilateral forebrain dysfunction has been proposed as the pathophysiologic basis for respiratory apraxia. The patient with respiratory apraxia is unable to take a deep breath or hold a breath on specific command such as may be seen in the patient with acute unilateral CVA who has bihemispheral dysfunction. In addition, voluntary swallowing may also be impaired in patients with respiratory apraxia.

Posthyperventilation apnea is the most common abnormality of breathing seen in patients with unilateral cerebral infarction. The second most frequent abnormal respiratory pattern in patients with unilateral cerebral vascular disease is CSR. Abnormal respiratory patterns are usually intermittent in these patients and occur more often in the presence of marked neurologic deficits, i.e., hemiplegia. Depression of sensorium is especially sensitive in unmasking the abnormal respiratory pattern.[12] If the neurologic basis of CSR depends on an increased sensitivity to carbon dioxide, then bilateral hemispheral dysfunction is necessary for the production of CSR. How then does unilateral cerebral vascular disease lead to a respiratory pattern known to be associated with bilateral structural lesions in the cerebrum? This may be explained by the phenomenon known as "cerebral diaschisis" in which there is depression of cerebral activity with associated decreased cerebral blood flow in the hemisphere opposite to that in which the vascular lesion has occurred.[34-36] This would subsequently result in bilateral hemispheral dysfunction which is known to result in an increased sensitivity to carbon dioxide by the central respiratory control system and thus allow for the production of CSR.

SUMMARY

Respiratory patterns vary with the degree and cause of alteration in consciousness. These patterns bear some relationship to the anatomic location of the CNS lesions. Although breathing is automatic when one is conscious, voluntary control can be superimposed. In the comatose state breathing is wholly automatic. The rate, depth, and rhythm may be a reflection of the anatomical level of nervous system dysfunction. A change from one pattern of respiration to another is an observation of extreme importance because it denotes that the level of neural function has altered. A patient may pass from normal to Cheyne-Stokes pattern as cerebral function is altered. This may be followed by rhythmic hyperventilation as the central pontine area is released from higher controls, and by periodic cluster breathing as structures in the lower brain stem are no longer influenced by rostral mechanisms. Finally, ataxic respiration may occur when medullary drive persists exclusively. This entire pattern typifies the respiratory deterioration associated with any supratentorial lesion which compromises brain stem function in a progressive and more or less orderly fashion

In contrast, lesions of the posterior fossa may compress the brain stem rapidly and change the respiratory pattern from normal to ataxic within a matter of minutes. Therefore, disorders of the posterior fossa are potentially more dangerous and often constitute greater emergencies than do supratentorial disturbances.

Abnormalities in respiratory patterns in patients suffering cerebrovascular accidents can aid the physician in the localization of the neurologic lesion. Most often these patterns of breathing rarely occur alone and frequently periodic respirations of the Cheyne-Stokes type is seen intermixed with either Cheyne-Stokes variants or CNH. Apneustic breathing is often overshadowed by Cheyne-Stokes or periodic respirations or ataxic breathing. Controversy exists over whether periodic breathing or apneusis with CNH is more common in vascular lesions of the pons. Infarction of the medulla may cause failure of automatic respirations, but because of bilateral vertebral supply to this area, infarction of only the medulla rarely leads to abnormalities in respiration. Arterial blood gases may be helpful in determining the prognosis of patients with acute cerebrovascular accidents. Alkalosis with depression of arterial carbon dioxide tension appears to be associated with a poor prognosis.

Acknowledgment

The author would like to express his gratitude to Dr. Arthur C. Klassen, Professor of Neurology, University of Minnesota Hospitals for sharing his experience in this field and for his most helpful comments during preparation of this manuscript.

REFERENCES

1. Sahs, A.L.: Cooperative study of intracranial aneurysms and subarachnoid hemorrhage. *Stroke* **5**: 550–601, 1974.
2. Hutchinson, E.C., and Acheson, E.J.: *Strokes: Natural History, Pathology, and Surgical Treatment.* Major Problems in Neurology, Vol. 4. Philadelphia, W.B. Saunders Co., 1975, pp. 90–91.
3. Adams, R.A., and Victor, M.: Cerebrovascular diseases. In *Principles of Neurology* 28. New York, McGraw-Hill Book Co., 1977, pp. 541–547.
4. Marie, P.: Des foyers lacunaires de desintegration et de differents autres cavitaires du cerveau. *Rev. Med. (Paris)* **21**: 281–292, 1901.
5. Fisher, C.M.: Small, deep cerebral infarcts. *Neurology* **15**: 774–784, 1965.
6. Plum, F., and Posner, J.B.: *Diagnosis of Stupor and Coma*, 2nd Ed. Philadelphia, F.A. Davis Co., 1972, pp. 15–17.
7. Plum, F., Brown, H.W., and Snoep, E.: The neurological significance of post-hyperventilation apnea. *J.A.M.A.* **181**: 1050–1055, 1962.

8. Plum, F.: Neurologic integration of behavioral and metabolic control of breathing. In Porter, R.J. (ed.): *Breathing; Hering-Breuer Centenary Symposium,* Ciba Symposium. New York, Longman, Inc., 1970, pp. 159–181.
9. Heyman, A., Birchfield, R.I., and Sieker, H.O.: Effects of bilateral cerebral infarctions on respiratory sensitivity. *Neurology* **8**: 694–700, 1964.
10. Eyster, J.A.E.: Clinical and experimental observations upon Cheyne-Stokes respiration. *J. Exper. Med.* **8**: 565, 1906.
11. Cheyne, J.: A case of apoplexy in which the fleshy part of the heart was converted to fat. *Dublin Hosp. Rep.* **2**: 216–223, 1818.
12. Brown, H.W., and Plum, F.: The neurologic basis of Cheyne-Stokes respiration. *Am. J. Med.* **30**: 849–860, 1961.
13. Comeau, W.J.: Cheyne-Stokes respiration and auriculoventricular conduction. *N. Eng. J. Med.* **219**: 977, 1938.
14. Karp, H.R., Sieker, H.O., and Heyman, A.: Cerebral circulation and function in Cheyne-Stokes respiration. *Am. J. Med.* **30**: 861–870, 1961.
15. Lee, M.C., Klassen, A.C., Heaney, L.M., et al.: Respiratory rate and pattern disturbances in acute brain stem infarction. *Stroke* **7**: 382–385, 1976.
16. Plum, F., and Swanson, A.G.: Central neurogenic hyperventilation in man. *Arch. Neurol. Psychiat.* **81**: 535–549, 1959.
17. Plum, F., and Brown, H.W.: The effect on respiration of central nervous system disease. *Ann. N.Y. Acad. Sci.* **109**: 915–929, 1963.
18. Lee, M.C., Klassen, A.C., and Resch, J.A.: Respiratory pattern disturbances in ischemic cerebral vascular disease. *Stroke* **5**: 612–616, 1974.
19. Rout, M.W., Lane, D.J., and Wollner, L.: Prognosis in acute cerebrovascular accidents in relation to respiratory pattern and blood gas tensions. *Br. Med. J.* **9**: 7–9, 1971.
20. Pitts, R.F.: The function of components of the respiratory complex. *J. Neurophysiol.* **5**: 403–413, 1942.
21. Plum, F., and Alvord, E.C.: Apneustic breathing in man. *Arch. Neurol.* **10**: 101–112, 1964.
22. Haymaker, W.: *Bing's Local Diagnosis in Neurologic Disease.* St. Louis, C.V. Mosby Co., 1969, pp. 41–42.
23. Hoff, H.E., and Breckenridge, C.G.: Regulation of Respiration. In Fulton, J.F. (ed.): *A Textbook of Physiology,* 17th Ed. Philadelphia, W.B. Saunders and Co., 1955, Chap. 43.

24. Plum, F., and Swanson, A.G.: Abnormalities in central regulation of respiration in acute and convalescent poliomyelitis. *Arch. Neurol. Psychiat.* **80**: 267–285, 1958.
25. McKissock, W., Richardson, A., and Walsh, L.; Spontaneous cerebellar hemorrhage: A study of 34 consecutive cases treated surgically. *Brain* **83**: 1–9, 1960.
26. Richardson, A.E.: Spontaneous cerebellar hemorrhage. In Vinken, P.J., and Bryun, G.W. (eds.): *Handbook of Clinical Neurology,* Vol. 12. Amsterdam, North Holland Publishing Co., 1972, pp. 54–67.
27. Fisher, C.M., Picard, E.H., Polack, A., et al.: Acute hypertensive cerebellar hemorrhage; diagnosis and treatment. *J. Nerv. Ment. Dis.* **140** (1): 38–57, 1965.
28. Levin, B.E., and Margolis, G.: Acute failure of automatic respirations secondary to a unilateral brain stem infarct. *Ann. Neurol.* **1**: 583–588, 1977.
29. Devereaux, M.W., Keane, M.W., and Davis, R.L.: Automatic respiratory failure associated with infarction of the medulla. *Arch. Neurol.* **29**: 46–52, 1973.
30. Jackson, J.H.: Superior and subordinate centres of lowest level. *Lancet* **1**: 476–478, 1895.
31. Fluck, D.C.: Chest movements in hemiplegia. *Clin. Sci.* **31**: 383–388, 1966.
32. Ross, G.F., and Brodal, A.: Corticofugal fibers to the brain stem reticular formation. An experimental study in the cat. *J. Anat.* **90**: 42–62, 1956.
33. Delgado, J.M.R., and Livingston, R.B.: Some respiratory vascular and thermal responses to stimulation of orbital surface of frontal lobe. *J. Neurophysiol.* **11**: 39–55, 1948.
34. Skinhφj, E.: Bilateral depression CBF in unilateral cerebral diseases. *Acta Neurol. Scand.* **41 (Suppl. 14)**: 161–163, 1965.
35. Meyer, J.S., Kanda, T., Fukuuchi, T., et al.: Diaschisis resulting from acute unilateral cerebral infarction. *Arch. Neurol.* **23**: 241–247, 1970.
36. Paulson, O.B.: Cerebral apoplexy (stroke): Pathogenesis, pathophysiology and therapy as illustrated by regional blood flow measurements in the brain. *Stroke* **2**: 327–360, 1971.
37. Sambrock, M.A., Hutchinson, E.C., Aber, G.M.: Metabolic studies in subarachnoid hemorrhage and strokes. *Brain* **96**: 171–190, 1973.

8

Respiratory Disease and Seizures

Donna Bergen, M.D.

Aside from diaphragmatic myoclonus (dealt with elsewhere in this book), respiratory dysfunction at first would appear to have no direct cause or effect relation with the paroxysmal cerebral discharges which cause clinically apparent seizures. Nevertheless, seizures and pulmonary disease often occur in the same patient, one of these conditions or its treatment giving rise to the other—sometimes predictably, more often as an idiosyncratic response or because of unusual combinations of synergistic factors. This chapter will describe and discuss some of these circumstances, under two general categories: seizures as a consequence of pulmonary disease and its treatment, and respiratory dysfunction as a complication of seizures and anticonvulsants.

RESPIRATORY DISEASE OR DYSFUNCTION CAUSED BY SEIZURES AND ANTICONVULSANTS

Postictal Pulmonary Edema

Mild to severe pulmonary edema has been observed following generalized convulsions.[1-4] This appears to be a relatively rare occurrence, and awareness of its existence is desirable mainly to be able to differentiate the condition from postictal aspiration pneumonia, a well-known and common complication of generalized seizures.

The condition has been reported most often in young epileptics, and often recurs in the same individual.[2] The symptoms of dyspnea, hemoptysis, and tachypnea may appear after an episode of status epilepticus, but most patients have had only a single generalized convulsion ("grand mal" fit) before developing pulmonary edema. Early reports of postictal pulmonary edema record high mortality rates (four out of 11 patients in Shanahan's original series),[5,6] but most of the more recent cases have shown only mild to moderate symptoms; in some cases the patients have recovered without any therapy at all.[3]

Chest x-rays typically show diffuse or multilobar, patchy infiltrates, often more pronounced on one side.[2] The x-ray changes are much more severe than those associated with aspiration pneumonia, in which a localized lobar infiltrate, usually in an upper lobe, is seen. The patient with postictal pulmonary edema is usually only mildly to moderately symptomatic, and typically responds readily to oxygen therapy alone. Occasionally positive pressure breathing may be helpful.[4]

Both the symptoms and the x-ray abnormalities tend to clear quickly, often within several hours. The chest x-ray may less frequently continue to show some changes for several days.[2] The course of postictal pulmonary edema thus differs from that of postictal aspiration pneumonia, in which the patient with a favorable outcome is usually ill for 24 to 48 hours and in which x-ray abnormalities persist for two to three weeks.[7]

The pathophysiology of postictal pulmonary edema is a matter for speculation. One possibility rests on the observation that increased intracranial pressure can be accompanied by pulmonary edema, and that generalized convulsions may cause increased intracranial pressure.[8,9] The chain of events would then be convulsions leading to intracranial hypertension leading to pulmonary edema. Against this hypothesis is the fact that the occurrence of pulmonary edema does not correlate with the number of seizures, and that the disease often recurs in the same patient, as though idiosyncratic or constitutional factors are a major contribution to this particular response to grand mal fits.

The latter observation in fact is more in keeping with the hypothesis that pulmonary edema results from ictal activation of autonomic neuronal circuits. Other positive autonomic phenomena such as flushing, tachycardia, and sweating are well-recognized ictal events, usually from seizure foci in the temporal lobes.[10] Similar discharges, with activation of the sympathetic nervous system to produce vasoconstriction of peripheral blood vessels and redistribution of blood to the heart and pulmonary bed, could conceivably produce transient heart failure and pulmonary congestion.[10] Sympathetically mediated dilatation of pulmonary blood vessels could also contribute.[3] Details of the patient's usual seizure pattern and the location of any EEG spike foci might offer a clue to such a mechanism (since psychomotor seizures and temporal lobe spikes might be expected to occur), but are generally not reported. The cause of pulmonary postictal edema thus remains unknown.

Anticonvulsant Toxicity

In 1959 Moore reported a single patient without symptoms of pulmonary disease, who was found to have marked, diffuse x-ray changes most compatible with interstitial fibrosis.[11] She had been taking phenytoin or methylphenylethyl hydantoin (Mesantoin) for four years before the severe x-ray abnormalities were found; they remained unchanged for 16 months. Apparently no pulmonary function tests were done. Moore then did chest x-rays on 31 other asymptomatic patients with long histories of hydantoin use, and claimed that 27 showed evidence of "diffuse pulmonary fibrosis" or "accentuated bronchovascular markings."

Certainly such dramatic findings are not within the experience of neurologists who see hundreds of such patients. Moore's finding was conclusively and convincingly rebutted shortly afterwards.[12,13]

The question of hydantoin toxicity involving the lungs has recently been raised again with the demonstration of reduced steady-state diffusing capacities and abnormal blood gas tension during exercise in 18 of 40 patients tested.[14] Abnormalities were particularly common in patients who had started phenytoin before the age of eight. In view of phenytoin's demonstrated capacity to stimulate fibroblast proliferation and collagen deposition, an effect typified by the gingival hyperplasia caused by the drug, the development of pulmonary fibrosis would not be a surprising finding, especially in children exposed to the drug during a final stage of alveolar development.[15]

Aspiration Pneumonia and Lung Abscess

Aspiration pneumonia is probably the most frequent pulmonary complication of epilepsy, yet considering the generalized flaccidity characterizing the postictal state, and the usual presence of saliva and blood (from a lacerated tongue) which accumulates in the pharynx during a generalized fit, it is only surprising that aspiration pneumonia is not commoner. Gastric contents may also be aspirated under these conditions.[7] Treatment consists of broad-spectrum antibiotics and corticosteroids.[17]

Patients with pyorrhea are notoriously prone to develop lung abscesses, presumably following aspiration of small amounts of pyogenic material in sleep.[17] Epileptic patients with pyorrhea are at similar risk, or perhaps greater, since aspiration during a postictal state is frequent, and such cases have been reported.[18]

Changes in Respiration During Seizures

The most dramatic respiratory changes occur of course during a generalized tonic-clonic convulsion. The initial tonic phase of such an attack consists of a violent and sustained contraction of striated muscles, including laryngospasm, causing total apnea. Apnea continues during the following clonic phase of the attack, and even during the initial part of the postictal period. The total apneic period thus may be well over a minute, and marked cyanosis is the rule. Abnormal muscle activity probably cannot account for the continuing postictal apnea; central neurogenic mechanisms may well be involved.[49] Hyperventilation characterizes the subsequent postictal state, although the obstructive effect of accumulated upper airway secretions (and often blood from tongue-biting) further delays adequate ventilation. The efects of ictal hypoxia on the brain are discussed in the next section.

Respiratory irregularities or apneic periods can also occur during petit mal absences or during some psychomotor seizures.[47] Such events are not generally a clinically significant or even noticeable component of these seizures.

Respiratory changes are, however, not only an important element of some neonatal seizures, but they may be the only clinical sign of a fit in the newborn infant. The immature brain of even the full-term neonate is incapable of producing the fully-organized grand mal or petit mal attack, so that fragmentary patterns are the rule. Premature infants demonstrate the most primitive and limited ictal signs; brief apnea may be accompanied by posturing of a limb, eye deviation, grimacing or chewing, and proper diagnosis may require EEG confirmation.[50]

SEIZURES AS A RESULT OF RESPIRATORY DISEASE

Anoxia and Fits

Undoubtedly the most common way in which pulmonary disease causes seizures is through hypoxia. Hypoxia and hypercarbia have distinctly different effects on neuronal activity, and the effect varies again if ischemia is added. Pure hypoxia causes an initial increase in the discharge frequency of neurons, probably caused by a decrease in the resting membrane potential as sodium leaks into the cell from the intercellular space. Further hypoxia is accompanied by progressive abnormalities of action potential formation and finally by a reduction of electrogenesis and cell death. The effects of pure hypercarbia are more complex, neurons in various areas showing either abnormal inhibition or excitation. Mammalian cortical cells primarily show an inhibitory effect, caused by a reduction of excitatory postsynaptic potentials, membrane hyperpolarization, and a reduction of repetitive spike generation.[45,16]

Of course the usual clinical case includes elements of hypoxia *and* of asphyxia (hypercarbia), and this is certainly true of patients with respiratory failure. The nature of the electrical activity induced by such abnormalities depends on the interaction between their excitatory and inhibitory effects.

It is impossible to state pO_2 or pCO_2 levels at which seizures are usually provoked, since other factors are also involved. For example, an arterial pO_2 which is adequate for normal cerebral metabolism in a normotensive person may no longer be sufficient if cerebral perfusion falls because of systemic hypotension. Blood glucose levels have similar effects, since cerebral metabolism depends almost entirely upon the aerobic oxidation of a continuous glucose supply; anoxia and hypoglycemia act synergistically, causing more dependence on the less efficient anaerobic metabolism of glucose, and therefore a critical reduction in the adenosine triphosphate so necessary for the maintenance of neuronal membrane potentials.[20] Finally, acidosis may play a contributing role in the effects of respiratory failure on the brain.[45]

Seizures which occur in the context of hypoxic pulmonary disease are usually generalized tonic-clonic convulsions. Obviously the primary goal of therapy is to remove the cause of the seizures, namely the hypoxia, but it should always be remembered that repeated generalized *or* focal seizures can themselves cause brain damage. This is particularly true in the event of status epilepticus. The metabolic load which convulsions put on neuronal tissue is tremendous, and eventually cannot be met even if the usual normal blood levels of glucose, pO_2, and systemic blood pressure are maintained.[46] Cerebral edema and the resultant regional or global reduction in central blood flow also contribute to the disparity between supply and demand. Since it is impossible in any one case to determine whether or not the critical levels of glucose and oxygen are being supplied to the convulsing brain, the safest and indeed the only reasonable course is to stop the seizures.

Generalized status epilepticus is best treated with intravenous diazepam. Ten to twenty mg is usually sufficient, with hypotension the main dose-limiting side effect. Respiratory depression also occurs, but is usually not a problem in these patients who are often already receiving assisted ventilation. Phenytoin is probably the next drug of choice.

When treating status epilepticus the drug usually must be given parenterally, and this means intravenously, since it is erratically and imperfectly absorbed from intramuscular injection sites.[24] To get an immediate effect, a loading dose of 600 to 1000 mg of the drug is given intravenously at a rate of 50 mg per min,[25] while monitoring the EKG and blood pressure. When cardiac arrhythmias or hypotension occur, they usually respond simply to slowing the rate of infusion of phenytoin.[25]

If repeated seizures respond to diazepam, they will usually start again within half an hour, owing to the short half-life of the drug. Thus a loading dose of a longer-acting anticonvulsant should be given and maintenance doses continued, until the threat of further seizures is judged to have passed. Phenytoin is the usual choice.[48]

The presence of *focal* seizures, with or without subsequent generalization of the fit, is a sign of possible focal cerebral pathology. The possibility of localized cerebral ischemia, infarction, or abscess should be considered, and investigated appropriately. Older patients with previous symptomatic or clinically silent cerebral infarcts may have such focal seizures in the absence of any signs of active focal cerebral disease, although computerized tomography often demonstrates their presence.

Comatose patients with postanoxic encephalopathy often demonstrate multifocal myoclonus, which may be spontaneous or induced by tactile stimuli or sound.[21] This type of myoclonus usually reflects profound, diffuse brain injury, and does not respond well to anticonvulsant therapy.

Finally, Lance and Adams first described a delayed and often permanent effect of anoxia on otherwise functional survivors of respiratory or cardiac arrest, so-called "action myoclonus."[22] This consists of repetitive, often violent, jerking of a limb only on attempted movement. It is a moot point whether such a disorder should be classified as a type of reflex epilepsy, with brief motor fits triggered by voluntary movement. The EEG does usually show concomitant spike discharges over the Rolandic areas. Some observers postulate that damage to serotonergic neuronal systems cause postanoxic myoclonus, since improvement is seen with serotonin precursors tryptophan (with a monoamine oxidase inhibitor) and 5-hydroxytryptophan.[23,41] The anticonvulsant clonazepam is also reported to reduce or abolish this type of myoclonus.[41]

Encephalopathy with Treatment of Chronic Respiratory Failure

The authors of several recent reports have tried to define a special type of cerebral dysfunction following treatment of chronic respiratory failure.[26,28] Typically, a patient with chronic lung disease is treated aggressively for recent pulmonary decompensation. Blood gases are corrected, but the patient acutely deteriorates, becoming comatose, having focal or multifocal seizures, and occasionally demonstrating focal neurologic abnormalities on examination.[26] The mortality rate is high, and autopsy findings are not distinctive.[27]

Giroud and his colleagues postulate that an abrupt "therapeutic" drop in pCO_2 and alkalosis may cause sudden cerebral vasoconstriction and resultant hypoxia.[28] Faden pointed out that nearly all patients with the syndrome were the unintentional victims of a certain combination of treatments and circumstances, primarily alkalosis, hypotension, and aminophylline therapy (see below).[26] This theory seems plausible, and it appears likely that this "encephalopathy" is simply the result of cerebral anoxia coupled with the analeptic effect of aminophylline.

Drug-Induced Seizures

Two drugs frequently used in the treatment of pulmonary disease have epileptogenic properties. The first, aminophylline, has long been known to produce generalized fits if given in toxic doses.[31] The second, isoniazid, is such a powerful convulsant at high doses that isoniazid-induced fits are a commonly studied experimental seizure model.[32]

As discussed above, in the section on *Encephalopathy*, most patients receiving high-dose aminophylline therapy usually are also subjected to other conditions which may cause seizures (primarily hypoxia), so that in any single case it may be difficult or impossible to place blame accurately when such a patient convulses. Clinical evidence is quite convincing, however, that large doses of intravenous aminophylline, and perhaps the orally administered drug as well, are likely to cause convulsions as a toxic effect.[29,30] Both generalized and focal seizures have been reported, the latter often in patients with other evidence of old or new focal cerebral pathology.[29,30] Toxic blood levels of aminophylline are found in such patients (10-20 μg/ml being the recommended therapeutic level).[33] Monitoring the blood level of aminophylline in all patients receiving the drug, particularly those on intravenous therapy, is essential both for preventing seizures and for diagnosing their cause when they do occur.

Isoniazid in large doses can lower the photo-convulsive threshold: a rapidly flickering light provokes facial myoclonus which spreads into generalized body jerks and eventually triggers a grand mal convulsion.[42] Self-administered overdose of isoniazid has been reported to cause generalized seizures, sometimes with a prodrome of headache and vomiting but often occurring without warning.[43] Treatment with anticonvulsants (with phenytoin as first choice) is necessary only if there are multiple fits; the usual course is spontaneous recovery within 24 hours.[43]

It is also claimed that isoniazid may produce seizures in nonepileptic patients even when given in fairly standard dosages.[39] Caution should certainly be exercised when prescribing the drug for epileptic patients. Scrupulous maintenance of anticonvulsant blood levels at the high end of the therapeutic range should be achieved.

The mechanism behind the convulsant action of isoniazid is not entirely clear, but probably involves the drug's effect on the metabolism of gamma-amino-butyric acid (GABA), an important inhibitory neurotransmitter. Isoniazid inhibits glutamic acid decarboxylase (GAD) and GABA-aminotransferase (GABA-T), enzymes which, respectively, enable the synthesis and degradation of GABA. Direct correlations between whole brain levels of GAD, GABA, or GABA-T with isoniazid-induced convulsions in animals have not been demonstrated. Woods and Peesker, in a series of papers, argue that inhibition of GAD at GABA-ergic nerve endings is the critical factor, and that inhibition of GABA-T with resultant rises in GABA occurs in a subcellular compartment (?mitochondria) relatively far removed from GABA's site of action, the synaptic cleft.[34,43] The net effect is therefore a reduction of the inhibitory transmitter GABA at its active cellular site, and a resultant increase in cerebral excitability with convulsions. Withdrawing the drug is sufficient treatment of this unusual side effect.

Isoniazid given to some patients already taking phenytoin can cause phenytoin toxicity by inhibiting metabolism of the drug.[40] The usual signs are ataxia, dysarthria, and incoordination. Blood levels of phenytoin are elevated beyond 20 to 25 μg per ml.

Seizures with Hyperbaric Oxygen Therapy

The mechanism of the toxic effect of high-pressure oxygen on the central nervous system is entirely conjectural.[35,36] It has been observed, however, that generalized seizures are reliably and immediately induced whenever oxygen is breathed at pressures over 3.5 atmospheres absolute,[37] but they have also been reported with repeated exposure to as little as 2.5 atmospheres absolute.[38] No anticonvulsant treatment is necessary; the seizures stop if the hyperbaric chamber is decompressed, and do not recur.

REFERENCES

1. Sarhar, T.K., Munshi, A.T.: Postictal pulmonary edema. *Postgrad. Med.* **61**:281–285, 1977.
2. Archibald, R.B., and Armstrong, J.D.: Recurrent postictal pulmonary edema. *Postgrad. Med.* **63**:210–213, 1978.
3. Bonbrest, H.L.: Pulmonary edema following an epileptic seizure. *Am. Rev. Resp. Dis.* **91**:97–100, 1965.
4. Bloom, S.: Pulmonary edema following a grand mal epileptic seizure. *Am. Rev. Resp. Dis.* **97**:292–294, 1968.
5. Shanahan, W.T.: Acute pulmonary edema as a complication of epileptic seizures. *N.Y. Med. J.* **87**:54, 1908.
6. Ohlmucher, A.P.: Acute pulmonary edema as a terminal event in certain forms of epilepsy. *Am. J. Med. Sci.* **139**:417, 1910.
7. Mendelson, C.L.: The aspiration of stomach contents into the lungs during obstetric anesthesia. *Am. J. Obstet. Gynecol.* **52**:191–205, 1946.

8. Ducher, T.B., and Simmons, R.L.: Increased intracranial pressure and pulmonary edema. 2. The hemodynamic response of dogs and monkeys to increased intracranial pressure. *J. Neurosurg.* **28**:118, 1968.
9. White, P.T., Brant, P., Mosier, J., et al.: Changes in cerebral dynamics associated with seizures. *Neurology* **11**:354–361, 1961.
10. Sarnoff, S.J., and Sarnoff, L.C.: Neurochemodynamics of pulmonary edema. *Circulation* **6**:51–54, 1952.
11. Moore, M.T.: Pulmonary changes in hydantoin therapy. *J.A.M.A.* **171**:1328–1333, 1959.
12. Low, N.L., and Yahr, M.D.: The lack of pulmonary fibrosis in patients receiving diphenylhydantoin. *J.A.M.A.* **174**:1201, 1960.
13. Livingston, S., Whitehouse, D., and Pavli, L.: Study of the effects of diphenylhydantoin on the lungs. *N. Eng. J. Med.* **264**:648, 1961.
14. Hazlett, D.R., Ward, G.W., and Madison, D.S.: Pulmonary function loss in diphenylhydantoin therapy. *Chest* **66**:660–664, 1974.
15. Shafer, W.G.: Effect of dilantin sodium on growth of human fibroblast-like cell cultures. *Proc. Soc. Exp. Biol. Med.* **104**:198, 1960.
16. Siegel, G.J., Albers, R.W., Katzman, R., and Agranoff, B.W.: *Basic Neurochemistry,* 2nd Ed. Boston, Little, Brown & Co., 1976.
17. Thorn, G.W., Adams, R.D., Braunwald, E., Isselbacher, K.J., Petersdorf, R.G. (eds.): *Harrison's Principles of Internal Medicine,* 8th Ed. New York, McGraw-Hill Book Co., 1977.
18. Levine, M.M., Ashman, R., and Heald, F.: Anaerobic (putrid) lung abscess in adolescence. *Am. J. Dis. Childh.* **130**:77–81, 1976.
19. Tower, D.B.: *Neurochemistry of Epilepsy.* Springfield, Ill., Charles C Thomas, 1960.
20. Tower, D.B.: Neurochemistry of epilepsy. In Vinken, P.J., and Bruyn, G.W. (eds.): *Handbook of Clinical Neurology,* Vol. 15, *The Epilepsies.* Amsterdam, North-Holland, 1974.
21. Plum, F., and Posner, J.B.: *The Diagnosis of Stupor and Coma.* Philadelphia, F. A. Davis Co., 1972.
22. Lance, J.W., and Adams, R.D.: The syndrome of intention or action myoclonus as a sequel to hypoxic encephalopathy. *Brain* **86**:111–136, 1963.

23. Van Woert, M.H., Rosnaum, D., Howelson, J., et al.: Long-term therapy of myoclonus and other neurologic disorders with L-5 hydroxytryptophan and carbidopa. *N. Eng. J. Med.* **296**:70–75, 1977.
24. Wilenski, A.J., and Lowden, J.A.: Inadequate serum levels after intramuscular administration of diphenylhydantoin. *Neurology* **23**:318–324, 1973.
25. Cranford, R.E., Leppik, I.E., Patrick, B., Anderson, C.B., and Kostick, B.: Intravenous phenytoin: Clinical and pharmacokinetic aspects. *Neurology* **28**:874–880, 1978.
26. Faden, A.: Encephalopathy following treatment of chronic pulmonary failure. *Neurology* **26**:337–339, 1977.
27. Rotheram, E.B., Safar, R., and Robin, E.D.: CNS disorder during mechanical ventilation in chronic pulmonary disease. *J.A.M.A.* **109**:993, 1964.
28. Giroud, M., du Grés, B., and Martinez-Almoyna, M.: Accidents neurologiques au cours de la reventilation d'insuffisants respiratoires chroniques en décompensation aiguë. *Ann. Anesth. Franc.* **9**:681–688, 1968.
29. Yarnell, P.R., and Chir, N.-S.: Focal seizures and aminophylline. *Neurology* **25**:819–822, 1975.
30. Matthay, R.A., Matthay, M.A., and Weinberger, M.M.: Grand mal seizure induced by oral theophylline. *Thorax* **31**:470–471, 1976.
31. Editorial. Intravenous aminophylline. *Lancet* **2**:950, 1973.
32. Purpura, D.P., Penry, J.K., Tower, D.B., Woodbury, D.M., Walter, R.D. (eds.): *Experimental Models of Epilepsy.* New York, Raven Press, 1972.
33. Nicholson, D.P., and Chick, T.W.: A reevaluation of parenteral aminophylline. *Am. Rev. Resp. Dis.* **108**:241–247, 1973.
34. Wood, J.D., and Peesker, S.J.: Development of an expression which relates the excitable state of the brain to the level of GAD activity and GABA content, with particular reference to the action of hydrazine and its derivatives. *J. Neurochem.* **23**:703–712, 1974.
35. Felig, P., and Lee, W.L.: Protective effect of alkalinizing agents in oxygen toxicity in rats. *Aerospace Med.* **35**:265, 1964.
36. Ward, J.D., Watson, W.J., and Stacey, N.E.: A comparative study of hyperbaric oxygen-induced and drug-induced convulsions with particular reference to gamma aminobutyric acid. *J. Neurochem.* **13**:361, 1966.

37. Bert, P.: Barometric pressure. In *Researches in Experimental Physiology,* trans. by M.A. Hitchcock and F.A. Hitchcock. Columbus, Ohio, College Book Co., 1943.
38. Krishnamurti, S., and Wadhawan, M.L.: Central nervous system toxicity with hyperbaric oxygen: Case reports. *Clin. Aviation Aerospace Med.* **45**:782–784, 1974.
39. Goodman, L.S., and Gilman, A. (eds.): *The Pharmacological Basis of Therapeutics,* 5th ed. New York, Macmillan, 1975.
40. Kutt, H., Winters, W., and McDowell, F.H.: Depression of parahydroxylation of diphenylhydantoin by antituberculosis therapy. *Neurology* **16**:594–602, 1966.
41. Chadwick, D., Hallett, M., Harris, R., Jenner, P., Reynolds, E.H., and Marsden, C.D.: Clinical, biochemical and physiological features distinguishing myoclonus responsive to 5-hydroxytryptophan, tryptophan with a monoamine oxidase inhibitor, and clonazepam. *Brain* **100**:455–487, 1977.
42. Reilly, R.H., Killam, K.F., Jenney, E.H., Marshall, W.H., Tausig, T., Apter, N.S., and Pfeiffer, C.C.: Convulsant effects of isoniazid. *J.A.M.A.* **152**:1317-1321, 1953.
43. Wood, J.D., and Peesker, S.J.: A correlation between changes in GABA metabolism and INH. *Brain Res.* **45**:489–498, 1972.
44. Meyer, J.S., and Marx, P.W.: The pathogenesis of EEG changes during cerebral anoxia. In Magnus, O. (ed.). *Handbook of EEG and Clinical Neurophysiology,* Vol. 14A. Amsterdam, Elsevier, 1972.
45. Plum, F., Howse, D.C., and Duffy, T.E.: Metabolic effects of seizures. *Res. Publ. Assoc. Nerv. Ment. Dis.* **53**:141–157, 1974.
46. Fischgold, H., and Arfel-Capdevielle, M.: Modifications respiratoires dans les paroxysmes epileptiques. *Electroenceph. Clin. Neurophysiol.* **7**:165–178, 1955.
47. Record, K.E., Rapp, R.P., Young, A.B., and Kostenbauder, H.B.: Oral phenytoin loading in adults: rapid achievement of therapeutic plasma levels. *Ann. Neurol.* **5**:268–270, 1979.
48. Gastaut, H., Broughton, R., Rogers, J., and Tassinari, C.A.: Generalized convulsive seizures without focal onset. In Magnus, O., and Lorentz de Haas, A.M. (eds.): *Handbook of Clinical Neurology,* Vol. 15, *The Epilepsies.* Amsterdam, Elsevier, 1974.
49. Lombroso, C.T.: Seizures in the newborn period. In Magnus, O., and Lorentz de Haas, A.M. (eds.): *Handbook of Clinical Neurology,* Vol. 15, *The Epilepsies.* Amsterdam, Elsevier, 1974.

9

CENTRAL DISTURBANCES OF RESPIRATION IN MULTIPLE SCLEROSIS

Dusan Stefoski, M.D., and Floyd A. Davis, M.D.

Respiratory failure of unspecified cause in patients with multiple sclerosis (MS) accounted for three out of 85 deaths in McAlpine's series of 840.[1] McIntyre and McIntyre[2] described the causes of three deaths in their 55 MS-patients only as bulbar palsy, and at least one of the three died of respiratory paralysis. Lumsden's report[3] revealed 12 percent of 60 consecutive deaths from MS as the result of bulbar palsy (without more specific details about the clinical manifestations). Carter et al.[5] reported no instances of respiratory control failure as the cause of death in 49 autopsy-verified cases of MS. Other descriptions[6,7] of fulminant and fatal cases of MS often refer to signs of respiratory difficulties in even vaguer terms (dyspnea, hypoventilation) which prevents the reader from identifying the possible presence and extent of involvement of the central respiratory system.

To a relatively small number of these cases, one can add only a few which describe in greater detail clinical aspects of central failure of ventilation in MS. Guthrie et al.[8] had experience with four such patients (two had transient failure and two died), Boor et al.[9] with one patient (who recovered at least from the first episode), and we treated successfully one young woman with a similar problem. Obviously this type of abnormality is not common.

Relatively infrequent encounters of significant involvement of the respiratory control system by central nervous system (CNS) diseases leads to the assumption that these systems function with a great safety factor. This enables the functions of the system to remain satisfactory in most cases of even severe CNS damage, at least temporarily. Empirical evidence exists that chronic CNS diseases with a potential for afflicting the respiratory controls can be compensated for much better than acute conditions. Spatial and temporal dissemination of demyelination plaques, as seen in MS, is likely to involve the respiratory pathways. However, the clinical experience with MS as a cause of central respiratory control failure is so rare that it still merits publication of individual cases. In the same context, it seems reasonable to limit a discussion of this topic to what has been reported rather than examining theoretical possibilities.

The types of respiratory failure in MS which can be termed peripheral (pneumonia, atelectasis) will not be dealt with here. Putative failure of the central control system will be discussed.

ANATOMICAL AND PHYSIOLOGICAL CONSIDERATIONS

The concept of dual systems of respiratory control seems to be well established and accepted.[10-12] The automatic system differs significantly from the other, termed voluntary or behavioral, in topographical representation, physiology, and in signs reflecting malfunctions. The evidence of medullary localization of automatic respiration is ample.[13-15] Both observations from animal experiments and the clinical-pathological ones in humans have ultimately led to the discovery (Merill[15]) of primary respiratory neurons in the dorsolateral reticular formation of the medulla oblongata near the nucleus ambiguus. In it the chemoreceptor, vagal, pontine and proprioceptive afferent impulses are integrated and blood-gas and acid-base homeostasis is regulated. The automatic system functions at the rate corresponding to metabolic conditions.[16] In the cat the efferent axons cross the midline at the level of obex and descend within ventral reticulospinal tracts in the ventral portion of the lateral columns of the spinal cord, just medial to the spinothalamic tracts. Additional crossing of fibers occurs between the two reticular spinal tracts.[17] The fibers synapse with spinal respiratory neurons.[12] Damage to the automatic respiratory system abolishes automatic respiration and diminishes the response to carbon dioxide.[10,11,24] The latter phenomenon could (at least partially) explain the lack of subjective breathlessness, which in turn causes apnea in not fully alert patients with such damage—they simply forget to breathe and require mechanical respiratory assistance, particularly during sleeping hours, similarly to what occurs in "Ondine's Curse."[20,11] Plum,[11] Deveraux,[18] and Boor[9] described patients with such symptoms.

The voluntary or behavioral system also mediates control of respiratory functions, is necessary for production of voice, and is involved in preparation for imminent changes in metabolic demands (physical activity) and for adaptation to behavioral acts.[10] It originates primarily in the cortical (somatomotor) and limbic system structures of the cerebrum and projects in part to the medullary automatic system, while its greater portion projects through the corticobulbar and corticospinal pathways to spinal respiratory neurons. It functions only when the cerebrum is fully activated (such as in wakefulness). Damage to the voluntary respiratory system results in a loss of volitional control of breathing with preserved, but fixed-rate, automatic respiration. This condition has been described in infarction of the base of the medulla oblongata which destroyed both pyramids.[19]

CLINICAL MANIFESTATIONS

Three of the four MS patients described by Guthrie et al.[8] had signs of lower brain stem and/or high cervical cord lesions—quadraparesis, and certain signs of brainstem damage including gaze paralysis, nystagmus and facial weakness. Two of the three recovered well with the help of a respirator and one died. The fourth patient had right palatal weakness, absent gag and cough reflexes, right facial paresis, painless dyspnea, dysphonia, and weakness in both legs and one arm. Subsequently he became unconscious and shortly thereafter died. At autopsy plaques of new demyelination were found in the cerebrum, spinal cord, mesencephalon and pons, whereas none was present in the medulla. None of the four patients had clear clinical signs of direct damage to the respiratory control system. Their respiratory difficulties were described as shallow breathing, dyspnea, and minimal excursion of the respiratory musculature. The authors concluded that the best explanation for their patients hypoventilation was severe skeletal muscle weakness. Fever listed as a sign in three of the four patients in this group probably had a significant role in determining the degree of severity of the presenting symptoms.

Boor et al.[9] treated a middle-aged, newly diagnosed male for clinically and laboratory proven MS manifested mainly by posterior fossa symptoms and signs, attributable to the pons, medulla and the cerebellum. No signs of corticospinal system involvement were present. Immediately following recovery from an apparently noncardiac respiratory arrest early in the course of the disease, the patient developed irregular spontaneous respirations, episodes of apnea during periods of relaxation which were completely devoid of subjective breathlessness, and profound loss of proprioception with pseudoathetosis of the fingers. The patient would stop breathing unless reminded to do so, necessitating the use of a respirator. Within a week the proprioception deficit and nystagmus receded and respiration became regular. The ensuing 13-month period was characterized by the waxing and waning signs of ataxia, dysmetria, hemiparesis, diplopia, nystagmus, proprioception deficit and hypnagogic confusion terminating in the patient's death during sleep. Postmortem examination revealed a large area of demyelination and gliosis with some perivascular lymphocytic cuffing on its periphery and slight axonal loss in its center extending from the midolivary level to the fourth cervical cord segment. The lesion occupied most of the dorsomedial region of the lower medulla and the dorsal columns of the cervical spinal cord. Most of the pyramids were spared. Plaques of demyelination were also seen scattered in the cerebrum, cerebellum, optic chiasm, and lower cervical spinal cord. Clinical pathological correlation in this case is rather impressive and merits emphasizing 2 points. One is the fact that the clear-cut dissociation of respiratory functions provides further support for the theory of dual respiratory control in humans; the automatic control was impaired whereas voluntary functions remained intact due to sparing of the pyramids which enabled the patient to continue breathing during wakefulness by employing learned behavioral patterns. The second point is the combination of severe proprioception deficit and automatic respiration arrest as a result of proximity of the lemniscal and respiratory system decussations. Boor postulated that profound and diffuse proprioception loss with pseudoathetosis could be a warning sign of impending respiratory arrest.

We had an opportunity to care for a young woman (born in 1955) who had first noticed paresthesiae in her legs in middle 1973 at age 18. Over the ensuing few years this was followed by recurrent episodes of dizziness, balancing difficulties, blurred vision in the left and right eye at different times, right facial numbness, bilateral leg weakness and emotional disturbances. Most of the symptoms were of a fluctuating intensity. In 1975 a presumptive diagnosis of MS was established in a hospital in Utah where laboratory testing, including CSF examinations, proved nondiagnostic. A number of other signs and symptoms, waxing and waning in character, occurred during 1975. These included hand and arm weakness, incoordination, dysarthria, urinary incontinence, euphoria, worsening of the lower paraparesis, paraesthesiae in legs and occasional fecal incontinence. Several courses of ACTH and prednisone treatments during 1974 and 1975 brought about partial relief of symptoms

In the last week of November 1975, she was brought to the Emergency Room because she could be barely aroused the morning after what appeared to be a usual night of sleep. On physical examination she was found to be stuporous with only equivocal response to strong auditory stimuli. Upon noxious stimulation of either side she reacted by tonically extending both arms in pronation with inner rotation, extending both legs, retroflexing the neck and head and slightly arching the back. Blood pressure was 120/90, pulse 100 and regular, respirations 16 and irregular, temperature 98.8°F. Eyes were conjugately and tonically deviated to the left. Cold water stimulation of both ears elicited tonic deviation of the eyes toward the stimulated side. Anisocoria of 0.5 mm was noted with the left pupil larger and sluggish in response to light. Funduscopically both optic discs appeared to be somewhat atrophic with pale temporal halves. A mild right central facial palsy was present. All four extremities revealed rigidity. Bilateral ankle clonus was easily elicited. No spontaneous movements were observed. The tendon stretch reflexes were very brisk symmetrically. Plantar response was extensor bilaterally.

Normal laboratory data at the time of admission included CBC, SMA-18 serum biochemistry profile, blood coagulation studies, autoimmune disease profile, chest x-ray, EKG, screen for psychoactive drugs and lumbar CSF, (opening pressure 110 mm H_2O, protein 41 mg/dl with 9.4% gamma globulin, glucose 88 mg/dl, 5 RBC, 5 lymphocytes, negative bacteriological tests). CT brain scan revealed multiple lucencies in both cerebral hemispheres, including some periventricular ones. One in the right hemisphere increased in density following Hypaque infusion. There was also a slight enlargement of the left frontal horn and a questionable mass effect on the right frontal horn. Radiosiotope brain scan revealed an ill-defined area of increased uptake in the right hemisphere. Electroencephalogram consisted of diffuse theta and delta rhythms with only sparse 7-9 cps waves. Four vessel cerebral angiogram was normal. Respirations became increasingly irregular and shalow, slowing to about 6 to 10 per minute in two hours, and soon apneustic episodes necessitated fully automated mechanical assistance of ventilation. Several attempts to reactivate the patient's spontaneous automatic respiration failed. She was not even triggering the respirator. On the next day the patient remained in a coma with decerebrate posturing on noxious stimulation. Neurologically she remained without change remaining on the respirator for the next 23 days. During that time she was found to have normal CSF findings on two additional lumbar punctures. Sterile bacteriological cultures of the CSF, sputum and urine and low nondiagnostic titers for encephalitis-meningitis group of viruses and EB virus titers were reported. Repeated EB virus titers did not rise and EB virus IgM was negative. T3, T4, and cortisol levels were normal, and so were porphyrins, urophophyrins and coproporphyrins.

Two subsequent EEGs revealed marked diffuse slowing with delta and theta range activity. CT brain scan 16 days after admission revealed no change. Temperature varied between 99° and 101°F without a demonstrable cause except for a small transient area of atelectasis in the left lung. The patient received a 14-day course of dexamethasome (16 mg per day) which was then slowly tapered. Twenty-five days after admission she was seen to blink occasionally in response to light and to trigger the respirator. Two days later spontaneous conjugate eye movements toward a light source were observed and 31 days after admission, she could follow simple verbal commands for gaze directions, could swallow fluids, and was breathing spontaneously for the most part, using the ventilator to assist inspirations. EEG on that day showed improved background with predominance of 4-6 cps activity. Thirty-six days following admission, mechanical assistance of respiration was discontinued, she was able to sit up and speak, but the arms were still tonically extended in inner rotation and pronation although minimal voluntary movements were possible. A CT brain scan now showed a great deal of bilateral periventricular lucencies which did not enhance with Hypaque infusion.

A pseudobulbar type of emotional lability was observed. Jaw jerk was hyperactive. Forty-four days after entering the hospital she could bend and raise her legs off the bed and the tonic extension of the arms subsided. Plantar responses were extensor. Muscle strength improved more proximally than distally and more in the arms than in the legs. Position and vibration sensation were moderately diminished in all four limbs. She was discharged to a rehabilitation hospital. Since that time she has received three additional course of ACTH, each time for exacerbation of multiple sclerosis-related symptoms manifested mainly by deterioration of motor and cerebellar functions. She did not have further respiratory dysfunction. Based upon clinical observations it was felt that an area of demyelination at the level of medulla and the lower pons was the direct cause for the episode of coma, decerebration and respiratory arrest.

COMMENT

It is possible that the usual small chronic plaques[3] of demyelination in MS, even when present in the medulla, involve an insufficient number of axons to cause a significant deficit within the respiratory system. This is especially true for the voluntary system since it has a rather wide spatial distribution of fibers. Different effects might be seen, however, with a fresh plaque which has a significant inflammatory component (edema, cellular infiltration), hence transiently causing dysfunction within a larger area than it does in its chronic phase. Obviously this increases the likelihood of central respiratory distress when fresh plaques appear in the medulla, and not necessarily within the respiratory pathways.

In view of the basic pathophysiology of multiple sclerosis, which is axonal conduction impairment through the demyelinated segments (borderline normal, slowed or blocked), a sudden deterioration of a once stabilized symptom which is not related to disease process activity (i.e., to fresh demyelination) poses a serious threat in cases where respiratory distress constituted a part of an earlier exacerbation. A condition which can precipitate such sudden exacerbations of MS-related symptoms is increased body temperature.[22] Recently, other conditions with similar net effects were described.[23] Also, Davis and Schauf have stressed that a number of demyelinated axons conduct marginally and with markedly lower safety factors than normal axons, and that even the slightest further insult (e.g., fever) can result in the block of conduction. Such a mechanism could have been responsible for the death of Boor's patient, particularly in view of the fact that the postmortem histological examination showed no significant activity within the medullary plaque thought to have caused respiratory distress earlier in the course of the disease.

Failure of central respiratory control occurs infrequently in multiple sclerosis. Accurate clinical observation of respiratory function is often difficult in situations when MS patients develop complications such as quadraplegia, pneumonitis, sepsis, and kidney failure. However, in these situations it is more likely that the embarrassment of ventilation is a secondary phenomenon. Only when clinical signs indicate the presence of MS pathology in the medulla oblongata (bulbar signs and symptoms) prior to the acute respiratory decompensation, can the etiology of the latter be labeled central with reasonable certainty.

REFERENCES

1. McAlpine, D., and Comston, N.: Some aspects of the natural history of disseminated sclerosis. *Quart. J. Med.* **21**: 135–167, 1952.
2. McIntyre, H.D., and McIntyre, A.P.: Prognosis in multiple sclerosis. *Arch. Neurol. Neurosurg. Psychiat.* **50**: 431–439, 1943.
3. Lumsden, C.E.: The neuropathology of multiple sclerosis, In Vinken, P.J., and Bruyn, G.W. (eds.): *Multiple Sclerosis and Other Demyelinating Diseases. Handbook of Clinical Neurology,* Vol. 9. Amsterdam, North Holland, 1975, pp. 217–309.
4. McAlpine, D., Lumsden, C.E., and Acheson, E.D.: *Multiple Sclerosis: A Reappraisal.* Baltimore, Williams and Wilkins, 1965, pp. 163–164.
5. Carter, S., Sciarra, D., and Merritt, H.H.: The course of multiple sclerosis as determined by autopsy proven cases. *Res. Nerv. Ment. Disord.* **28**: 471–511, 1956.
6. Riser, P., Geraud, J., and Lavitry, S.: La Sclérose en plaques aiguë. *Presse Med.* **46**: 1193–1196, 1938.
7. Castaignc, P., and Escourollc, R.: Comas transitoircs avcc hyperthermic au cours de la sclerose en plaques. *Rev. Neurol.* **114**: 147–150, 1966.
8. Guthrie, T.C., Kurtzke, J.F., and Berlin, L.: Acute respiratory failure in multiple sclerosis and its management. *Ann. Intern. Med.* **37**: 1197–1203, 1952.
9. Boor, J.W., Johnson, R.J., and Canales, L.: Reversible paralysis of automatic respiration in multiple sclerosis. *Arch. Neurol.* **34**: 686–689, 1977.
10. Plum, F.: Neurological intergration of behavioral and metabolic control of breathing. In *Breathing: Hering-Breuer Centenary Symposium.* London, J. and A. Churchill, Ltd., 1970.
11. Plum, F.: Breathlessness in neurological disease: The effects of neurological disease on the act of breathing. In Stowell, J., and Campbell, E. (eds.): *Breathlessness.* Philadelphia, F.A. Davis Co., 1966, pp. 203–222.
12. Nathan, P.W.: The descending respiratory pathway in man. *J. Neurol. Neurosurg. Psychiat.* **26**: 487–499, 1963.
13. Burns, D.B.: The central control of respiratory movements. *Br. Med. Bull.* **19**: 7–10, 1963.
14. Salmoiraghi, G.C., and Burns, D.B.: Localization and patterns of discharge from respiratory neurons in the brainstem of cat. *J. Neurophysiol.* **23**: 2–13, 1960.

15. Merrill, E.G.: The lateral respiratory neurons of the medulla. *Brain Res.* **24**: 11–18, 1970.
16. Salmoiraghi, G.C.: Functional organization of the brainstem respiratory neurons. *Ann. N.Y. Acad. Sci.* **109**: 571–585, 1963.
17. Cohen, F.: Effects of various lesions on crossed and uncrossed descending inspiratory pathways on the cervical spinal cord of the cat. *J. Neurosurg.* **39**: 589–595, 1973.
18. Devereaux, M.W., Keane, J., and Davis, A.: Automatic respiratory failure associated with infarction of the medulla. *Arch. Neurol.* **29**: 46–52, 1973.
19. Meyer, M.S., and Herndon, R.: Bilateral infarction of the pyramidal tracts in man. *Neurology* **12**: 637–642, 1962.
20. Mellins, R.B., Balfour, S.T., Turino, G., et al.: Failure of automatic control of ventilation (Ondine's Curse). *Medicine* **49**: 487–504, 1970.
21. Davis, F.A., and Schauf, C.L.: Pathophysiology of multiple sclerosis. In Klawans, H. (ed.): *Models of Human Neurological Diseases.* Amsterdam, North Holland Press, 1974.
22. Davis, F.A., Schauf, C.L., Reed, B.J., et al.: Experimental studies of the dependence of conduction in normal and demyelinated nerve on extrinsic factors. I. Temperature. *J. Neurol. Neurosurg. Psychiat.* **39**: 441, 1976.
23. Schauf, C.L., and Davis, F.A.: The occurrence, specificity, and role of neuroelectric blocking factors in multiple sclerosis. *Neurology* **28**: 34–39, 1978.
24. Korczyn, A.D., Carel, R.S., and Bruderman, I.: Ventilatory response to carbon dioxide in multiple sclerosis. *J. Neurol.* **215**: 67–71, 1977.

10

NEUROTOXINS AND RESPIRATORY DYSFUNCTION

Christopher G. Goetz, M.D.

Most toxic/metabolic encephalopathic states exhibit changes in respiratory patterns that are a result of systemic acid-base alterations. Occasionally, however, toxins themselves may cause direct stimulation or depression of brain stem respiratory centers. Prominent findings of shared neurologic-respiratory dysfunction should suggest the possibility of neurotoxins affecting brain stem physiology. These instances of toxic, centrally-mediated respiratory acidosis or alkalosis are usually medical emergencies, and offer immediate and practical examples of the close interaction between neurology and pulmonary medicine. Two examples will be discussed, narcotic and salicylate intoxications.

NARCOTICS

The narcotic agents, whether naturally occurring or synthetically prepared, are associated with a variety of neurologic respiratory complications. Morphine is the most widely used opiate medically, and heroin, its diacetyl derivative, has become the major opiate of illicit drug abuse. Other opiate derivatives, pantopan, dihydromorphinone (Dilaudid), levorphenol (Dromoran), meperidine (Demerol), and methadone share the general toxic properties of the opiate group, but vary in their onset and duration of toxic signs. It must be emphasized that opiate drug abusers may often be exposed to many other toxic agents including septic conditions and drug adulterants, as well as alcohol or hallucinogens. For this reason, some neurotoxic syndromes, especially in the case of heroin abuse, should be viewed as potential hazards of drug abuse and its life style rather than primarily due to the pharmacologic agent itself. These secondary abuse syndromes include subacute bacterial endocarditis with multiple emboli and abscess formation, osteomyelitis and various infections, but since they do not have specific accompanying respiratory alterations they will not be discussed.

The strict structural requirements of opiates, their high potency and their stereospecificity suggest that narcotics may in fact act at specific opiate receptor sites.[1] Such opiate binding sites have been demonstrated in the central nervous system specifically in those regions felt to be associated with pain transmission, and with brain stem visceral reflexes including respiration.[2] Opiates additionally alter the activity of known neurotransmitter systems centrally, although consistent changes and a unifying concept of interaction have not been established.[3] Hypotheses linking together opiates and neurotransmitters have been suggested to explain narcotic tolerance on the basis of denervation hypersensitivity.[4] The following discussion focuses on the neurologic-respiratory hazards of narcotic abuse with primary reference to morphine and heroin.

Morphine

Morphine overdose is especially common in circulatory collapse where the drug is administered more than once; while the patient is in shock, the drug remains at the site of the injection, but, once the blood pressure is reestablished, large amounts of morphine are suddenly absorbed and toxic signs may develop. Initially there is a sensation of warmth and comfort progressing to a dreamy confusion. The face flushes but within approximately one hour, it pales as the pulse begins to slow. Lethargy progresses, reflexes are lost, and the muscles relax and become flaccid. The pupils constrict to pinpoint size and fail to react to light although terminally they dilate. As the pulse slows, skin temperature declines, cyanosis becomes evident and secondary anoxic seizures may develop, especially in children.[5]

Respiratory complications of morphine relate primarily to its direct suppressive effect on brain stem respiratory centers.[6] The respiratory depression is evident even when the doses are too small to alter the level of consciousness, and abnormal respiratory patterns have been reported after therapeutic doses of the drug. These therapeutic doses actively suppress multiple respiratory parameters including rate, minute volume and tidal volume. The patterns of abnormal breathing range from slow but regular to periodic and eventually irregular after the dose becomes higher.[7] In man, death from morphine intoxication is almost invariably due to respiratory arrest.

Maximal respiratory depression occurs within seven minutes after intravenous morphine administration, but peaks at approximately 30 minutes after intramuscular and 90 minutes after subcutaneous administrations. The sensitivity of the respiratory center returns towards normal after two to three hours, although even after therapeutic doses, respiratory minute volume remains considerably below normal for four to five hours.[8] The mechanism of respiratory depression relates to two major factors. First, narcotics cause a direct depression of both pontine and medullary respiratory centers so that rhythmicity and automaticity are disturbed.[9] This effect appears to be primary to the brain stem and not related to depressed afferent input since even electrical stimulation of the brain stem centers fails to elicit normal responses. Second, the brain stem chemoreceptivity declines so that increases in pCO_2 fail to induce reflex hyperventilation.[10] This loss of chemosensitivity is selective and hypoxia remains at least a partly effective respiratory stimulant. This fact has therapeutic significance in that the hypoxic drive may be the only factor maintaining automatic respiration in a patient; inadvertant over-oxygenation will remove this drive and may cause total apnea.

The combined effects of these two depressant factors, direct brain stem depression and loss of chemosensitivity, are life threatening. An additional, less understood, factor that aggravates respiratory compromise in morphine-intoxicated patients is an alteration of voluntary control of breathing. After large doses of morphine, patients breathe if instructed to do so, but if left unstimulated, they become relatively apneic. The pathophysiology of this effect relates presumably to the drug's preferential activity on brain stem centers with descending cortical influences left predominantly intact. These cortical areas have been discussed already in the section on Respiratory Neuroanatomy (Chapter 1). Natural sleep also produces a decrease in medullary center pCO_2 sensitivity, so that the effects of morphine and sleep are additive.[11] These pharmacologic findings help to explain the historical treatment of morphine intoxication which included forced arousal, constant and deliberate reminding of the patient to breathe, and above all, prevention of sleep.

Not all narcotic agents are equivalent to morphine in their effects on respiratory depression. Death from respiratory depression is exceedingly rare after codeine administration, while heroin is felt to be even more potent in its depressive effects on respiration than morphine. No natural or synthetic narcotic is free of respiratory depressive effects and all are dangerous to varying degrees. Other morphine effects not directly respiratory but which may secondarily compromise ventilation include the induction of central vomiting and suppression of the cough reflex. Both increase the risk of aspiration and subsequent inadequate ventilation.[12] Opiates as a class have an additional bronchoconstrictive effect.

During recovery from morphine overdose, there is gradual improvement in respiration and the depression of consciousness. Coma will lighten into a prolonged sleep lasting hours, interrupted by waking periods where the patient is lucid but often complains of headaches. Relapses may occur and are felt to be due to reabsorption of morphine previously excreted into the intestinal tract. The ordinary fatal dose of morphine is generally considered to be 120 to 240 mg, although individual responses vary: death from therapeutic doses has occurred while some addicts tolerate up to one gram of morphine daily.

Present treatment of morphine overdose centers on the use of the narcotic antagonist naloxone, 1 cc (0.4 mg) given intravenously at five-minute intervals until the patient awakens. Failure to obtain significant improvement after three doses suggests that other nonopiate drugs have also been administered or that other concomitant disease processes may be active.[13]

Heroin

Heroin is synthetically prepared by acetylation of both hydroxyl groups of morphine, resulting in diacetyl morphine. It is utilized in large amounts principally for its euphoric effects and is often the drug most sought by addicts. The analgesic and euphoric properties of heroin are greater than those of morphine and excitement often accompanies the euphoric state; respiratory depression, however, is also greater and is a continual and predictable hazard of heroin abuse. The drug is rapidly absorbed from the mucous membranes, hydrolyzed completely in the body and excreted as morphine. Heroin crosses the blood-brain barrier more rapidly than morphine with brain levels peaking 15 minutes after intravenous administration.[14] Once within the brain, heroin is metabolized to morphine.

The most serious neurologic-respiratory complication of heroin abuse is the acute toxic narcotic syndrome that accounted for more than half of the deaths in narcotic users reported for New York City in 1974. Clinically, the syndrome is characterized by severe hypoventilation with increasing lethargy, coma, constricted pupils and massive pulmonary edema.[3]

The pathophysiology of this catastrophic syndrome remains obscure. Formerly considered to relate exclusively to overdosage, it appears that multiple factors are probably important. Overdosage in the strict sense does occur especially with long-acting methadone where the user readministers the drug because there are no acute effects. When the drug finally does peak, the patient is exposed to a double dose with the dangerous hazards of respiratory toxicity. However, not all respiratory complications can be explained by high central nervous system narcotic levels. Addicts are sometimes found with injection needles still in place and witnesses have described very rapid, fatal responses over a few minutes. These descriptions suggest an allergic or hypersensitive reaction to heroin or its adulterants. A vasculopathy similar to polyarteritis nodosa has been described in patients dying after combined use of heroin and metamphetamine.[15]

Severe respiratory depression is a hallmark of heroin intoxication and the pathophysiology of this picture in the case of overdosage appears similar to that seen with morphine. High central nervous system levels of drug suppress respiratory functions by direct brain stem depression as well as depressed chemosensitivity to changes in pCO_2. Additionally, however, the acute toxic reaction seen with heroin addiction is accompanied by a profound degree of pulmonary edema. The minimal respiratory efforts that continue to exist are often enough to whip the pulmonary fluid into an obstructive froth that exudes from the mouth and nose. Hemoptysis may be present and severe. Several hypotheses have been proposed to explain the pulmonary edema. Abnormal stimulation of autonomic or limbic system structures in the brain can induce pulmonary edema and because of the other known neurologic effects of heroin, centrally mediated pulmonary edema has been suggested.[16] Hypoxia, acute allergic reactions, or direct toxic effects at the alveolar membrane have also been proposed.[17,18] The pulmonary edema may be a species-specific reaction in man since intravenous injection of "street" heroin in several species of animals including primates induces predictable coma and hypoventilation but never pulmonary edema.[19]

Treatment of the acute toxic syndrome involves judicious oxygenation, treatment of the pulmonary edema and naloxone 1 cc (0.4 mg) every five minutes until the patient awakens. Further neurologic manifestations including seizures and increased intracranial pressure may complicate the patient's medical condition and require further treatment. The seizures characteristically are generalized and usually do not recur after recovery from the acute syndrome.[20] Following the acute reaction, patients often enter a transient delirium with hallucinations and extreme agitation lasting hours to days. Rarely, a chronic dementia follows and probably relates to hypoxic brain damage.[5] Instances of cerebrovascular accidents without evidence of emboli are reported but strokes associated with infectious endocarditis are more common.

Heroin abuse has been associated with an additional gamut of neurologic disorders including chronic myopathies, transverse myelopathy, neuropathies and Guillain-Barré syndrome. All of these can affect the ascending and descending pathways necessary to effective respiration. The details, however, on heroin's pharmacologic activity at the level of the spinal cord, nerve and muscles are not well established. The general poor health of heroin abusers and their chronic exposure to septic needles and utensils appear to play significant roles in many syndromes seen in narcotic abusers. Myelopathies, neuropathies, and myopathies remain nevertheless important diagnostic considerations in heroin abusers who may demonstrate signs of respiratory compromise. The general pathophysiology of toxic myopathies and neuropathies relative to the respiratory system is discussed in other chapters.

SALICYLATES

Because of their ready availability in almost all households, salicylates represent a common source of intoxication, accounting for the largest yearly number of serious childhood poisonings.[21] In acute intoxication, the prominent neurologic and respiratory signs may immediately suggest the correct diagnosis and direct prompt and appropriate intervention. The neurologic manifestations of salicylate toxicity include a rapid and dramatic alteration in consciousness and global function with convulsions and coma.[5] Confusion and restlessness are seen early, leading within a few hours to excitability, tremor, incoherent speech and often delirium or hallucinosis. This phase has been referred to as "salicylate jag" to indicate its similarity to alcoholic inebriation, although euphoria and elation are conspicuously absent with salicylates.[22] After this phase, a gradual depression in the level of consciousness occurs with a rapid lapse into coma. Seizures are especially common in children and are as a rule generalized.[23] The pathophysiology of the convulsions appears to relate to the combined effects of metabolic and respiratory disturbances as well as hypoglycemia.[24] Salicylates additionally inhibit the synthesis of gamma-amino-butyric acid (GABA), a putative neurotransmitter in the central nervous system. Since depressed levels of GABA have been suggested to relate to the lowering of seizure threshold, salicylates may induce convulsions by this mechanism.[25] In infants, salicylate intoxication induces a marked hypoglycemia and seizure activity is especially hazardous in this young age group. Diplopia, dizziness, and decreased visual acuity can also be seen with salicylate intoxication. Involvement of the audiovestibular (8th cranial) nerve can lead to tinnitus, vertigo, and complete deafness. This complication is more common with chronic salicylate intoxication and is seen especially in patients treated for arthritic or headache conditions where aspirin or salicylate compounds are ingested daily.[26] Inadvertant acute intoxication in elderly patients being treated with salicylates for medical conditions carries an especially high mortality rate estimated at 25 percent.[27]

The respiratory complications of salicylate toxicity are of paramount importance since they contribute to a severe acid-base disturbance. Salicylates stimulate respiration by three basic mechanisms, direct brain stem activation, enhanced central chemosensitive response mechanisms, and a compensatory hyperventilation stimulated by metabolic increases in CO_2. The earliest change is the latter effect, since salicylates increase oxygen consumption and CO_2 production in skeletal muscle as a result of uncoupling or oxidative phosphorylation.[28] Respiratory depth reflexly increases with only a slight increase in rate. This respiratory effect is not specific to salicylates, but should be considered a compensation for peripheral increases in CO_2 production.

As salicylate gains access to the medulla, it directly stimulates the respiratory center and induces a marked hyperventilation, with both an increase in depth and rate of breathing. Respiratory rates may increase tenfold to drive the pCO_2 below 18 mmHg.[29] This effect is independent of the early compensatory phenomenon. Moreover, there is no evidence that this effect is due to a primary cerebrospinal fluid (CSF) acidosis, since direct application of a low concentration of salicylate to the medulla or the cerebral ventricle is followed by prompt and dramatic hyperventilation, a fall in alveolar pCO_2, a rise in arterial pH, but no fall in CSF pH.[30] The central effect of salicylate is clearly not a stimulation of increased central CO_2 since CO_2 stimulates depth more than rate, whereas salicylates stimulate rate more than depth. The precise localization of brain stem activation by salicylates appears to involve both the medullary as well as pontine centers.[6]

The final stimulatory effect of respiratory mechanisms involves a heightened sensitivity of chemoreceptors to ambient pCO_2 fluctuations.[31] This effect is linked to the primary brain stem stimulation and is considered by some authors to be a result or consequence of that phenomenon as opposed to a separate entity.

These phenomena combine to induce a pronounced early respiratory alkalosis. This picture is seen in adults and in children acutely, although subsequent changes in acid-base balance will occur in children to involve more complicated metabolic disturbances. Salicylates gradually will induce a depressant effect on brain stem function after high doses or after prolonged exposure. The picture begins as a predominately uncompensated respiratory acidosis, but this situation merges into a combined respiratory and metabolic acidosis as three metabolic acid groups accumulate. First, salicylate acid derivatives dissociate at toxic doses and can displace 2 to 3 mEq/L bicarbonate. Second, vasomotor depression occurs in salicylate toxicity and although the mechanism underlying this effect is not clearly understood, the consequences of such depression include impaired renal function with poor clearance of sulfuric and phosphoric acids. Finally, organic acids accumulate from salicylate effects on carbohydrate metabolism inducing ketosis as well as acidosis.[21]

This sequence from primary respiratory alkalosis to respiratory acidosis to combined respiratory-metabolic acidosis forms the hallmark of salicylate intoxication in infants and young children. In school-aged children, respiratory alkalosis and respiratory acidosis are seen, while in adults the respiratory alkalosis is the prominent feature with depression of breathing being seen only with very high levels of toxic products. Although the mechanism of this maturational resistance to metabolic acidosis remains unclear, the consistent respiratory-metabolic patterns of the different age groups assist in the acute management of these patients. Furthermore these patterns serve especially to alert the physician to the possibility of more than one ingested toxic substance when the clinical picture deviates from the expected age-related sequence. These instances would include adults who attempt suicide with multiple drugs and children who invade the medicine chest where more than one toxic compound is available.

Treatment of salicylate toxicity involves minimizing drug absorption, hastening drug elimination, correcting acid-base disturbance and treating existing neurologic or medical complications.[32] Induced emesis in the awake patient is the most effective means of emptying the stomach. Enhanced elimination is effected by alkalinization of the urine or by peritoneal or hemodialysis. Careful fluid and electrolyte management are tantamount and depend on the age of the patient and the stage of intoxication. The complications of hypoglycemia in infants must be anticipated and prevented. Seizures are usually treated with dilantin and phenobarbitol.

There is poor correlation between the serum salicylate levels and the clinical severity of intoxication.[32] Despite apparently adequate treatment and progressive lowering of toxic plasma salicylate levels, sudden and unexplained deaths are not rare. Experimental studies demonstrate that animals dying from salicylate overdose may show wide variance of plasma salicylate concentrations but have consistent brain salicylate levels.[34] These data suggest that brain and potentially CSF levels of salicylate may be of more critical prognostic value in the management of salicylate-intoxicated patients.

SUMMARY

This discussion has focused on two examples of neurotoxins manifesting prominent respiratory signs. Although the toxins have other systemic effects, the major respiratory alterations can be traced to neurologic dysfunction. The two agents typify the spectrum from pathologic brain stem depression to pathologic over-activation. Various other drugs and neurotoxins similarly affect central respiratory function. The neurologic signs may differ from one agent to another, but the basic pathophysiologic respiratory mechanisms discussed for narcotics and salicylates will remain applicable.

REFERENCES

1. Snyder, S.H., and Pert, C.B.: Membrane receptor. In Snyder, S.H., and Matthysse, S. (eds.): *Opiate Receptor Mechanisms.* Cambridge, Mass., MIT Press, 1975.
2. Hiller, J.M., Pearson, J., and Simon, E.J.: Distribution of stereospecific binding of the potent narcotic analgesic etorphine. *Res. Com. Chem. Path. Pharm.* **6**: 1052, 1973.
3. Pearson, J., and Richter, R.W.: Neurologic aspects of addiction opiates. In Vinken, P.J., and Bruyn, G.W. (eds.): *Handbook of Clinical Neurology.* Amsterdam, North Holland Press, 1979.
4. Jaffe, J.H., and Sharpless, S.K.: Pharmacologic denervation supersensitivity in the CNS. *Res. Pub. Ass. Res. Nerv. Ment. Dis.* **46**: 226, 1968.
5. Goetz, C.G., Klawans, H.L., and Cohen, M.M.: Neurotoxic agents. In Baker, A.B., and Baker, E.L. (eds.): *Clinical Neurology.* Hagerstown, Md., Harper and Row, 1980.
6. Pentiah, P., Reilly, F., and Borison, H.L.: Interaction of morphine sulfate and sodium salicylate on respiration in cats. *J. Pharm. Exp. Ther.* **154**: 110–118, 1966.
7. Goodman, L.S., and Gilman, A.: *Pharmacological Basis of Therapeutics,* 4th Ed. New York, Macmillan, 1970.
8. Nichols, J.R.: How opiates change behavior. *Scient. Amer.* **212**: 80–88, 1965.
9. Florez, J., McCarthy, E., and Borison, H.L.: A comparative study in the cat of the respiratory effects of morphine. *J. Pharm. Exp. Ther.* **163**: 448–455, 1968.
10. Eckenhoff, J.E., and Oech, S.R.: Effects of narcotics upon respiration and circulation in man. *Clin. Pharm. Ther.* **1**: 483–524, 1960.
11. Lasagna, L.: Clinical evaluation of morphine and its substitutes as analgesics. *Pharm. Rev.* **16**: 47–83, 1964.
12. Chakravarty, N.K., Matallana, A., Jensen, R., and Borison, H.L.: Central effects of antitussive drugs on cough and respiration. *J. Pharm. Exp. Ther.* **117**: 127–135, 1956.
13. Fultz, J.M., and Senay, E.C.: Guidelines for the management of hospitalized narcotic addicts. *Ann. Intern. Med.* **82**: 815–818, 1975.
14. Mansky, P.A.: Opiate action. In Synder, S.H. (ed.): Opiate receptor mechanisms. *Neurosciences Res. Prog. Bull.* **13**: 13–17, 1975.

15. Citron, B.P., Halpern, M., McCarron, M., Lundberg, G.D., McCormick, R., Pincus, J., Tatter, D., and Haverback, B.J.: Necrotizing angiitis associated with drug abuse. *N. Eng. J. Med.* **283**: 1003–1011, 1970.
16. Moss, G., Staunton, C., and Stein, A.A.: Cerebral etiology of shock syndrome. *J. Trauma* **12**: 885–890, 1972.
17. Frand, V.I., Shim, C.S., and Williams, M.H.: Heroin-induced pulmonary edema. *Ann. Intern. Med.* **77**: 29–35, 1972.
18. Heurich, A.E., Shim, C.S., Richter, R.W., and Lyons, H.A.: Management of drug overdose and pulmonary edema. In Richter, R.W. (ed.): *Medical Aspects of Drug Abuse.* Hagerstown, Md., Harper and Row, 1975, pp. 134–147.
19. Reichman, L.B., Shim, C.S., Baden, M.M., and Richter, R.W.: Development of tolerance to street heroin in addicted and non-addicted primates. *Am. J. Pub. Health* **63**: 801–803, 1973.
20. Bruun, B., Baden, M.M., Challenor, Y.B., Pearson, J., and Richter, R.W.: De neurologiske komplikatiuner ved heroin-misbrug. *Ugesk. Lae.* **134**: 88–93, 1972.
21. Done, A.K.: Salicylate intoxication. *J.A.M.A.* **192**: 770–772, 1965.
22. Graham, J.O.P., and Parker, W.A.: The toxic manifestations of sodium salicylate therapy. *Quart. J. Med.* **17**: 150–156, 1945.
23. Done, A.K.: *Salicylates, An International Symposium.* Boston, Little, Brown & Co., 1963.
24. Limbeck, G.A., Ruvalcaba, R.H.A., Samols, E., and Kelley, V.C.: Salicylates and hypoglycemia. *Am. J. Dis. Child.* **109**: 165–167, 1965.
25. Symonds, C.: Excitation and inhibition in epilepsy. *Brain* **82**: 133–146, 1959.
26. Myers, E.N., Berstein, J.M., and Fostriopolous, G.: Salicylate ototoxicity, a clinical study. *N. Eng. J. Med.* **273**: 587–590, 1965.
27. Anderson, R.J., Potts, D.E., Gabow, P.A., Rumack, B.H., and Schrier, R.W.: Unrecognized adult salicylate intoxication. *Ann. Intern. Med.* **85**: 745–748, 1976.
28. Smith, M.J.H., and Smith, P.K.: *The Salicylates: A Critical Bibliographic Review.* New York, John Wiley, 1966.
29. Cochran, J.B., and Ramsey, A.G.: The hyperpnea produced by i.v. administration of salicylates. *Br. J. Pharmacol. Chemother.* **11**: 364–378, 1956.

30. Lambertsen, C.J.: Drugs and respiration. *Ann. Rev. Pharmacol.* **6**: 327–378, 1966.
31. Tenney, S.M., and Miller, R.M.: The respiratory and circulatory actions of salicylates. *Am. J. Med.* **19**: 498–508, 1955.
32. Done, A.K.: Treatment of salicylate intoxication. *Clin. Toxicol.* **1**: 451–467, 1968.
33. Done, A.K.: Salicylate intoxication; significance of measurements of salicylate in blood in cases of acute ingestion. *Pediatrics* **26**: 800–807, 1960.
34. Hill, J.B.: Experimental salicylate poisoning; observations of the effects of altering blood pH on tissue and plasma salicylate concentrations. *Pediatrics* **47**: 658–655, 1971.

11

Respiratory Reflexes

William C. Koller, M.D., Ph.D.

This chapter will discuss the anatomy, pathophysiology, etiology, clinical manifestations, and treatment of hiccups. Other types of respiratory movements including yawning, myoclonus, and sneezing will also be discussed.

HICCUPS

Hiccups or singultus, hiccups' more formal medical name, stated simply is a single or repeated spasm of the diaphragm, which results in a sudden inspiration, which is abruptly terminated by closure of the glottis, which produces the characteristic audible sound.[1] Isolated or transient hiccups is a common perhaps universal human experience. While hiccups are usually benign and self-limited, representing only a minor annoyance, when they persist they may become a serious threat to health. Hiccup as medical symptom dates back to the time of Hippocrates.[2] While hiccups are an infrequent symptom in the context of medical illness, they may become intractable and present significant management problems.[3,4] Not withstanding this, medical textbooks have generally ignored discussion of this topic and only scanty information is available regarding hiccups.

Anatomy

The diaphragm is the major structure involved in the genesis of hiccups. While the importance of the diaphragm is unmistaken, little research has been done to delineate its exact anatomy. The diaphragm is dome-shaped and in mammals separates the abdominal and thoracic cavities. It is known that the diaphragm is predominately a muscular tissue (70%). Musculofibrous bundles are found through the muscle. They are localized posterior and lateral to the midline.[6] Each half of the muscular part of the diaphragm is divided into three parts: sternal, costal, and lumbar. The three parts are inserted into the central tendon.

The diaphragm is the most important muscle of respiration. It descends when it contracts, and draws the central tendon downward with it. The volume of the thorax is thereby increased and intrathoracic pressure decreased. The volume of the abdominal cavity is decreased, however, and intra-abdominal pressure is raised.

The costal part of the diaphragm raises and everts the costal margin. The movements of the diaphragm are also important in the circulation of the blood. The decreased intrathoracic pressure and increased abdominal pressure that accompany the descent of the diaphragm facilitates the return of blood to the heart.

Each half of the diaphragm has a separate nerve supply, and paralysis of one half does not affect the other half. However, the two halves of the diaphragm usually contact synchronously. The diaphragm is under voluntary control only to a certain extent. No one can voluntarily hold his breath to the point of asphyxiation.

Each half of the diaphragm is innervated by the phrenic nerve which arises mainly from the fourth cervical segment. Abnormalities in phrenic trunk formation (e.g., thick root from cervical root three) exist but the percentage is unknown.[7] The phrenic nerve in its course is in close relationship to the deep musculature of the neck, the first portion of the subclavian artery, subclavian vein, internal mammary artery, the root of the lung, and the pericardium. The left phrenic nerve is in proximity to the left vagus and the arch of the aorta. The phrenic nerves also communicate with the sympathetic system in the chest.[8] An accessory phrenic nerve occurs in 20 to 30 percent of cases.[9] The nerves pass through the diaphragm in branches and innervation occurs mainly on the inferior surface. The phrenic nerves carry both efferent and afferent fibers. Branches of the intercostal nerves also innervate the diaphragm and are thought to supply motor fibers only. In the area of interdigitation between the lower costal branches of the diaphragm and the transverse abdominis muscle, innervation is supplied by the lower thoracic nerves. The crura may be innervated by the lower thoracic and the upper two lumbar nerves.[9,10] Sympathetic nerve supply is conveyed from the celiac ganglion through the phrenic plexus with which the phrenic nerves communicate. There is also a series of intercommunicating fibers between the phrenic, vagus, and sympathetic chain in the cervical region.[5,11] The laryngeal branches of the vagus innervate the glottis. Thus, while the phrenic nerve is the main motor nerve of the diaphragm, it is clear that other nerves also contribute and that all these structures most likely play some role in the genesis of hiccups.

While the anatomy of the peripheral nerves is well known, the knowledge of central nervous system structures involved in respiration and hiccup remains fragmentary. Although the precise anatomy and physiology of central respiratory centers need further clarification we know that respiratory centers are located in the brainstem in the medulla and pons. Kuntz,[9] in 1947, stated that a special hiccup center in the brainstem was improbable and no new data have established the presence of such a structure. It is more likely that the combined action of respiratory and phrenic centers together with hypothalamic sympathetic centers all play a role in the central nervous system generation of hiccups.

Physiology

The neural mechanisms in the control of hiccups are complex and poorly understood. A simplified pathway for hiccups is illustrated in Figure 1. Receptors located in the larynx, trachea, and bronchi as well as the pleura and stomach, transmit stimuli via the vagus nerves to centers in the medulla. Afferents from receptors in the pericardium and

FIGURE 1

PATHWAY OF HICCUPS

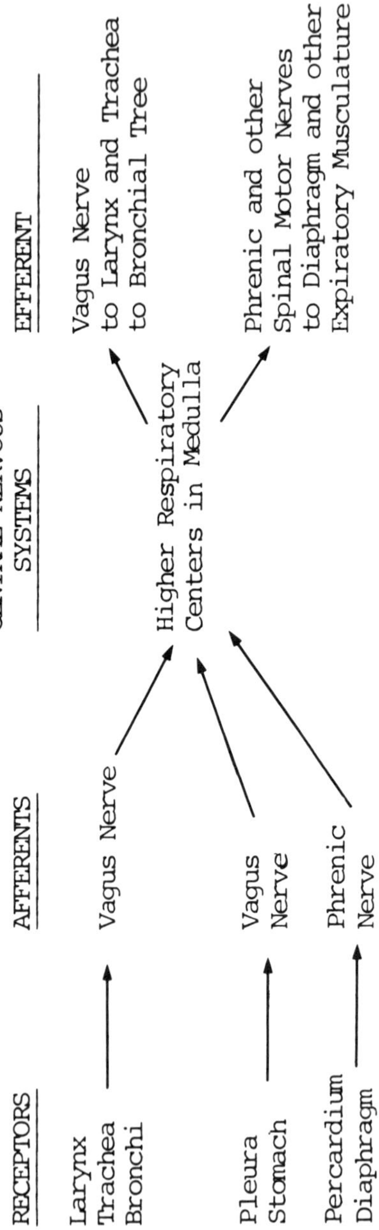

diaphragm are supplied by the phrenic nerve to the medullary respiratory centers. Efferents to the larynx and tracheobronchial tree are located within the vagus nerve, while the phrenic nerve and other spinal motor nerves provide the efferent innervation to the diaphragm and other expiratory musculature. An abnormal stimulus which may affect these nerves at their origin or in their course may induce hiccups.[12,13] Unlike vomiting, which utilizes a similar pathway, hiccups appear to serve no useful physiologic purpose.

Physiologic investigations of hiccups are indeed rare. However, J. Newson Davis[14] has studied in some detail the electrophysiology of persistent hiccups in humans. While such studies in humans are difficult, he has shown in three patients that the diaphragm is not the only muscle involved and that the hiccup has in fact only a minimal effect on ventilation. Each spasm consists of synchronous bursts of activity in the diaphragmatic and external (inspiratory) intercostal muscles with inhibition of expiratory intercostal activity. The glottis is closed from just after hiccups to after its completion, thus explaining the lack of effect on ventilation. Breath holding (a remedy sometimes successful in terminating hiccups) and increasing pCO_2 were both found to reduce the frequency but not the amplitude of hiccups. Davis also concluded that hiccups are influenced by supraspinal mechanism distinct from the pathways for normal respiration.

Clinical Manifestations

Hiccups may occur at any period of life, from infancy to old age. It may vary in degree from a mild temporary discomfort to a prolonged exhausting, and even fatal disorder. Most cases lie somewhere between these two extremes. Hiccoughing may be slow or as rapid as 50 to 100 a minute, and may rarely be so rapid and violent as to interfere with breathing. Pain, usually centered around the chest and along the line of attachment of the diaphragm, may occur during the attack presumably due to ischemia and increased lactate production within this muscle. If it is intractable and prolonged, exhaustion may follow. If not hysterical in etiology, hiccups may persist at night and seriously disturb and disrupt sleep. Hiccups, however, are usually superimposed on a normal respiratory cycle. Most investigators have found that the majority of hiccups are unilateral, more often confined to the left hemidiaphragm.

A careful history should be taken from all patients with persistent hiccups including the number of previous attacks, duration and frequency of attacks and previous attempted treatment. Careful attention should be given to the psychological status of the patient because of the high incidence of hysterical hiccups, especially in females. The diagnosis of hiccups is not difficult. Examination should include visual inspection of the costal arches during spasms. When hiccups persist, fluoroscopic examination should become part of the evaluation.

In addition, the phrenic circle test may be performed as described by Samuels.[7] A small pillow is placed under the patient's neck producing a slight anterior arching. The first two fingers of the right hand are placed at the posterior border of the sternomastoid muscle immediately above its clavicular insertion. The fingers are pushed medially and posteriorly at an angle of 30 degrees until the resistance of the scalenes and the transverse cervical processes can be felt. Pressure is then made directly posteriorly by bending the terminal phalanges. Pressure should be gentle and steady and should not exceed two minutes. Spasm usually ceases on the side on which the pressure is excited within one minute. Testing one side after the other simplifies the determination of uni- or bilateral spasm. In all cases in which bilateral spasm is found, spasm is observed to be greater on one side than the other. This has been termed the pacemaker side. Samuels,[7] using fluroscopic data, offered the following classification of hiccups:

1. Single complete unilateral contraction of the whole diaphragm.
2. A single complete spasm followed by one to three smaller spasms in quick succession.
3. Contraction of one or more segments of the diaphragm, all unilateral without complete spasm.
4. Unilateral complete spasm with segmental spasm of the opposite side.
5. Complete bilateral spasm, which may or may not be followed by smaller spasms (rare).

Etiology

The causes of hiccups are extremely diverse. As stated above, hiccup is thought to be a reflex excited by stimulation of sensory nerves, especially the phrenic and vagus nerve. Irritation in the brainstem or anywhere along the pathway of these nerves may result in the pathological condition known as hiccups. A classification of causes of hiccups according to anatomic location is presented in Table 1.

Hiccups may be a result of a variety of insults to brainstem structures. Infectious causes such as meningitis and encephalitis may elicit hiccups. Hiccups were not an infrequent symptom in encephalitis lethargica (von Economo encephalitis).[15] Infarcts of the lateral medulla due to occlusion of the posterior inferior cerebellar artery (Wallenberg's syndrome) can cause hiccups. While this may be a distressing symptom, it usually does not persist. Tumors of the brainstem may also cause hiccups. Various types of seizure disorders, hydrocephalus, and pontine hemorrhage have also been associated with hiccups. While it is clear that hiccups may be a part of the symptom complex of central nervous system disease, there are several reports of it being the initial and presenting complaint of what later is diagnosed as serious central nervous system pathology.[16,17]

A variety of different disease states in the thoracic cavity may result in hiccups.[18] Infectious processes including perihepatitis, subphrenic abscess, mediastinitis, pleuritis, tuberculosis, pneumonia, and laryngotracheobronchitis may be associated with hiccups. Tumors of the lung, mediastinum, or diaphragm can also give rise to hiccups. Aortic aneurysms can also cause singultus. There is also a case report of obstinate hiccups as a prodromal symptom in thoracic herpes zoster.[19]

Hiccup is a dangerous potentially fatal complication of coronary artery disease.[20,21] Hiccups occur in the setting of acute myocardial infarction although there is a disagreement as to whether this represents a poor prognostic sign.[20,22] In the cases reported no specific location of infarction appears to be related, although posterior wall infarction would be expected to be more likely to produce excitation of the diaphragmatic pleura. Hiccups occurring

TABLE I
Classification of the Causes of Hiccups

I. CENTRAL NERVOUS SYSTEM DISEASE
- Brainstem tumors
- Meningitis
- Encephalitis
- Hydrocephalus
- Central nervous system malaria
- Lateral medullary syndrome
- Seizure disorders
- Brainstem hemorrhage
- Lesion of the cervical cord

II. THORACIC CAVITY DISEASE
- Perihepatitis
- Subphrenic abscess
- Mediastinitis
- Pleuritis
- Lung cancer
- Mediastinal tumors
- Aortic aneurysms
- Diaphragmatic metastases
- Pneumonia
- Laryngotracheobronchitis
- Tuberculosis
- Herpes zoster

III. CARDIAC DISEASE
- Acute myocardial infarction
- Pericarditis
- Pacemakers

IV. ABDOMINAL DISEASE
- Dilatation and atony of the stomach
- Gastritis
- Enteritis
- Peritonitis
- Acute or chronic bowel obstruction
- Esophagospasm
- Pancreatitis
- Hepatitis
- Metastatic disease of the liver
- Strangulated hernia

TABLE I (Continued)

V. METABOLIC
- Renal failure
- Alcoholic intoxication
- Hepatic failure
- Acetonemia

VI. PSYCHOGENIC

VII. IDIOPATHIC

VIII. MISCELLANEOUS
- Immoderate laughter

only with exertion and relieved by rest or nitroglycerin have also been reported in one patient with coronary artery disease.[23] Because of the intercommunication between the cervical segments of the spinal cord, sympathetic ganglion, and the vagus nerves, it appears likely that hiccups in cornary artery disease is of reflex origin. Other cardiac causes of hiccup include pericarditis and irritation of the phrenic nerve by pacemaker wires.

Various abdominal ailments are common causes of hiccups. Hiccups in this setting are frequently seen in the general population, are usually not persistent, and are thought to be due mainly to indiscretion in diet or to too rapid extension of the stomach. Food that is too hot, too cold, or highly seasoned may cause hiccups. Dilatation or atony of the stomach is thought to be the mechanism of hiccups in infants during feeding and to play a role in the genesis of hiccups in the postoperative patient. More serious abdominal pathology, such as strangulated hernia, intestinal obstruction, ileus, carcinoma, appendicitis, peritonitis, or pancreatitis, may give rise to hiccups.

Uremia is the most common metabolic cause of hiccups.[24] The reason why the azotemic patient should be inclined to hiccup remains a mystery. It is also not known what degree of uremia is necessary to induce hiccups. Hiccups occur in hepatic insufficiency, although less frequently. The reason it occurs at all in liver failure is also unknown.

Psychogenic factors are fairly common causes of intractable hiccups. Theobor and McKesney[25] have reviewed psychogenic hiccups in some detail. They emphasized that all patients with intractable hiccups should be carefully screened for possible contributory psychosocial and emotional factors. A variety of psychological disorders may be responsible.

While hiccups may be associated with a variety of illnesses, it may be the only symptom in a healthy individual in whom no pathology is found. These cases are labeled idiopathic.

With regard to the frequency of the various etiologies mentioned, only one large study exists. Souadjian and Cain[4] investigated 220 patients with intractable hiccups at the Mayo Clinic. They found an overwhelming female preponderance and a significant increase with age. Most of the females (92%) were diagnosed as having psychogenic hiccups. These investigators also found that a majority of patients with intractable hiccups had multiple illnesses, any one of which could give rise to hiccups (cause irritation of the phrenic nerve or higher centers). They concluded that multiple conditions occurring concomitantly may be necessary to produce intractable hiccups.

Treatment

The treatment of hiccups, especially intractable hiccups, remains a difficult problem.[26,27] First of all, attention must be directed at discovering an etiology of the hiccups. If hiccups are idiopathic in origin or the underlying cause can not be corrected, a variety of popular and medical remedies are available. Modes of treatment can be divided into three categories: mechanical, pharmacological and surgical. The mutiplicity of measures advocated for the treatment of hiccups are testimony enough that no single effective therapy has yet been found.

Under the heading of mechanical therapy, techniques are included of which the average person is cognizant. Many lay treatments have been passed down for the therapy of hiccups. In ancient Greek literature, one finds Eryximacleus speaking of Aristophanes who is suffering from singultus during dinner, saying, "Let me advise you to hold your breath, and if this fails, gargle with a little warm water, and if the hiccup still continues, tickle your nose with something and sneeze, and if you sneeze once or twice, the most violent hiccup is sure to go."[2] Folk medicine also suggests sudden fright, taking a hot bath, ice packs on the side of the neck, and sneezing induced by pepper. Other home remedies include pressure on the upper lips or eyeballs, drinking cold water from the side of a glass, or tickling the nares with a feather. For trivial hiccups, other time-honored maneuvers include holding the breath, deep breathing, breathing in and out of a paper bag, drawing up the legs so as to compress the diaphragm, inhalation of smelling salts, firm traction on the tongue, and the induction of vomiting.

More scientific mechanical maneuvers have also been proposed. Galvanic sinusoidal current applied to the skin has been recommended but not universally successful.[28] Salem and his colleagues[29] have developed a technique of pharyngeal stimulation by the frictional movement of a nasal catheter whose tip is accurately situated in the pharynx opposite cervical segments two and three. They reported that 148 out of 150 patients were relieved by this purely mechanical means. However, the results were often only temporary.

Numerous pharmacologic agents have been used in the treatment of hiccups with varying degrees of success. Clearly, no one pharmacologic agent has proven effective. Assessment of individual agents in the treatment of hiccups suffers from the lack of any well controlled studies. Also, since most attacks of hiccups are short-lived and self-limited, evaluation of the efficacy of individual drugs proves difficult.

The two drugs with the most apparent success have been chlorpromazine and metaclopromide.[26] Chlorpromazine should be the first drug administered for the control of intractable hiccups. While this drug is generally considered effective, disagreement exists concerning the route of administration.[30,31] An intravenous bolus of 50 mg is stated to be effective. Friedgood and Lipstein[32] claimed an 80 percent permanent cure and a 10 percent temporary effectiveness in 50 patients with various medical and surgical diagnoses. Side effects are usually restricted to sedation, dermatitis, and transient postural hypotension. Extrapyramidal side effects can also occur. No serious side-effects occurred during short term treatment. Metaclopromide has been used with a certain amount of success.[33,34] A dose of 10 mg orally four times a day is given for a 10-day course. There are no data comparing the efficacy of different routes of administration. Like chlorpromazine, metaclopromide may cause extrapyramidal side effects and these drugs should not be used together.

Other centrally acting drugs that have been used include phenytoin, 200 to 400 mg a day,[35,36] haloperidol,[37] 15 mg a day, and amphetamine, 30 mg a day. Orphenadrine is another agent with some efficacy.[38,39] Barbiturates are recommended by some authors; however, no data support their effectiveness and these drugs and other sedatives are probably best avoided. Conflicting data exist concerning methylphenidate.[40,41] A dose of 20 mg, intravenously, has been reported to be very effective. However, Gregory and Way[41] reported on a double blind study of 51 patients with hiccups under anesthesia. Eighteen of 24 patients responded within three minutes to intravenous methylphenidate; 15 of 27 patients who received saline solution also had cessation of their hiccups.

A variety of other drugs whose action is not primarily on the central nervous system have been used in the treatment of hiccups. Antispasmodics, nitroglycerin, and amyl nitrate, are drugs which possess only limited efficacy.[42,43] Quinidine sulfate, at a dose of 200 mg four times a day, has been successful in stopping hiccups in some patients.[44] Such doses may cause cardiac side-effects. A proposed mechanism of action is that the drug renders the motor endplate insensitive to the action of acetylcholine.

Granulated sugar, swallowed dry, was immediately successful in 19 of 20 patients.[45] However, not all of the patients had intractable hiccups. The mode of action is thought to be related to increased input to the afferent limb of the hiccup reflex, so counteracting the effects of the original stimulus.

The uses of various gases, carbon dioxide and oxygen, have been recommended.[46] These gases appear to be more efficacious if used early in the treatment of hiccups. Periods of inhalation should not exceed 10 minutes. Most authors recommend gas administration only by a competent anesthetist.

A host of other pharmacologic agents have been stated to be effective in single case reports but these findings have not been confirmed and there is no need to list these drugs.

When hiccups represent serious morbidity and when all other therapeutic maneuvers have failed, and no underlying etiologic factors can be corrected, then surgical intervention should be considered. These procedures usually involve direct attack on the phrenic nerve, and included traction,[47] electrical stimulation,[48] injection with local anesthesia,[49,50] and crushing and avulsion.[51] Before any surgical procedure, fluoroscopic examination should be performed to document which diaphragmatic leaves are involved. Because of the existence of accessory phrenic nerves in some cases, it is essential to repeat fluoroscopy after the surgical procedure.

Phrenic nerve block can be attempted by injection of procaine or other local anesthesias which will cause a temporary paralysis.[27] Injection should be done two fingerbreadths above the clavicle at the anterior border of the sternomastoid at the depth of 2 to 4 cm, allowing several days interval between the injection of the two sides. If permanent relief is not achieved by phrenic nerve block, then it may be necessary to crush one or both of the phrenic nerves. The blocking of nerves beforehand permits prior knowledge of the effect the procedure will have on pulmonary function. Respiratory function tests should be performed before attempting to paralyze the phrenic nerve. The left side should be blocked first to evaluate the effect on hiccup and respiratory function. Left-sided diaphragmatic contraction is more distressing to the patient and block on this side alone is often successful in stopping hiccups. If a unilateral block is effective in causing temporary cessation of the hiccups, both sides may be done at the same time or preferably at two separate operations, several weeks apart. This procedure is contraindicated in patients with pre-existing respiratory disease, such as emphysema. Phrenic nerve crush is preferred to phrenectomy since permanent phrenic paralysis from nerve section is unwarranted and the duration of the effect of phrenic crush is almost always sufficient for permanent relief of hiccups. Unilateral paralysis of the diaphragm produces no symptoms. Bilateral paralysis results in dyspnea on exertion and some times even when the patient is at rest. Moreover, in bilateral paralysis coughing and straining at stool are often poorly performed. Chronic congestion at the base of the lungs may also result. However, some patients tolerate bilateral phrenic crush very well.[51] Accurate assessment of the overall effectiveness of surgical procedures is difficult since the number of patients treated by these procedures is very small. It should also be noted the hiccups may persist after bilateral phrenic nerve crush.

In summary, the treatment of hiccups requires first the correction of any identifiable cause, then various breath holding maneuvers and other home remedies should be attempted. Mechanical means, such as nasogastric tubes and pharmacologic agents, e.g., chlorpromazine or metaclopromide, should be used next if hiccups persist. When all these methods have failed, phrenic nerve block and then crush should be considered. Williamson and MacIntyre (1977)[26] have suggested a protocol for treating hiccups which is illustrated in Table II.

It happens in some cases that hiccups remain refractory to all modes of treatment. The case of Jack O'Leary illustrates both the intractibility of hiccups and the various possibilities of treatment. This poor individual hiccoughed from June 1948 to June 1956 (the longest case on record).[52] He received over 60,000 suggestions for cures of which only apparently worked, a prayer to St. Jude, the patron saint of lost causes.

YAWNING

Yawning is another respiratory reflex. It is an involuntary paroxysmal action consisting of a deep inspiration associated with a wide open mouth. While it is a commonplace phenomenon in human experience, the scientific and medical community has generally ignored any discussion of the topic. Textbooks of physiology and medicine rarely contain more than a short paragraph concerning yawning. The basic anatomy and physiology of yawning remains unelucidated.

TABLE II

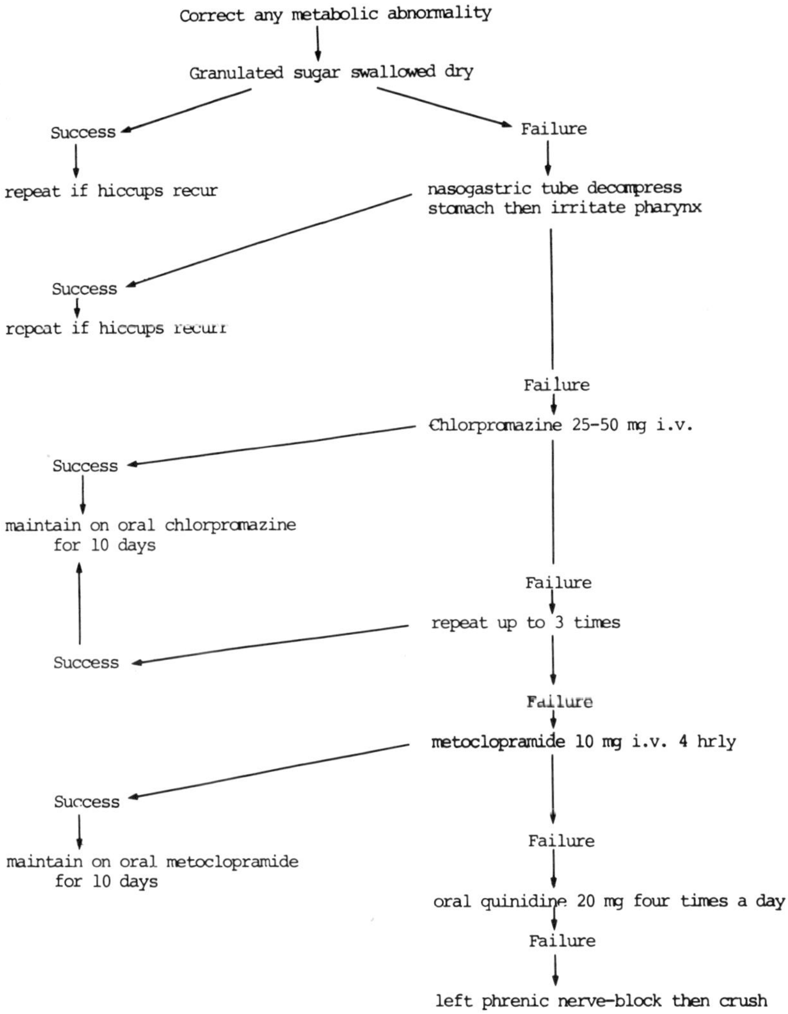

Table 2. Proposed treatment plan for intractable hiccups. (Taken with permission from Williamson, W.A., and MacIntyre, I.M.: Management of intractable hiccups. *Br. Med. J.* **2**:501–503, 1977.)

Yawning is also known by such synonyms as pandiculation, oscitation and chasma. Yawning is derived from the English verb *ganien* which means an "opening," in the sense of "to gape." Pandiculation comes from the Latin verb *pandiculare*, meaning to stretch oneself. While the act of stretching is frequently associated with yawning, the term pandiculation has apparently become synonymous with yawning.[53] Chasma and oscitation are also Latin derivatives meaning "a cleft" and "an open mouth" respectively.[54] Yawning appears to be a universal act. The occurrence of yawning throughout the animal kingdom is widespread.[55] Humans begin to yawn as neonates and continue this behavior throughout their lives.

The specific anatomy of yawning is unknown. It can be stated with some certainty that there is no specific center in the central nervous system that subserves yawning. Stimulation of brain areas has not produced isolated yawning, although yawning may be associated with stimulation of structures which induce sleep.[56] Because of the relationship of yawning to sleep it is thought that the brainstem reticular formation plays some role in yawning. It has been suggested that yawning is controlled in the medulla oblongata in close vicinity to the respiratory and vasomotor centers. However, there are few data to support these logical deductions.

The act of yawning can be divided into three phases which may invariably be distinguished. The first phase consists of a progressive opening of the mouth, dilatation of the pharynx, larynx, and thorax, descent of the diaphragm and widening of the chest. There is elevation of the ali nasa and soft palate, and a downward and backward displacement of the tongue and abduction of the vocal cords. The mouth usually opens very slowly and the mouth is still half open when the dilatation of the pharynx and larynx is at its maximum. Observation will reveal a lowering of the neck's air axis with lowering of the thyroid cartilage. A radiograph taken at this time will show that the body of the hyoid bone, which stands at rest at the level of the C2-C3 vertebra, goes down to C6-C7, and explains the tongue movement as it is pulled back and downward, the tip going well away from the teeth. The dilatation of the glottis and the abduction of the vocal cord can easily be visualized by laryngoscopic examination. Radiographs also show that the dilatation of the pharynx is enormous, increasing three to four times its normal size. The trachea and the bronchial tree also appear to dilate. While the opening of the mouth and the deep inspiration may be observed in many instances apart from yawning, the marked expansion of the pharynx with the lowering of the hyoid bone and tongue is limited to the act of yawning. The second phase of yawning corresponds to the acme of the mouth's opening and to that of the pharyngeal and thoracic dilatation. Facial modifications now begin to occur. There is contraction of the lip dilators, which exaggerates the mouth's opening, and contraction of the eyelids, which causes a partial or total occlusion of the eyes. The nostrils dilate. The skin at the base of the nose wrinkles and the eyebrows are lifted. Tonic contraction of the extensor muscles of the neck and trunk may occur. There may also be hyperextension of the limbs. The stretching, which is far from constant, has the result of increasing the thoracic capacity. The number and distribution of muscles recruited in the stretch reflex are subjected to variation and may be modified by voluntary control. Other phenomena observed include the secretion of tears and saliva. The third phase is a passive expiratory one. Inspiration ceases abruptly. Expiration is slow and noisy, sometimes followed by a sound generated in the larynx. The pharynx returns to its normal size, the mouth closes itself, and the face resumes its normal configuration. This final stage of yawning may be accompanied by a subjective sense of satisfaction. An average yawn lasts from 4 to 7 seconds.[57] Once yawning is initiated it cannot be suppressed; however, the varied manifestations outlined above can be voluntarily modified. Yawning appears to be infectious in that yawning in one individual tends to induce yawning in others. The idea that yawns are catching can be traced back to Mayer (1921)[58] who believed that some individuals have a low threshold for this so-called psychologically released yawning. There appears to be no adequate explanation for this fascinating phenomenon.

Stretching is frequently associated with yawning. Infants and children tend to yawn and stretch together more frequently than adults who tend to yawn and stretch independently. Yawns have a tendency to occur before one goes to sleep, and stretching often occurs upon waking. There is no evidence to support a yawn-stretch reaction as a primitive reflex.

The etiological causes of yawning can be divided into three categories: physiologic, pathological, and psychogenic. The physiologic heading includes most common etiologies of yawning, which are boredom and drowsiness. Boredom from any of a variety of sources will induce yawning. Those in the academic community know well from personal experience that a dull lecture will readily induce this reflex and that the ability to suppress yawning in this setting is difficult. Yawning is also a frequent occurrence when one is sleepy. Yawning is observed both in humans and other animals preceding sleep. Yawning is also sometimes seen when one emerges from sleep. Other physiological causes of yawning are said to include weariness and hunger.[59] Yawning has also been associated with drowsiness after a heavy meal.

Pathological causes of yawning are harder to define. Exactly what constitutes morbid yawning is unclear, although the incidence may be more than we assume owning to the general neglect of the topic. Yawning associated with disease states is almost exclusively limited to disease of the central nervous system. In most of these cases, the brainstem appears to be the anatomic area of the nervous system involved. Severe brainstem hemorrhage is not infrequently associated with yawning as well as many other neurological signs.[57] Paroxysmal yawning is seen in encephalitis, again along with varied other neurologic symptoms.[60] Expanding lesions of the posterior fossa, including brainstem tumors, cerebellar tumors and abscesses appear to induce yawning. Nash (1942)[61] suggested that these lesions cause irritation of brainstem structures resulting in afferent impulses to the medullary respiratory centers which modify its rhythmic activity. In the above cases it has not been possible to ascribe yawning to proven lesions at a particular location in the nervous system. In rare cases yawning may be an aura in epileptic patients.[62,63] Wilson (1940)[62] thought that yawning as an aura is associated with periventricular or visceral epilepsy wherein the yawn is followed by voiding of urine, giddiness, headaches, and sometimes vomiting. Penfield and Jasper (1954)[64] reported two cases where yawning was an element of automonic diencephalic seizures. One case was that of a young woman who had a large astrocytoma occupying the whole left temporal lobe and the lower portion of the corpus striatum, whose fits started abruptly with occipital pain accompanied by yawns and hiccups, while at the same moment the left arm and left side of the mouth became numb. The fit ended with a need to urinate. Heusner (1946)[54] has suggested that patients with Huntington's disease have a propensity for yawning and stretching. However, this is not the experience of others (Weiner, personal communication). There has also been one reported case where fits of yawning were a sign of myasthenia gravis.[65] Prostigmine was reported to stop the yawning; however, this must be an exceedingly rare event. It has also been noted that patients with hemiplegia will often yawn and that this may be accompanied by stretching movements of the paralyzed limb. There is some speculation that yawning may be a symptom of disease outside the nervous system, particularly in the digestive tract.[59] However, there is little information to support this. At this time, it is not possible to comment on the possible significance of excessive yawning as an isolated symptom. As a pathological condition it appears to be associated with other signs of brainstem disease.

The third classification of yawning is psychogenic. Since the time of Charcot, yawning has been recognized as a manifestation of hysteria. However, there has been no study documenting the incidence or characteristics of psychogenic yawning.

Yawning is a behavioral phenomenon which has no known physiological significance. It may have psychological meaning since it shows those around us that we are indifferent and have a lack of interest. Simply stated, yawning appears to be a symptom of boredom, and only rarely is associated with pathological process. The neural mechanisms which trigger and control this reflex remain to be determined. Numerous hypotheses concerning the mechanism and significance of yawning have been proposed, although there are no data or experimental work to support any of these theories. Russel[66] in 1891 suggested that yawning was an automatic impulse caused by bad air in the lungs. Other hypotheses, no more advanced than the first theory, suggest that yawning is an expression of cerebral fatigue or is a transient disorder of the respiratory center.[67,68] Clearly our knowledge is rudimentary on this topic. Of the few experimental studies, there have been two reports in which yawning has been induced in animals by pharmacologic means. A stretching-yawning syndrome was induced in cats by the intracisternal injection of adrenocortotrophic (ACTH) and melanotrophic (MSH) hormones.[69] Urba-Holmgren and coworkers (1971)[70] found that physostigmine would induce yawning especially in young animals when injected intraperitoneally. This action was blocked by centrally acting muscarinic anticholinergics. However, how these studies relate to the basic mechanisms of yawning is not clear.

MYOCLONUS

Myoclonus is a descriptive term for involuntary, brief, jerking movements of a muscle or limb which may occur in a symmetrical, focal, rhythmical or irregular manner. When myoclonus affects the palate, larynx, pharynx, or diaphragm, there may be consequences to pulmonary function. Myoclonus occurs in the setting of many dissimilar pathological states. These movements are seen in various epilepsies, lipid-storage diseases, viral encephalopathies, toxic-metabolic conditions, particularly uremia, and in postanoxic brain damage.[71-73] Myoclonus can be classified under two headings: arrhythmical and rhythmical (segmental).[74] Arrhythmical is the more common form and includes the disorders mentioned above. Segmental or rhythmical myoclonus is characterized by synchronous rhythmic, jerking movements localized to muscles innervated by either a single segment or several contiguous segments of spinal cord or brainstem. This form of myoclonus is usually unaffected by sensory stimulation or voluntary activity and persists during sleep and even coma. The main structures involved are the palate, pharynx, larynx, diaphragm, and intercostal muscles. Since myoclonus of these muscles is more likely to escape attention than myoclonus of superficial structures, less is known about them.

Palate myoclonus has been the best studied of the segmental group. Pulitzer, an otolaryngologist, is credited with the first documentation of palatal myoclonus in 1862. Gallet[75] in 1927 summarized 37 proven cases, many of whom had myoclonus of structures of the oropharynx besides the palate.[5] In 1931, Guillain and Mollaret[76] reviewed the topic in the neurological literature and made pathological correlation. Since that time myoclonus of structures of the oropharynx has become a well defined entity that is not infrequently observed.

Myoclonus of the oropharynx and respiratory structures can clinically be divided according to the muscles involved. Many cases involve only the palate. These cases can be divided according to whether involvement is unilateral or bilateral. Unilateral palatal myoclonus may become bilateral.[77] Most patients with segmental myoclonus tend to be older with 70 percent of cases occurring after 40 years of age. Frequently, palatal myoclonus will be asymptomatic. In other cases, contraction of the muscles about the orifices of the eustachian tube produces a sudden opening of the tube with a resultant click which is audible to the patient and, at times, to bedside observers. The rate of contraction of the palate varies between 50 and 240 with the majority of cases having a rate between 140 to 180 contractions per minute. Observation day to day in the same patient may reveal variation in the rate of contraction.[78] The movement of the palate is upward and downward with contraction of the pillars. In palatal myoclonus other movements of the oropharynx are seen.[79] The uvula may move up or to one side. The posterior pharyngeal wall, vocal cords, and the entire larynx may be involved. Other muscles, especially those of the eye may demonstrate abnormalities.[80,81] Likewise, muscles about the angle of the mouth and chin, and muscles of the neck may show various degrees of involvement. While the movements are remarkably constant they are suspended or diminished during swallowing or vocalizations. The most common associated symptom was cerebellar dysfunction which occurred in as many as 40 percent of cases.[78] Other less frequent symptoms include headache, difficulties with speech, third nerve palsy, and dysphagia. Myoclonus of the palate and structures of the oropharynx tend not to disappear. It can even spread progressively to involve other muscles. These abnormal movements are unique in that they persist during sleep.[80] Almost all other types of involuntary movements, especially those due to dysfunction of the extrapyramidal system, will cease during sleep.

The etiology of most cases of myoclonus of the oropharynx is vascular disease. In almost all series the causative factor has been acute brainstem infarction.[80,81] Rarer causes include multiple sclerosis, trauma, tumor, and encephalitis.[81] Diagnostic evaluation of these patients should include a computerized tomogram of the brain and brain radionuclide scan. These tests may reveal evidence of brainstem pathology although they may be normal. Electroencephalography usually shows no abnormalities.

In rhythmical myoclonus of the palate, pharynx, and associated structures, lesions have been found in the pontine tegmentum or in the dentate nucleus of the cerebellum. There are usually structural alterations in the inferior olive on the same side as the pontine lesion and opposite the cerebellar damage.[82,83] This consists of the so-called "pseudohypertrophy." The olivary nucleus appears swollen but shows degeneration of nerve cells on microscopic examination.[84] Both lesion and stimulation experiments of these structures in animals produce a syndrome similar to palatal myoclonus. From these observations the concept of the Guillian-Mollaret triangle arose in which a lesion within the triangle between the central tegmental tract, the ipsilateral inferior olive, the contralateral dentate nucleus, and the ipsilateral red nucleus would cause myoclonus in the opposite side of the body.

The pathophysiological mechanisms responsible for the production of myoclonus are not well understood. Various animal models of myoclonus have been investigated which involve either the injection of toxic chemicals administered intravenously or lesions placed in the mesial thalamus.[85,86,87] Animal models of segmental myoclonus are produced by the direct local effect on the spinal cord such as the local application of penicillin or injection of Newcastle disease virus.[88,89] More recent clinical and laboratory investigations have suggested a relationship between brain serotonin metabolism and certain types of myoclonus.[90] Serotonin is a central nervous system neurotransmitter that is thought to have inhibitory functions. It is synthesized from the essential amino acid tryptophan. Injections of hydroxtryptophan, the precursor of serotonin, produced myoclonus in the guinea pig.[91] However, other experimental models in which serotonin activity was decreased also produced myoclonus.[92]

Myoclonus is notoriously resistant to suppression by drugs. Since some consider myoclonus an epileptic variant, most of the anticonvulsant drugs have been tried in myoclonus.[92] Although myoclonus may respond to any of the established anticonvulsants, most patients respond erratically, if at all. Of the anticonvulsants the benzodiazepenes particularly diazepam and clonazepam appear to have the most efficacy.[93] The mechanism of action of these drugs in myoclonus had not been established. A new anticonvulsant agent diproplyacetate (sodium valproate) has been used successfully to treat the myoclonic epilepsies, as well as other forms of epilepsy. Dipropylacetate elevates gamma-aminobutyric acid (GABA) levels presumably by inhibiting GABA-transaminase. Whether this effect is relative to its antimyoclonic action remains to be determined. In view of recent clinical and animal data suggesting a relationship between brain serotonin metabolism and certain types of myoclonus, attempts have been made to alter serotonin levels pharmacologically. Van Woert and co-workers have used 5-hydroxytryptophan (5-HTP) and a peripheral dopa decarboxylase inhibitor (carbidopa) to successfully treat post-anoxic intention myoclonus.[92] Other myoclonic disorders have also shown some but less striking improvement. Most of the drug studies have been on patients with generalized, nonsegmental myoclonus. The few studies of therapy of palatal myoclonus reveal that anticonvulsants are of little worth. Serotonin precursor therapy, (5-HTP and carbidopa) has been reported to be of benefit in some patients but not in others.[93,94] Dipropylacetate has not been studied in palatal myoclonus to date. It can be stated at this time that there is no proven effective therapy for myoclonus of the oropharynx structures. Further clinical trials may demonstrate the effectiveness of serotonin precursor therapy.

SNEEZING

Sneezing is another respiratory reflex. It is a commonplace experience, and only rarely does it represent a significant medical problem, although intractable paroxysmal sneezing does occur. Medical literature makes little reference to the subject, even in textbooks of allergy, the subspecialty where this symptom most frequently occurs. Simply stated, sneezing or sternutation is a reflex that results in a spasmodic inspiration followed by a spasmodic expiration.[95,97] Historically, the act of sneezing had varying significance. The ancient Greeks and Romans viewed sneezing as a good omen and a sign of good fortune.[95] The Talmud called sneezing a "pleasure sent from God," and Pope Gregory the Great (540–604) introduced the expression, "God bless you," to be said to a person after he had sneezed. This pope reigned during the years of epidemic plague and sneezing was a common feature of this fatal disease. The benediction would have been better translated as, "God help you." Likewise, the Germans responded to sneezing by saying, Gesundheit, or good health to you.

The anatomic pathways and physiology of the sneeze reflex are complex. The sneeze can be viewed as consisting of two phases, the nasal and the respiratory. Both are reflex in character, consisting of afferent nerves, a central mechanism, efferent nerves and responding organs. The sneezing reflex is usually initiated by stimulation of the receptors in the anterior part of the nose. However, other stimuli besides nasal irritation can also produce sneezing.[98,99] Holmes and associates[99] have compiled the following list of sneeze-evoking stimuli; contact with infectious agents, inhalation of irritant dusts and chemical fumes, strong odors and bright lights, chilling of body surface, inhalation of pollens and other substances to which the subject is sensitive, menstruation and pregnancy, stimuli provocative of sexual excitement, life experiences provocative of conflict, resentment, and frustration. Everett[100] studied, in detail, sneezing in response to light (photic sneeze reflex) and suggested that hereditary factors predisposed to the reflex. He proposed that parasympathic overactivity was the responsible physiological mechanism. The nasal phase is initialed by nasal irritants, which produce an afferent impulse conducted via the fifth cranial nerve (trigeminal) to the trigeminal sensory ganglia in the brainstem. Efferent connections are carried by the parasympathetic portions of the seventh cranial nerve to the lacrimal glands and the vessels of the nasal mucosa via the nervous intermedius, greater superficial petrosal nerve, vidian nerve, sphneopalatine ganglion, and postganglionic palatine nerve.[95,97] The duration of the nasal phase is variable but results in nasal secretion and vascular congestion. The nature of the secretion is that of a slightly viscid mucus. The congestion and secretions initiate the more rapid respiratory phase. Afferent impulses are again sent to the trigeminal sensory neurons. Brainstem centers for inspiration, closure of the nasopharynx, and expiration are then activated. The respiratory phase consists of an initial large sudden inspiration followed by a sudden forcible expiration. Before expiration the palate is raised and the superior constrictor of the pharynx contracts so that the respiratory passages are shut off from the nose. Contraction of the diaphragm and abdominal muscles cause the intrapulmonary pressure to rise. The nasopharynx is forced open and air is driven out. Involuntary closing of the eyes also seems to be a part of the reflex. The noise of the sneeze appears to originate in the mouth. Occasionally there is some incoordination of palatal movements and a "pharyngeal sneeze" results in which the blast of air comes out of the nose. A characteristic feature of the sneeze is a highly atomized naso-oral discharge; nose droplets have been found to be of 0.1 to 0.2 mm in diameter and are expelled at a velocity of 30 m/sec or greater to a distance of 0.5 to 1.6 mm.[96,97] Sneezing seems to be without purpose. As a reflex behavior it is said to be protective, with its object to remove an irritant in the nose; however, with a sneeze the expulsion of air is through the mouth.

Symptomatically, sneezing is usually of minor importance and only when sneezing persists is it brought as a complaint to a physician. Sometimes the cause of sneezing is easily found, such as a foreign body in the nose or ear, nasal polyps, or other local nasal pathology.[101] Frequent sneezing may also accompany various infectious diseases such as pertussis or measles. Patients with sneezing should receive a complete examination of the ears, nose and throat as well as a neurological examination.

Intractable persistent sneezing is an extremely rare disorder with only 12 cases reported.[96-98,101-106] In these cases there were nine females and three males, with ages ranging from 11 to 40 years. However, the majority of the cases were teenagers. One half the patients had a history of allergy. The final diagnosis in 10 of 12 cases was psychogenic sneezing. In the two other cases sneezing was attributed to a seizure disorder[98] and to tuberculosis cervical lymphadenitis.[104] The patient with seizures had temporal lobe spikes and was said to stop sneezing after anticonvulsant therapy. The relationship of seizure activity to sneezing is a dubious one. However, Penfield and Jasper[107] reported one patient who was undergoing brain surgery for a temporal lobe arteriovenous malformation in whom electrical stimulation of the temporal area produced sneezing and chewing movements. The patients with psychogenic sneezing responded to various forms of psychotherapy. There is no known effective pharmacologic treatment for stopping sneezing, except for the rare case where seizure activity may be involved in which anticonvulsants should be used.

In summary, sneezing is a reflex that results in a spasmodic inspiration followed by a spasmodic expiration. Intractable persistent sneezing is a very rare medical entity and generally is psychogenic in origin.

REFERENCES

1. Wilson, S.A.K.: *Clinical Neurology.* Baltimore, Williams and Wilkins, 1955, pp. 1804–1805.
2. Riddell, W.R.: Hippocrates and hiccup. *Med. J. Anat. Rec.* **40**:132–138, 1930.
3. Fabrocamt, N.D.: The distressing hiccup. *Eye, Ear, Nose, Throat Monthly* **41**:215–218, 1962.
4. Souadjian, J.V., and Cain, J.C.: Intractable hiccups. *Postgrad. Med.* **43**:72–77, 1968.
5. Gray, H.: *Anatomy, descriptive and applied.* Longman, London, 1926.
6. Alexander, J.: *The Surgery of Pulmonary Tuberculosis.* Philadelphia, Lea and Febiger, 1925, p. 176.
7. Samuels, L.: Hiccups. *Canad. Med. J.* **67**:315–322, 1952.
8. Cunningham, H.: *Manual of Anatomy.* Baltimore, Williams and Wilkins, 1947.
9. Kuntz, A.: *The Autonomic Nervous System.* Philadelphia, Lea and Febiger, 1947, p. 214.
10. Siwe, S.A.: Correlative anatomy of the diaphragm. *Am. J. Anat.* **48**:479–482, 1931.
11. Grant, J.C.: *Grant's Atlas of Anatomy.* Baltimore, Williams and Wilkins, 1962.

12. Bellinghan-Smith, E.: The significance and treatment of obstinate hiccough. *Practitioner* **135**:166–171, 1938.
13. Bailey, H.: Persistent hiccup. *Practitioner* **150**:175–178, 1943.
14. Davis, J.N.: An experimental study of hiccup. *Brain* **93**:851–872, 1970.
15. Baker, A.B.: *Clinical Neurology.* New York, Hoeber, 1955.
16. Stotka, V.L., Barcay, S.J., Bell, S.H., and Clare, F.B.: Intractable hiccough as the primary manifestation of brainstem lesion. *Am. J. Med.* **32**:313–315, 1962.
17. Kozia, M., and Onsianonska, T.: Persistent hiccoughing as the predominant symptom with a tumor of the medulla oblongata. *J. Neurol.* **212**:91–93, 1976.
18. Noble, E.C.: Hiccups. *Canad. Med. Ass. J.* **31**:38–41, 1934.
19. Efrati, P.: Obstinate hiccup as a prodromal symptom in thoracic herpes zoster. *Neurology* **6**:601–602, 1956.
20. Rubin, C.H., Albright, L.F., Bornstein, P.K., and Scheimmer, O.: Hiccup in coronary thrombosis, relieved with phrenic crush. *J.A.M.A.* **146**:1418–1420, 1950.
21. Swan, H.R., and Simoson, L.H.: Hiccups complicating myocardial infarction. *N. Eng. J. Med.* **247**:726–728, 1952.
22. Weiss, M.M.: Hiccoughs as a complication of acute coronary artery occlusion. *Am. Ind. Med.* **13**:187–190, 1939.
23. Chavany, J.A., and Haganmiller, P.: Sur un cas de loquet chronique. *Presse. Med.* **58**:721–725, 1950.
24. Beeson, R.A., and McDermott, W. (eds.): *Textbook of Medicine.* Philadelphia, W.B. Saunders Co., 1967.
25. Theobar, C., and Mekegney, F.A.: Hiccups of psychogenic origin. A case report and review of the literature. *Comprehens. Psychiat.* **11**:377–384, 1970.
26. Williamson, W.A., and MacIntyre, I.M.: Management of intractable hiccups. *Br. Med. J.* **2**:501–503, 1977.
27. Gigot, A.F., and Flynn, P.A.: Treatment of hiccups. *J.A.M.A.* **150**:760–764, 1952.
28. Barnard, F.G.: Treatment of severe singultus. *Am. J. Surg.* **77**:230–234, 1949.
29. Salem, M.R., Baraka, H., Ratterburg, C.C., and Holiday, D.A.: Treatment of hiccups by pharyngeal stimulation in anesthetized and conscious subjects. *J.A.M.A.* **200**:126–130, 1967.
30. Bendensky, G., and Baren, M.: Hypnosis in the termination of hiccups unresponsive to conventional treatment. *Arch. Int. Med.* **104**:417–420, 1959.

31. Ikram, H., Orchard, R.T., and Read, S.E.C.: Intractable hiccuping in acute myocardial infarction. *Br. Med. J.* **2**:504–505, 1971.
32. Friedgood, C.E., and Ripstein, C.B.: Chlorpromazine (Thorazine) in the treatment of intractable hiccups. *J.A.M.A.* **157**:309–311, 1955.
33. Middleton, R.S.W.: Treatment of intractable hiccups. *Postgrad. Med. J.* **49**:90–93, 1973.
34. Modonogopolen, N.: Metroclopromide in hiccup. *Current Med. Res. Opinion* **3**:371–374, 1975.
35. Prineas, J.: Treatment of hiccup. *Science* **178**:760–761, 1972.
36. Davis, J.N.: Diphenylhydantoin for hiccups. *Lancet* **1**:997, 1974.
37. Lalanabe, T., and Okazade, H.: Hiccups. *Lancet* **2**:509, 1973.
38. Gibbs, A.E.: Two cases of persistent hiccup treated with orphenadrine. *Practitioner* **191**:646–648, 1963.
39. Finch, J.W.: Rapid control of persistent hiccups by orphenadrine citrate. *Med. Times* **94**:485–486, 1966.
40. Macris, S.C., Macus, G.J., Cavouri, A.A., and Karapiperis, S.M.: Intravenous methylphenidate for treatment of singultus. *Anesth. Analg.* **42**:440–446, 1963.
41. Gregory, G.H., and Way: Methylphenidate for the treatment of hiccups during anesthesia. *Anesthesiology* **31**:89–93, 1969.
42. Raute, C.S., Powers, J.M., and Suzehr, E.: Drug treatment of hiccups. *Arch. Neurol.* **30**:29–32, 1973.
43. Dubois-Dalen, M., Schumacher, E., and Sever, J.: Hiccups. *Lancet* **2**:1408–1409, 1973.
44. Bellet, S., and Nadler, C.S.: Use of quinidine sulphate in hiccup: Preliminary report. *Am. J. Med. Sc.* **216**:680–686, 1958.
45. Engleman, E.G., Lankton, J., and Lankton, B.: Granulated sugar as treatment for hiccups in conscious patients. *N. Eng. J. Med.* **285**:1489–1490, 1971.
46. Bailey, H.: Persistent hiccup. *Practitioner* **173**:178, 1943.
47. Slemmer, R.E.: Phrenic nerve traction for persistent hiccough (singultus) *Arch. Surg.* **71**:927–928, 1955.
48. Korczyn, A.D.: Hiccups. *Br. Med. J.* **2**:591–592, 1971.
49. Pitkin, G.P.: Anesthesia. Philadelphia, J.B. Lippincott Co., 1953.
50. Sornoff, S.J., and Sornorr, L.E.: Hiccups. *Anesthesia.* **12**:270–273, 1953.

51. Campbell, M.F.: Malignant hiccup with report of a case following transurethral prostate resection requiring bilateral phrenicetomy for cure. *Am. J. Surg.* **48**:449–455, 1940.
52. McWhirter, N., and McWhirter, R.: *The Guinness Book of Records.* London, Guinness Superlative, 1965.
53. Dorland, W.A.H.: *The American Illustrated Medical Dictionary.* Philadelphia, Saunders Co., 1976.
54. Heusner, A.P.: Yawning and associated phenomena. *Physiol. Rev.* **26**:156–168, 1946.
55. Cramer, F.: Über Sodbrennen and Gahnen. *Arch. f. Verdauungskr.* **35**:149–153, 1924.
56. Hess, W.R.: *Das Zwischenhirn und die Regulation von Kreislauf und Ahnung.* Vol. I. Leipzig.
57. Bartizat, J.: Yawning. *J. Neurol. Neurosurg. Psychiat.* **21**:203–207, 1958.
58. Mayer, O.: Physiologie und Pathologie des Gahnen. *Ztschr. Bri.* **73**:101, 1921.
59. Schrliver, S.: Über das Magengahnen. *Arch. f. Verdauungskr.* **43**:378–385, 1928.
60. Appenzeller, O.: *The Autonomic Nervous System.* New York, North Holland Publishing Co., 1970, p. 93.
61. Nash, J.: *Surgical Pathology.* Springfield, Ill., Charles C Thomas Publishing, 1942, p. 92.
62. Wilson, S.A.K.: *Textbook of Neurology.* Baltimore, Williams and Wilkins, 1940.
63. Penfield, W., and Erickson, T.C.: *Epilepsy and Cerebral Localization.* Springfield, Ill., Charles C Thomas Publishing, 1941.
64. Penfield, W., and Jasper, H.: Epilepsy and the functional anatomy of the human brain. New York, Churchill, 1954, p. 417.
65. Salmon, A.: *Presse Med.* **56**:739, 1948.
66. Russell, A.: Yawning. *The Delsarte Series.* Mp/ 1. New York, U.S. Book Co., 1891.
67. Wiggers, G.T.: *Physiology in Health and Disease,* 3rd Ed. Philadelphia, Lea and Febiger, 1939.
68. Peiper, A.: Das Gahnen. *Deutsch. Med. Wochenschr.* **58**:693, 1932.
69. Gessa, G.L., Vargin, L., and Ferrari, W.: Stretchings and yawning induced by adrenocorticotrophic hormones. *Nature* **211**:426–432, 1966.
70. Urba-Holmgren, R., Gongoly, R.M., and Holmgren, B.: Is yawning a cholinergic response? *Nature* **287**:201–206, 1977.

71. Unverricht, H.: *Die Myoclonic.* Liepzig, Franz Deutsche, 1891, p. 128.
72. Hunt, F.R.: Dyssynergia cerebellaris myoclonia. Primary atrophy of the dentate system, a contribution to the pathology and symptomatology of the cerebellum. *Brain* **44**:490–583, 1921.
73. Lance, J.W., and Adams, R.D.: The syndrome of intention or action myoclonus as a sequel to hypoxic encephalopathy. *Brain* **86**:111–136, 1963.
74. Krebs, E.: Les myoclonics etude semarologique. *Rev. Neurol.* **86**:549–566, 1953.
75. Gallet, S.: Le nystagmus du voile: le syndrome myoclonique de la calitte protuberantielle. Thése de Paris, 1927.
76. Guillaim, G., and Mollaret, P.: Deux cas de myoclonies synchrones at rythmées velo-pharyngo-laryngo-diaphragmatiques. *Rev. Neurol.* **2**:545, 1931.
77. Swanson, P.D., and Luttrell, C.N.,; Magladery. Myoclonus—A report of 67 cases and review of the literature. *Medicine* **41**:339–356, 1962.
78. Riley, H.A., and Brock, S.: Rhythmic myoclonus of the muscles of the palate, pharynx, larynx, and other regions. *Arch. Neurol. Psychiat.* **29**:726–741, 1933.
79. Dobson, J.I., and Riley, H.A.: Rhythmic myoclonus: a clinical report of six cases. *Arch. Neurol. Psychiat.* **45**:145–150, 1941.
80. Hermann, C.J., and Brown, J.W.: Palatal myoclonus, a reappraisal. *J. Neurol. Sci.* **54**:373–377, 1967.
81. Erickson, T.C., and Ablin, G.: Palatal myoclonus in association with posterior fossa neoplasms, two cases. *Trans. Am. Neurol. Ass.* **78**:201–206, 1953.
82. Guilliam, G.: The syndrome of synchronous and rhythmic palato-pharyngo-laryngo-oculo-diaphragmatic myoclonus. *Proc. Roy. Soc. Med.* **31**:1031–1038, 1938.
83. Bender, M.B., Nathanson, M., and Gordon, G.G.: Myoclonus of muscles of the eye, face, and throat. *Arch. Neurol. Psychiat.* **67**:44–58, 1952.
84. Wilson, W.C., and Magoun, H.W.: Functional significance of the inferior olve in the cat. *J. Comp. Neurol.* **83**:69–77, 1945.
85. Alvord, E.C., and Fiorted, M.G.F.: A comparison of generalized reflex myoclonic reactions elicitable in cats under chloralose anesthesia and under strychnine. *Am. J. Physiol.* **176**:253–261, 1954.

86. Carmichael, E.A., Feldberg, W., and Fleischauer, K.: The relation between seizure discharge and myoclonus during perfusion of the cerebral ventricles with tubocararine. *J. Physiol.* **164**:301–317, 1962.
87. Milhorat, T.H.: Experimental myoclonus of thalamic origin. *Arch. Neurol.* **17**:365–378, 1967.
88. Luttrell, C.N., Bang, F.B., and Luxenberg, K.: Newcastle disease encephalomyelitis in cats. *Arch. Neurol. Psychiat.* **81**:258–291, 1959.
89. Kao, L.I., and Grill, W.E.: Penicillin-induced segmental myoclonus. Motor responses and intracellular recording from motor neurons. *Arch. Neurol.* **26**:156–162, 1972.
90. Munsat, T.L.: Sertonin and myoclonus seizures. *N. Eng. J. Med.* **296**:101–102, 1977.
91. Klawans, H.L., Goetz, C., Westheimer, R., and Weiner, W.J.: 5-Hydroxytryptophan induced behavior in intact guinea pigs. *Res. Commun. Chem. Pathol. Pharmacol.* **5**:555–559, 1973.
92. Van Woert, M.H., and Hwang, E.C.: Biochemistry and pharmacology of myoclonus. *Clinical Neuropharmacology,* Vol. 3. In Klawans, H.L. (ed.): New York, Raven Press, 1978, pp. 167–184.
93. Huang, C.Y., McLeod, J.G., Sampson, D., and Hensley, W.J.: Clonazepam in the treatment of epilepsy. *Med J. Aust.* **2**:5–8, 1974.
94. Magnussen, I., Dupont, E., Prange-Hansem, A., and Olivarius, B.: Palatal myoclonus treatment with 5-hydroxytryptophan and a decarboxylase inhibitor. *Acta Neurol. Scand.* **55**:251–253, 1977.
95. Brubaker, A.: The physiology of sneezing. *J.A.M.A.* **73**:585–587, 1919.
96. Schenley, C.: Intractable sneezing. Case report and literature review. *Arch. Neurol.* **36**:111–112, 1979.
97. Birch, C.: Sneezing. *Practitioner* **182**:122–124, 1959.
98. Kofman, O.: Paroxysmal sneezing. *Can. Med. Ass. J.* **91**:154–157, 1964.
99. Holmes, T., Goodell, H., and Wolf, S.: *The Nose.* Springfield, Ill., Charles C Thomas Publisher, 1950, pp. 4–52.
100. Everett, H.: Sneezing in response to light. *Neurology* **14**:483–490, 1964.
101. Kaplan, M., and Lanoff, G.: Intractable paroxysmal sneezing: A clinical entity defined with case reports. *Ann. Allery* **28**:24–27, 1970.

102. Shilkret, H.: Psychogenic sneezing and yawning. *Psychosom. Med.* **11**:127–128, 1949.
103. Murray, N., and Bierer, J.: Prolonged sneezing. *Psychosom. Med.* **13**:56–58, 1851.
104. Kammermire, R., Cited by Shapiro, S.L.: Paroxysmal sneezing. *Eye, Ear, Nose Throat Monthly* **46**:15–32, 1967.
105. Elkins, M., and Milstein, J.: Hypotherapy of pseudosneezing. A case report. *Am. J. Clin. M. Hypn.* **4**:273–275, 1962.
106. School girl sneezes but feels fine. Cited by Kaplan, M., and Lanoff, G.: *Ann. Allergy* **28**:26, 1970.
107. Penfield, W., and Jasper, H.: *Epilepsie and the Functional Anatomy of the Brain.* Boston, Little, Brown and Co., 1954, p. 453.

12

RESPIRATORY DYSFUNCTION IN PEDIATRIC NEUROLOGIC DISORDERS

John G. Brooks, M.D., and
Charles N. Swisher, M.D.

NEUROLOGICAL MECHANISMS OF RESPIRATORY DYSFUNCTION IN NEWBORN AND YOUNG INFANTS

A wide variety of respiratory problems of the newborn and young infant result from or are associated with neurological disease or dysfunction, or are a consequence of deviations from normal patterns of neurological development. The major emphasis in the first part of this chapter is on abnormalities in the control of respiration which are relatively unique to the newborn and young infant. Respiratory function of young patients can also be affected by many other neurological diseases such as intracranial hemorrhage, myasthenia gravis, muscular dystrophy, diaphragmatic paralysis, familial dysautonomia, and seizures.

Development of The Control of Breathing

The understanding of normal and abnormal patterns of the development of respiratory control involves the integration of developmental neurophysiology, anatomy, physiology, and neurochemistry. The pattern of respiration and the total minute ventilation at any time are the results of modulation of several factors including the output of the central respiratory "pacemaker" neurons, afferent activity from central and peripheral chemoreceptors, a variety of receptors in the lungs, upper airway, and chest wall, and varying degrees of cortical influence.

"Breathing" movements can be detected by ultrasonography in the human fetus as early as 11 to 14 weeks gestation. These respiratory efforts which are mainly isometric (minimal tidal exchange of fetal lung fluid), are very irregular early in gestation, but become progressively more regular at rates of 30 to 70 per min with increasing fetal maturation, and indicate fetal well-being. The breathing activity is intermittent and is associated with rapid eye movements and high frequency, low-voltage EEG patterns. In addition, there may be a second pattern of low-frequency (one to three per min) gasping respirations which indicate fetal distress. Functional carotid bodies, central carbon dioxide chemoreceptors, pulmonary stretch receptors, and possibly intrapulmonary irritant receptors have been demonstrated in fetal animals, although their influence on the presence, absence, or pattern of fetal respiratory activity is markedly less than their influence on respiratory control in a mature animal.

The increase in ventilation which occurs in response to hypercarbia is mediated by pH changes which are sensed by chemosensitive cells near the ventral surface of the medulla. These central chemoreceptor cells are functionally distinct from the primary respiratory neurons. The hypercapneic ventilatory response of the premature newborn, the full-term newborn, and the adult are remarkably similar in terms of sensitivity (change in ventilation per kilogram body weight per change in CO_2) and threshold (pCO_2 at which ventilation begins to increase). The sensitivity to CO_2 is slightly less in the premature than in the full-term newborn and adult, and threshold is slightly lower in newborn infants than in adults. The sensitivity differences may be largely due to changes in lung mechanics with growth, while the threshold changes probably reflect slightly lower serum bicarbonate levels in the newborn infant.

In contrast, the hypoxic ventilatory response, mediated primarily through the carotid bodies via the sinus nerve, changes markedly in the first month of life. During the first one to two weeks of life (possibly up to three weeks in prematurely born infants), the ventilatory response to hypoxia is biphasic. There is an initial one to two minute increase in ventilation followed by a return to control ventilation and then a fall of ventilation below control levels. This delayed ventilatory depression after three to five minutes of hypoxia is a reflection of decreased metabolic rate, so there is no associated elevation of pCO_2. The mechanism by which hypoxia depresses oxygen consumption in newborn infants is unknown. By one month of age, the normal adult hypoxic ventilatory response is seen, that is, sustained hyperventilation.

There are three types of vagally innervated mechanoreceptors in the lungs: (1) slowly adapting pulmonary stretch receptors, located within the airway smooth muscle, which inhibit inspiration in response to lung distention (Hering-Breuer reflex); (2) rapidly adapting pulmonary irritant receptors in the airway lining between epithelial cells, which cause rapid shallow breathing and/or cough in response to chemical or mechanical irritation, rapid changes in lung volume and probably lung deflation; (3) juxtapulmonary capillary receptors (J receptors), located in the wall of the pulmonary capillary, which may cause apnea in response to a variety of stimuli. The pulmonary stretch receptor-mediated inspiratory inhibition reflex (Hering-Breuer) increases in potency between 32 and 38 weeks post conception, and then wanes by one to four months after term to the relatively weak adult reflex which is not active during normal tidal breathing. Some of these apparent developmental changes may be due to the normal development of the mechanical properties of the lung and chest wall. Stimulation of pulmonary irritant receptors in premature human infants (less than 35 weeks post conceptional age) may cause a paradoxical slowing or cessation of respiration, in contrast to the stimulatory effect on ventilation seen in more mature subjects. Chest wall receptors (probably intercostal muscle spindles) which are probably involved in the increased respiratory effort response to respiratory loading, may have an absent or lesser effect on ventilation during the first one to two weeks of life. A variety of upper airway receptors, particularly those in the region of the larynx, have been identified which cause apnea, bradycardia and hypertension in response to chemical or mechanical stimulation, and have their afferent pathway through the superior laryngeal nerve or the trigeminal nerve. The apnea and bradycardia responses to chemical stimulation of the laryngeal receptors (probably free nerve endings in the epithelium) are more potent in the infant than in the adult animal, and, at least in some species, transiently increase in potency after birth before its decreasing to the adult reflex.[1-6]

Apnea of Prematurity

Recurrent apnea and periodic breathing are important clinical problems of premature infants. The incidence of apnea of prematurity is inversely related to birth weight, occurring in 25 percent of infants whose birth weight is less than 2,500 grams, and in 84 percent of infants whose birth weight is less than 1,000 grams. There are no absolute criteria for the diagnosis of apnea of prematurity, but characteristically, such infants are less than 36 weeks postconceptional age, and are between one day and two months' postnatal age. Most frequently, this clinical problem begins on the second or third day of life, and, when significant, is associated with bradycardia and often cyanosis. There are many causes of apnea in premature infants, and all specifically treatable causes must be ruled out before making a diagnosis of apnea of prematurity. The differential diagnosis includes sepsis, metabolic disorders (e.g., hypocalcemia, hypoglycemia, hyponatremia), seizure disorders, intracranial hemorrhage, congenital CNS anomalies, intermittent airway obstruction, hypoxia, abnormal body or environmental temperature, respiratory muscle weakness, congenital heart disease and iatrogenic causes such as oversedation or over or under hydration. The specific cause of apnea of prematurity is unknown although a variety of neurodevelopmental and neurochemical explanations have been suggested.

A reasonable approach to treating patients with apnea of prematurity, if it is associated with bradycardia or cyanosis, is first to measure arterial blood gases to insure that mild hypoxemia is not the cause, and to use tactile stimulation to re-initiate respiration. If recurrent episodes persist, some infants will respond to low levels (3-4 cm H_2O) of continuous positive airway pressure delivered by nasal prongs. There is some evidence that an oscillating waterbed may decrease the incidence of apnea in premature infants. If none of the above measures eliminates the apnea of prematurity, it is appropriate to initiate theophylline therapy (loading dose = 5.5 mg/kg, maintenance dose = 1.1 mg/kg per 8 hr). The theophylline should be discontinued every seven to ten days to determine whether the need still persists. Mechanical ventilation may be necessary in infants who do not respond to any of these measures, especially in very premature infants.[7,8]

Failure of Automatic Control of Ventilation (Ondine's Curse)

Failure of automatic ventilation can be either congenital or acquired. There are no clear-cut diagnostic criteria for this rare condition, but it generally is characterized by normal ventilation when the patient is awake and marked hypoventilation or apnea during sleep. In two reported infants the hypoventilation was limited to quiet sleep (Shannon et al.).[10] The only "successful" long-term therapy has been supportive mechanical ventilation during sleep. The use of aminophylline, doxapram, and long-term negative pressure ventilation, has not been successful. From the available literature, there is no evidence that congenitally affected infants will improve with age.[9,10]

Sudden Infant Death Syndrome

The Sudden Infant Death Syndrome (SIDS) is the largest single cause of postneonatal infant mortality, with an incidence of 1.5 to 2 per 1,000 live births in the United States, or a total of 5,000 to 10,000 deaths per year. There is a growing body of evidence which suggests that many SIDS deaths may be due to permanent or transient abnormalities of respiratory control.

The standard definition of SIDS is "the sudden death of any infant or young child, which is unexpected by history, and in which a thorough postmortem examination fails to demonstrate an adequate cause for death" (Second International SIDS Conference, 1969). Although this sounds like a diagnosis of exclusion, that is only partly so, since most cases of SIDS have a quite characteristic picture, as described below.

The epidemiology of SIDS has been reasonably well characterized. The most consistent characteristics (of key importance in assessing hypotheses of etiology) are the striking age distribution and the occurrence of the death during sleep. The great majority of SIDS deaths occur between two and four months of age. Ninety-one percent of these deaths occur in the first six months, yet only one percent occurs within the first two weeks of life. Since there is this striking postnatal increase in incidence before the incidence decreases after four months of age, the cause is not simple immaturity. Nearly all SIDS deaths occur during sleep, and more than 80 percent of them occur between midnight and 6 A.M. Other factors which are statistically associated with an increased risk of SIDS are male sex, low birth weight, low income, multiple births, and history of SIDS in a sibling. The incidence of SIDS decreases during the summer months.

A postmortem examination is essential in order to establish the diagnosis of SIDS, and to rule out the most common, non-SIDS etiologies for unexplained death in infancy such as meningitis, myocarditis, and intracranial hemorrhage. The SIDS victim is usually an apparently well-nourished, healthy infant, occasionally with a mild respiratory infection. The autopsy findings are mostly nonspecific, such as frothy fluid in the nares and mouth, pulmonary edema and/or vascular congestion, and sometimes mild pulmonary inflammation. The most consistent finding (reported in 87% of SIDS victims) is intrathoracic petechiae, especially on the surface of the thymus, pleura, and pericardium. The frequency of positive viral cultures taken at autopsy is higher than in a "control" population, with the recovery rate for nonpolio viruses of 23 to 42 percent in SIDS victims. In addition to the above-mentioned abnormalities which are evident on routine autopsy, findings consistent with recurrent or chronic hypoxemia prior to death have been identified through more detailed and specialized postmortem studies. Confirmed findings in SIDS victims include increased medial smooth muscle in pulmonary arterioles, increased retention of periadrenal brown fat, and increased extramedullary hematopoiesis.

More than one hundred etiologies for SIDS have been hypothesized but most have subsequently been repudiated. That the primary problem is a respiratory arrest followed by a secondary cardiac arrest is supported by the postmortem finding of very low oxygen tension in the blood of the left ventricle, and the finding of unclotted cardiac blood. Both of these findings indicate continued perfusion with extremely hypoxemic blood, suggesting that ventilation had ceased prior to loss of cardiac function. Currently, a great deal of interest is focused on several neurally mediated respiratory abnormalities, such as prolonged sleep apnea, decreased ventilatory sensitivity to carbon dioxide, upper airway obstruction, and intermittent, transient inhibition of respiratory drive as a result of stimulation of laryngeal chemoreceptors, as possible causes of SIDS. Steinschneider has described two infants with documented prolonged respiratory pauses during sleep, who subsequently were victims of SIDS. An increased frequency and duration of respiratory pauses during upper respiratory infections in apparently normal young infants has been documented in several studies. A decreased ventilatory sensitivity to inspired carbon dioxide has been reported in some patients with Nonfatal Apnea of Infancy (NAI), but this finding has not been confirmed. Upper airway obstruction from a variety of causes (e.g., choanal stenosis, cysts, vocal cord paralysis, small mandible, or a dynamic obstruction in infants with no apparent fixed upper airway narrowing) has been reported in apparently normal infants and those with a history of NAI. While some infants may experience apnea on the basis of mechanical or neurological mechanisms, the question remains as to why they would succumb to such a respiratory pause, rather than ultimately respond to the progressively increasing chemical drives to breathe. Studies in animals have shown that during REM sleep, the ventilatory response to CO_2 is depressed, as is the arousal response to hypoxia and hypercarbia. In addition, the respiratory inhibition which results from stimulation of laryngeal chemoreceptors is much more pronounced during REM sleep.

This laryngeal chemoreflex apnea originates in nerve endings around the larynx, its afferent pathway is via the superior laryngeal nerve, and the reflex response is apnea, bradycardia, hypertension, and swallowing. There is indirect evidence implicating this reflex, presumably stimulated by reflux of gastric contents, in the etiology of NAI and SIDS. Studies of this reflex in newborn animals have demonstrated its potentially fatal outcome as well as a postnatal increase and then decrease in its potency. Finally, however, it is important to re-emphasize that despite the existence of a number of plausible hypotheses, the etiology of SIDS has not yet been established.[11,12]

Nonfatal Apnea of Infancy

Because of its possible significance as a precursor of the Sudden Infant Death Syndrome, nonfatal apnea of infancy (NAI) ("near-miss SIDS", "aborted crib death") has recently become a subject of great interest. A recent task force of the American Academy of Pediatrics, preferring the designation "near-miss SIDS," has provided the following definition of this entity: "Cessation of breathing for 20 seconds or longer, or a briefer period associated with bradycardia, cyanosis or pallor." From the clinical standpoint, the pallor and cyanosis are most useful in many cases, since most of these spells occur out of the hospital where the heart rate is unknown, and the duration or presence of apnea is uncertain. Some infants included in this category may have had cyanosis without apnea, but all have had an episode which was frightening to the observers, whether lay or medical. The incidence of NAI is unknown, and its relationship to SIDS is unproven, although as a group these infants probably are at increased risk of succumbing to SIDS. Individual cases of NAI patients subsequently dying of autopsy-proven SIDS have been reported, and the concept of NAI as a precursor of SIDS is supported by the recent data indicating that SIDS victims have been exposed to chronic or recurrent hypoxemia prior to their death (see above).

The appropriate evaluation and therapy of infants with NAI is based on the types of diagnoses which have been directly or indirectly established in such patients (Table I). The minimal evaluation of such patients should include a

TABLE I
Possible Causes of Nonfatal Apnea of Infants

Laryngeal chemoreceptor apnea
Apnea of prematurity
Upper airway obstruction
Congenital heart disease
Seizure disorder
Breath-holding spells
Respiratory syncitial viral infection
Pertussis syndrome
Sleep apnea
Sepsis

careful history and physical exam with a complete and age-appropriate neurological exam, serum electrolytes, calcium, magnesium, glucose, complete blood count, chest x-ray, electrocardiogram and electroencephalogram. All patients should be continuously monitored for respiration and heart rate throughout their hospitalization. In addition, depending upon the clinical presentation, it is often appropriate to perform a variety of cultures, as well as arterial blood gases, laryngoscopy, barium swallow, echocardiogram, or esophageal pH monitoring.

Appropriate therapy for such patients has not been well established. It is clear that the families and other caretakers of all such patients should be instructed in mouth-to-mouth resuscitation, and that sympathetic counseling and emotional support must be provided for the families. Because of the possible contribution of chalasia to NAI, and the benign nature of the conservative treatment for chalasia, we have instituted elevation of the head of the bed (about 15 to 20 degrees depending on the age of the patient), and thickening of the formula in non-breast fed infants (up to 2 tablespoons of rice cereal per ounce of formula). When a specific cause or contributing factor, such as congenital heart disease, seizure disorder, anemia, and occasionally upper airway obstruction, is identified, appropriate specific therapy is instituted. Very rarely, surgical treatment of chalasia may be indicated. If there is no evidence of a seizure disorder, low-dose aminophylline therapy may be appropriate treatment for infants with apnea which appears to be due to laryngeal chemoreceptor stimulation, nonspecific sleep apnea or apnea of prematurity. Since there is a wide variability in the clearance rates of aminophylline in the age range of patients affected with NAI, relatively low doses (e.g., 1-2 mg per kilogram every 8-12 hours) should be used initially, especially in the younger patients. Home respiration and/or cardiac monitoring may be appropriate in selected, severely affected NAI patients, if an appropriate support system (medical, psychosocial, and technical) is readily available. It has not been clearly established that such home monitoring prevents deaths, although in most cases the families' reaction to the monitor has been very positive. The following are arbitrary criteria for home monitoring of patients with NAI when an appropriate support system is available (one of the following): (1) family history of SIDS or NAI, (2) recurrent apneic episodes requiring intervention, (3) extreme parenteral or physician anxiety. The incidence and severity of apneic episodes in these infants may be increased by infection (particularly respiratory infection), fever, immunization, and sleep deprivation or disruption of normal daily pattern. Arbitrary criteria for the discontinuation of home monitoring are (all of the following must be met): (1) the patient must be at least 6 months of age, (2) no significant apneic episode requiring intervention for at least two months, (3) the patient must have experienced an upper respiratory infection, and a DPT immunization without recurrence of clinically significant apnea. Finally, it is important to re-emphasize that the value of home monitoring has not been proven, and such a program should be undertaken only in centers prepared to provide appropriate support and collect and analyze relevant data to evaluate the efficacy of this mode of therapy. Similarly, it must be re-emphasized that there is no proof that most patients with NAI are at increased risk of SIDS.[13]

Vocal Cord Paralysis

Vocal cord paralysis can be unilateral or bilateral, congenital, or acquired. Vocal cord paralysis may occasionally be an isolated finding; however, it is associated more commonly with extralaryngeal abnormality, such as birth trauma, cerebral agenesis, severe retardation, or meningomyelocele. Unilateral vocal cord paralysis on the left may be due to intrathoracic problems causing irritation of or traction on the left recurrent laryngeal nerve. Vocal cord paralysis may present with varying degrees of inspiratory stridor or obstructive apnea. An artificial airway is usually required when the paralysis is bilateral, and only occasionally with unilateral paralysis. The diagnosis is established by direct laryngoscopy.

Patients with spina bifida and meningomyelocele may have bilateral vocal cord paralysis with intermittent apnea and cyanosis which are not eliminated by tracheotomy, indicating a central origin for the apnea. Such patients are also at increased risk for recurrent aspiration. Vocal cord paralysis may also occur in patients with Werdnig-Hoffman disease and patients with syringobulbia.[14,15]

NEUROLOGICAL MECHANISMS OF RESPIRATORY DYSFUNCTION IN CHILDREN FOLLOWING INFANCY

The second half of this chapter will be concerned with the spectrum of neurologic diseases and syndromes which produce respiratory dysfunction in child neurology. In considering the patterns of respiratory dysfunction in pediatric neurologic disorders, respiratory failure secondary to problems in the nervous system or neuromuscular system must be separated from both upper airway obstructive problems and cardiopulmonary failure. Upper airway obstruction includes such entities as choanal atresia, epiglottitis, laryngotracheitis, subglottic edema and stenosis, tracheal stenosis, avascular ring, foreign body aspiration, local neoplasm, or hypoplasia such as is seen in the Pierre Robin syndrome. Cardiopulmonary failure includes such conditions as status asthmaticus, bronchiolitis, cystic fibrosis, aspiration syndrome, near-drowning, inhalation burn, pneumonitis, pulmonary edema, hemorrhage, hypertension and contusion, and oxygen toxicity.[16] Without attempting an exhaustive treatment certain topics that are particularly illustrative of pediatric neurologic disorders will be discussed. Neuromuscular and peripheral nerve disorders are treated elsewhere in this book. An outline of the more common conditions contributing to respiratory dysfunction beyond the period of infancy is given in Table II.

In considering the neurologic causes of respiratory dysfunction in childhood it is of value to consider what clinical and laboratory criteria are relevant in assessing impending respiratory failure in infants and children. Table III illustrates these criteria (from Downes and Goldberg[16]). Close observation in an intensive care setting with the likelihood of endotracheal intubation or tracheostomy and ventilatory assistance is required for any child who meets their criteria.

Congenital Malformations

A number of congenital malformations produce characteristic disorders of respiration related to underlying neurologic mechanisms. The Arnold-Chiari malformation can produce intermittent apnea and cyanosis related to disruption in brainstem pathways. Likewise, the Dandy-Walker syndrome, a cystic fourth ventricle and hydrocephalus associated with agenesis of the cerebellar vermis, can also be associated with respiratory problems. This combination of abnormalities can produce interference with the medullary respiratory centers and can lead to respiratory failure as a cause of death. In addition, monitoring of respiration in a four-day-old infant with this syndrome demonstrated apneustic and cluster breathing and numerous apneic episodes, which suggested a lesion in the lower pons.[17]

A variant of this malformation has been reported to result in a pattern of periodic hyperpnea. One family has been described in which four affected siblings have partial

TABLE II
Conditions Contributing to Respiratory Dysfunction in Pediatric Neurology

Congenital malformities	Cerebral hypoxia
Trauma	Encephalopathy
Exogenous toxins	Breath holding and seizures
Infections	Neuropathy
Degenerative disorders	Tumors
Myopathy	Motor neuron disease
Dysautonomia	

TABLE III
Criteria of Respiratory Failure in Infants and Children With Neuromuscular Disease (Downes and Goldberg)

Clinical
- Weak to absent cough reflex
- Weak to absent gag reflex
- Incompetent swallowing mechanism
- Pooled oropharyngeal secretions

Physiologic
- Vital Capacity < 12 ml/kg
- $P_aO_2 < 60$ torr (IN AIR)

NOTE: Two clinical plus one physiologic criteria = impending respiratory failure.

Data taken with permission from Downes, J.J., and Goldberg, A.I.: Airway management, mechanical ventilation, and cardiopulmonary resuscitation. In Scarpelli, E.M., et al. (eds.): *Pulmonary Disease of the Fetus, Newborn and Child.* Philadelphia, Lea & Febiger, 1978.

or complete agenesis of the cerebellar vermis which is associated with episodic hyperpnea, abnormal eye movements, ataxia, and retardation. The episodes of hyperpnea lasted for 12 to 16 seconds and the respiratory rate ranged from 120 to 170 per minute alternating with 5 to 12 second periods of apnea. This breathing pattern resembled cluster breathing. Rotatory nystagmus was present on conjugate gaze and myoclonic movements and profound hypotonia were present. However, other cases of agenesis of the vermis have not been reported to have respiratory abnormalities.[18]

Another rare congenital malformation associated with respiratory dysfunction and brainstem pathology was observed by Axley and Swisher.[19] A full-term infant was noted to have the Moebius syndrome with absence of eye abduction, rigid closure of the jaw, and absence of facial, tongue and sternocleidomastoid activity. In addition, there was a bilateral talipes equinovarus deformity and partial syndactyly of the fingers of the right hand. Throughout the hospital stay, the child was noted to be cyanotic in room air without retractions. X-rays showed a bell-shaped configuration to the thorax and an absence of pulmonary pathology sufficient to explain the respiratory distress. The patient expired at 65 hours of life. At autopsy (Fig. 1), in addition to the congenital absence of the XII cranial nerves and hypoplasia of the hypoglossal nuclei, there was "pseudocalcium," extracerebral crystals, a mild astrogliosis and microgliosis which suggested that an intrauterine inflammatory process had occurred affecting the brainstem. Viral studies were negative.

In addition to congenital malformations involving brainstem structures within the posterior fossa, malformations of the cervical spine can also cause respiratory problems. A child has been reported with a 17q+ chromosomal abnormality and an associated severe atlantoaxial dislocation secondary to odontoid process hypoplasia. Transient respiratory arrests occurred because of cervical cord compression. Atlantoaxial malformation exists with a variety of skeletal dysplasias and must be searched for as a treatable cause of respiratory dysfunction in children with these syndromes.[20]

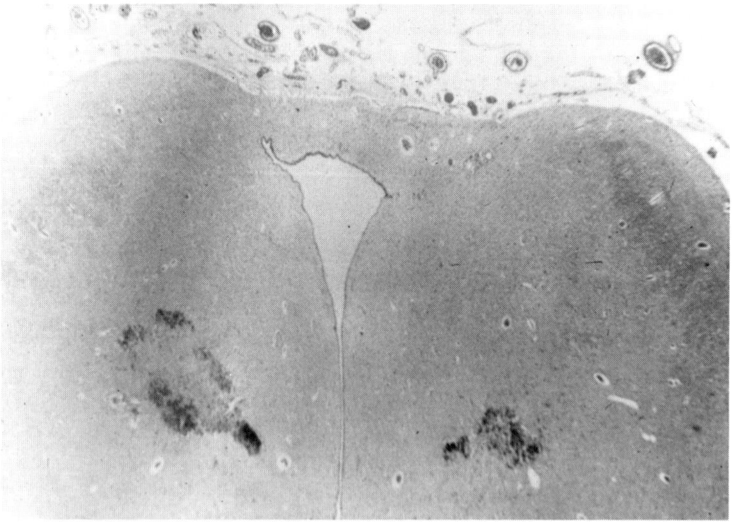

Figure 1. Section of brainstem in patient with Moebius syndrome and respiratory failure illustrating extracellular "pseudocalcium" in the tegmental areas of the rostral pons.

Trauma

A characteristic form of birth trauma associated with breech delivery and which affects respiration is injury to the spinal cord. This trauma appears to be related to unphysiologic forces on the fetus during the course of delivery, particularly longitudinal stretching, torsion, and excessive flexion of the neck. Intrauterine hyperextension of the head in breech position has been found to have a particularly ominous outcome as transection of the spinal cord occurred in 25 percent of these cases when vaginal delivery occurred.[21] Infants with a high cord transection demonstrate marked hypotonicity at birth with a weak cry and a diaphragmatic breathing pattern.

In addition to the classic pattern of injury associated with fracture-dislocation of the vertebrae in association with blunt trauma or extreme flexion or hyperextension of the neck, another form of spinal cord injury has been reported in childhood in association with minor trauma. This can present with a delayed syndrome beginning with flaccid weakness of both arms evolving to flaccid quadriplegia. Ischemic infarction of the cervical cord and low medulla has been demonstrated, presumably related to occlusion of the anterior spinal artery.[22] In addition to spinal cord injury, head injury can, of course, result in respiratory complications either as a result of direct involvement of brainstem structures or secondary vascular phenomena.

Reye's Encephalopathy

Reye's encephalopathy is a condition occurring in infancy and childhood characterized by a prodromal febrile illness frequently associated with epidemic influenza B or sporadic occurrence of varicella. There is an initial state of stupor and delirium, a later encephalopathic stage with coma, and a recovery phase. There is associated vomiting, delirium, coma, hepatomegaly, an SGOT over 50 μg/ml, an ammonia level over 125 μg/100 ml (although this varies), and a prolonged prothrombin time. Hyperventilation is very common and may precede the onset of coma. It has been observed in 85 percent of cases and is present in almost all children who progress to deep coma. Respirations are rapid, regular, and deep, resembling the breathing pattern of diabetic ketoacidosis. However, while the respiratory compensation for metabolic acidosis is a factor in some children, in the majority, the hyperventilation appears to be secondary to excessive direct stimulation of medullary respiratory centers, with development of respiratory alkalosis.[23] Death occurs by respiratory failure usually in association with profound cerebral edema and no CNS inflammatory response. Periodic breathing, ataxic breathing, or apneusis usually precedes the respiratory arrest.

In infants under six months of age, the clinical picture of Reye's encephalopathy is less characteristic. The most prominent clinical findings include marked respiratory abnormalities with tachypnea and apneic episodes. Vomiting is not the striking finding noted in older children, and there is a rather sudden onset of respiratory distress, usually tachypnea, followed rapidly by seizures and coma. In a review of 51 cases under 10 months of age, apneic episodes were noted in all but one of the infants during the acute phase of the illness.[24]

BREATH-HOLDING SPELLS AND SEIZURES IN CHILDHOOD

The relationship of breath-holding spells in children to underlying neurological phenomena is still a matter of some conjecture. The more severe of these spells are characterized by an initial episode of anger, fear, or injury followed by a cry. After the first few cries, the child gasps, begins holding the breath, and subsequently becomes either pallid or cyanotic. Following this, the child becomes rigid, suffers impairment of consciousness, and assumes an opisthotonic posture. Associated clonic activity is frequently seen. The duration of the episode is almost always brief, seldom lasting more than a minute. Episodes are rarely seen after age six.[25]

Proposed mechanisms for these episodes have included psychogenic factors, reduced cerebral blood flow secondary to increased intrathoracic pressure associated with a spontaneous Valsalva maneuver, glottic spasm, and cerebral anoxia associated with asystole. Additionally, a high familial incidence has been noted by several authors which might suggest some inherited pathophysiologic mechanism of cardiac or respiratory regulation. An experimental study of ocular compression in children with a past history of breath-holding spells compared to a group of age-matched controls has demonstrated a hypersensitive cardiac inhibitory reflex, presumably mediated via the vagus nerve.[26]

Seizures can be distinguished from breath-holding spells since seizures in childhood do not usually have a sharply delineated precipating factor, do not usually follow crying, are not associated with an early pattern of cyanosis, and are usually associated with a disordered EEG, while the EEG in breath-holding spells is almost always normal in the interictal period.[25]

Apneic seizures do occur in childhood and consist of attacks of intermittent respiratory arrest which may or may not be followed by other types of seizure activity. They are most frequently associated in the neonatal period with structural or metabolic disorders and may reflect immaturity of respiratory organization in the brainstem. Apneic seizures occurring in older children originate in the limbic system and often are interspersed with psychomotor seizures.[27]

Infections

The spectrum of respiratory dysfunction in central nervous system infections of childhood is a constantly changing one. While poliomyelitis was certainly the most prevalent CNS infection producing respiratory problems in children within the memories of many readers of this book, it has been relegated to the status of a medical curiosity at this time due to modern preventive medicine. It now appears in populations with religious objections to immunization or in immunized children with previously unrecognized immunodeficiency.

The syndrome of infant botulism and respiratory dysfunction has become more widely recognized. The clinical pattern of infant botulism is that of healthy infants who over a period of one to two days lose the ability to suck and swallow and become profoundly weak. Cranial nerve abnormalities include ptosis, a sluggish pupillary light reflex, and decreased extraocular motility. Of nine patients reported from California, three had respiratory arrests, but all recovered with appropriate supportive care. Extensive epidemiological studies have not identified any source of intoxication. Ingestion of ubiquitous *C. botulinum* spores appears to be the source of in vitro toxin production in the infant gut. It is recommended that specimens of blood and stool be sent for identification of botulinal toxin when the above polyneuropathic picture presents in infancy.[28]

Respiratory dysfunction can accompany encephalitis, meningitis, and brain abscess both by direct involvement of brainstem structures and by secondary pressure associated with cerebral edema. Likewise, spinal cord involvement can produce respiratory embarrassment either intrinsically in acute transverse myelitis or extrinsically as a result of a spinal epidural abscess. The Guillain-Barré syndrome has been discussed elsewhere in this volume and also occurs frequently in children, particularly in association with infectious mononucleosis. Brainstem encephalitis is a form of viral infection of the central nervous system in children with a particular predilection for the midbrain, pons, and medulla. Multiple cranial nerve signs, ataxia, and corticospinal tract signs occur in this condition which can resemble a pontine glioma in its signs, and even its radiographic appearance with medullary enlargement, but the history of onset is usually more acute and fulminant.[29] Full recovery is possible so supportive management should be aggressive, including respirator management of apnea.

Degenerative and Metabolic Disease in Childhood

Several disorders characterized by progressive loss of function in childhood have respiratory problems as a result of their pathophysiology. One rare form is progressive bulbar paralysis in childhood, or Fazio-Londe's disease. This condition results in a progressive dissolution of motor function in the brainstem which in the child usually signals a neoplasm. In this case, there is an underlying degeneration of motor nuclei of unknown cause, resulting in difficult respiration associated with stridor, paretic vocal cords, apnea, and generalized hypotonia. In addition to involvement of cranial nerve nuclei III, IV, VI, VII, X, and XII, there is diffuse degeneration of the neurons in the ventral horns of the cervical cord. This is a familial disease with autosomal dominant inheritance, and fortunately rare.[30]

While the pathophysiology of the degeneration in Fazio-Londe's disease is little understood, some understanding of the brainstem dysfunction in Leigh's encephalopathy (necrotizing encephalomyelopathy) is developing. This condition is characterized by the appearance in infancy of anorexia, diaphoresis, deafness, optic atrophy, abnormal pupillary responses and irregular eye movements, and spasticity. In a series of 50 cases, respiratory signs were noted in 40 percent. Respiratory abnormalities varied, including descriptions of dyspnea, apnea, tachypnea, Cheyne-Stokes respirations, central neurogenic hyperventilation, and ataxic respiration. These types of respiratory patterns are consistent with brainstem or thalamic disease or with a metabolic abnormality. Periods of hyperventilation appear to be the most common type of respiratory abnormality. Ondine's Curse has recently been noted as an associated finding.[31]

Respiratory studies have demonstrated, in the presence of profound sleep apnea, that expiratory volumes over time do not rise beyond the normal range in the face of an elevated pCO_2. Failure of respiratory drive is not due to CO_2 unresponsiveness. Lung compliance is normal. Theophylline produces no changes in physiological measurements or clinical state.[32] Of 86 cases reported of Leigh's encephalopathy, 78 were under 24 months of age and 52 under 12 months of age. The condition is known to involve an inborn error of metabolism involving thiamine utilization, and an inhibitor of thiamine pyrophosphate has been found in the body fluids of patients with the syndrome.[33]

Another metabolic disorder with a more delineated biochemical etiology is maple syrup urine disease, characterized by an abnormal metabolism of leucine, isoleucine, and valine. The clinical pattern is that of an infant who is normal at birth but who (with feeding of exogenous amino acids) by five or six days of age, develops feeding difficulties, a weak suck, diminished responsiveness, and within a few days is moribund. Shallow respirations and intermittent cyanosis are frequent, and respiratory arrest may occur. The urine has a striking maple syrup odor, and the underlying pathology is that of retardation of myelinization and a spongy degeneration affecting predominantly the white matter.[34]

Of the glycogenoses, or disorders characterized by the storage of glycogen, only Pompe's disease (Cori type II α 1,4 glucosidase deficiency) has striking respiratory failure. The infant progresses well for a month or more, and then loses motor skills. There is, in addition to decreased spontaneous movements and absent deep tendon reflexes by the fourth or fifth month, a progression to flaccid paralysis with pharyngeal pooling of saliva, cyanosis, and difficulty with feeding. Together with a weak cough, this leads to pneumonia with cardiac failure and death by the end of the first year of life. It is difficult to say how much of the respiratory problem may be solely due to the cardiac failure associated with storage of glycogen in cardiac muscle and how much may be due to the storage of glycogen in Clarke's column, the brainstem reticular formation, the olives, and other brainstem nuclei, as the glycogen storage is much less destructive to neurons than the lipid storage in the various lipidoses.[35] It should be noted that respiratory signs of neurologic origin appear to be less striking in the lipidoses despite the universal distension of neurons in the brain and spinal cord with lipid.

A storage disease where respiratory findings are more striking is Gaucher's disease, where glucocerebroside is deposited in neurons. However, Gaucher's is unique in that neuronal destruction is more pronounced than lipid storage, and loss of neurons is widespread through brainstem and cord and in particular the pontine tegmentum.[35] This loss of brainstem neurons in Gaucher's disease is associated with a variety of respiratory problems including laryngospasm, dyspnea, spastic coughing, and dysphagia.

Tumors

In contrast to the pattern in adults, primary intracranial tumors in childhood are predominantly infratentorial involving the cerebellum and brainstem. This leads to early aqueductal obstruction and brainstem dysfunction. As intracranial pressure increases, the central syndrome of herniation occurs with pressure exerted centrally on the diencephalon with initially frequent sighing respiration followed by ataxic breathing leading to apnea. A variety of specific breathing patterns can occur depending on the brainstem level affected, including central neurogenic hyperventilation, apneusis, and cluster breathing.[36] The association of such breathing patterns with medulloblastomas and pontine and cerebellar gliomas has been recognized. Recently, a child with tuberous sclerosis has been described with a hamartoma in the anterior inferior aspect of the pons demonstrated by pneumoencephalography. He demonstrated a persistent cyclic respiratory pattern consisting of prolonged apnea which occasionally triggered syncope or a generalized seizure, followed by hyperventilation. Increasing inspired CO_2 did not alter the respiratory pattern.[37]

Familial Dysautonomia

Familial dysautonomia is a condition characterized by poor feeding at birth, failure to produce overflow tears with the usual stimuli, absent or hypoactive deep tendon reflexes, an absent corneal reflex, postural hypotension, emotional lability, relative insensitivity to pain, and absence of fungiform papillae on the tongue. There is the laboratory finding of an absence of flare with intradermal histamine. Respiratory problems are aggravated by a dysphagia, with a primary defect in the functioning of the cricopharyngeus, similar to other patients with brainstem lesions.[38] The gag reflex is often absent or sluggish. Breath-holding is common in the first two years of life and is usually precipitated by emotional excitement. A relative insensitivity to hypoxia and hypercapnia has been demonstrated.[39] There is marked reduction in sympathetic postganglionic neurons and peripheral axons as well as norepinephrine, but pathologic findings are variable.

REFERENCES

1. Berger, A.G., et al.: Regulation of respiration. *N. Eng. J. Med.* **297**:93, 1977.
2. Wyman, R.J.: Neural generation of the breathing rhythm. *Ann. Rev. Physiol.* **39**:417–448, 1977.

3. Chernick, V.: Fetal breathing movements. *Sem. Perinat.* **1**:339–342, 1977.
4. Rigatto, H.: Respiratory control and apnea in the newborn infant. *Crit. Care Med.* **5**:2–9, 1977.
5. Woodrum, D.E., et al.: Development of respiratory control mechanisms in the fetus and newborn. In Hodson, W.A. (ed.): *Development of the Lung.* New York, Marcel Dekker, Inc., 1977, pp. 561–585.
6. Angell-James, J.E., and Daly, M.: Some aspects of upper respiratory tract reflexes. *Acta Otolaryng.* **79**:242–252, 1975.
7. Rigatto, H.: Apnea and periodic breathing. *Sem. Perinat.* **1**:375–381, 1977.
8. Naeye, R.L.: Neonatal apnea: Underlying disorders. *Pediatrics* **63**:8–12, 1979.
9. Mellins, R.B., Blafour, H.H., Jr., Turino, G.M., and Winters, R.W.: Failure of automatic control of ventilation (Ondine's Curse). Report of an infant born with this syndrome and review of the literature. *Medicine* **49**:487, 1970.
10. Shannon, D.C., Marsland, D.W., Gould, J.B., et al.: Central hypoventilation during quiet sleep in two infants. *Pediatrics* **57**:342–346, 1976.
11. Naeye, R.L.: The sudden infant death syndrome: A review of recent advances. *Arch. Pathol. Lab. Med.* **101**:165–167, 1977.
12. Valdes-Dapena, M.A.: Sudden unexplained death 1970–1975. An evolution in understanding. DHEW publication No. (HSA) 76-5255. Rockville, Md., 1978.
13. Kelley, D.H., et al.: Care of infants with near-miss sudden infant death syndrome. *Pediatrics* **61**:511, 1978.
14. Hollinger, P.C., et al.: Respiratory obstruction and apnea in infants with bilateral abductor vocal cord paralysis, meningomyelocele, hydrocephalus and Arnold-Chiari malformation. *J. Pediat.* **92**:368–373, 1978.
15. Cavanagh, F.: Vocal cord palsies in children. *J. Laryng. Otol.* **69**:399, 1955.
16. Downes, J.J., and Goldberg, A.I.: Airway management, mechanical ventilation, and cardiopulmonary resuscitation. In Scarpelli, E.M., et al. (eds.): *Pulmonary Disease of the Fetus, Newborn and Child.* Philadelphia, Lea and Febiger, 1978.
17. Krieger, A.J., et al.: Respiration in an infant with the Dandy-Walker syndrome. *Neurology* **24**:1064–1067, 1974.
18. Joubert, M., et al.: Familial agenesis of the cerebellar vermis. A syndrome of episodic hyperpnea, abnormal eye movements, ataxia, and retardation. *Neurology* **19**:813–825, 1969.

19. Axley, J.H., and Swisher, C.N.: Respiratory failure in the Moebius Syndrome. Read by title, Child Neurology Society meeting, Nashville, Tenn., October, 1973.
20. Todorov, A.B., and Lenn, N.J.: Atlantoaxial dislocation in a 17q+ child. Read by title. Child Neurology Society meeting, Monterey, Cal., October, 1976.
21. Bresnan, M.J., and Abroms, I.F.: Neonatal spinal cord transection secondary to intrauterine hyperextension of the neck in breech presentation. *J. Pediat.* **84**:734–737, 1974.
22. Ahmann, P.A., et al.: Spinal cord infarction following minor trauma in childhood. Read at Child Neurology meeting, Nashville, Tennessee, October, 1973.
23. Huttenlocher, P.R., and Trauner, D.A.: Reye's syndrome. In Vinken, P.J., and Bruyn, G.W. (eds.): *Handbook of Clinical Neurology,* vol. 29. Amsterdam, North Holland, 1977.
24. Huttenlocher, P.R., and Trauner, D.A.: Reye's syndrome in infancy. *Pediatrics* **62**:84–90, 1978.
25. Livingston, S.: Breathholding spells in children, differentiation from epileptic attacks. *J.A.M.A.* **212**:2231–2235, 1970.
26. Lombroso, C.T., and Lerman, P.: Breathholding spells (cyanotic and pallid infantile syncope). *Pediatrics* **39**:563–581, 1967.
27. Solomon, G.E., and Plum, F.: *Clinical Management of Seizures.* Philadelphia, W.B. Saunders Co., 1976.
28. Berg, B.O.: The syndrome of infant botulism. *Pediatrics* **59**:321–322, 1977.
29. Schain, R.J., and Wilson, G.: Brainstem encephalitis with radiologic evidence of medullary enlargement. *Neurology* **21**:537–539, 1971.
30. Gomez, M.R., et al.: Progressive bulbar paralysis in childhood (Fazio-Londe's Disease). *Arch. Neurol.* **6**:317–323, 1962.
31. Dooling, E.C., and Richardson, E.P.: Ophthalmoplegia and Ondine's curse. *Arch. Ophthal.* **95**:1790–1793, 1977.
32. Lott, I.T., and Shannon, D.C.: Central respiratory pathophysiology of Leigh's disease. Read by title, Child Neurology Society, Dillon, Col., September, 1978.
33. David, R.B., et al.: Necrotizing encephalomyelopathy (Leigh). In Vinken, P.J., and Bruyn, G.W. (eds.): *Handbook of Clinical Neurology,* vol. 28. Amsterdam, North Holland, 1976.
34. Moser, H.W.: Maple syrup urine disease. In Vinken, P.J., and Bruyn, G.W. (eds.): *Handbook of Clinical Neurology,* vol. 29. Amsterdam, North Holland, 1977.
35. Friede, R.L.: *Developmental Neuropathology.* New York, Springer-Verlag, 1975.

36. Plum, F., and Posner, J.B.: *The Diagnosis of Stupor and Coma,* 2nd Ed., Philadelphia, F.A. Davis Co., 1972.
37. Sackellares, J.C., et al.: "Apneic seizures" in a tuberous sclerosis patient with a pontine lesion. Read by title, Child Neurology Society meeting, Monterey, Cal., October, 1976.
38. Margulies, S.I., et al.: Familial dysautonomia: A cineradiographic study of the swallowing mechanism. *Radiology* **90**:107–112, 1968.
39. Filler, J., et al.: Respiratory control in familial dysautonomia. *J. Pediat.* **66**:509–516, 1965.

13

Respiratory Dysfunction in Neurosurgical Practice

Charles M. D'Angelo, M.D.

Most respiratory complications in neurological surgery present as atelectasis, pneumonia, and embolism. However, unlike other surgical specialties, small alterations in blood oxygen and carbon dioxide can produce dramatic devastating changes in the neurosurgical patient. Respiratory complications have been noted in more than 50 percent of patients with neuromedical and neurosurgical disorders.[34] This fact alone mandates an understanding of the interaction between respiratory function and neurosurgical disorders. An understanding of respiratory function also can assist neurological diagnosis and treatment. Neuroanatomic knowledge of the respiratory system often localizes the region of neurological dysfunction in patients with respiratory aberrations. The excellent correlation of respiratory patterns and neuraxis lesions by Plum and Posner[64] should be required reading for any physician caring for neurosurgical patients.

Physician manipulation of respiratory function is an important adjunct in neuroanesthesia and postoperative neurosurgical care. The pulmonary specialist must consider the special problems imposed by the neurosurgical patient. Injudicious use of intermittent positive pressure breathing can decrease jugular venous draining and increase intracranial pressure[74] in patients with head injury or contaminate the subarachnoid space with nasal pathogens in patients with basal skull fractures.[40]

In this chapter, respiratory dysfunction and complications encountered in the practice of clinical neurosurgery will be reviewed.

GENERAL CONSIDERATIONS

The rigid cranial vault has an approximate volume of 1200 to 1400 cc. The contents, 85 percent cerebral tissue and water, 10 percent cerebrospinal fluid, and 5 percent blood, are essentially noncompressible. If additional mass is added to the intracranial compartment, whether neoplasm, hematoma, or edema fluid, it is initially accommodated without increasing intracranial pressure by removal of cerebrospinal fluid or blood and normal intracranial pressure is maintained. Once maximum compensation is reached, further volume increases even if quite small, can cause a sudden increase in intracranial pressure.[18]

Pulmonary complications which produce increased intrathoracic pressure, hypoxia, or hypercapnea can increase intracranial pressure. Intracranial pressure monitoring has shown that pressure changes in the thoracic cavity are transmitted to the cerebral subarachnoid space.[45,74] Increased intrathoracic pressure increases intracranial pressure by reducing venous return in the jugular venous system. Variations in P_aco_2 cause profound changes in cerebral blood flow and intracranial pressure. As P_aco_2 levels are elevated by reduced ventilation, cerebral vasodilatation, cerebral blood flow, and cerebral vascular volume increase. The result is increased intracranial pressure. Reduced P_aco_2 also increases cerebral blood flow, which can result in increased intracranial pressure. When both P_aco_2 and P_ao_2 are reduced, low oxygen tension predominates and vasodilatation and increased intravascular volume occur.[15,39]

Normally, small increases in intravascular volume will not increase intracranial pressure. However, following trauma or when maximal compensation of an intracranial mass has already occurred, the small increase in intracranial volume produced by respiratory dysfunction can cause devastating neurological complications.

SUPRATENTORIAL DISORDERS

Supratentorial Mass Lesions

Although changes in respiratory rate and pattern have been reported with midline frontal and hypothalamic lesions,[4,77] the majority of neurosurgical supratentorial lesions affect respiration by increasing intracranial pressure.[82]

As supratentorial masses expand and cerebral shifts develop, there is progressive compromise of the diencephalon, pons, and medulla. With downward herniation of the diencephalon, as the patient becomes somnolent, the normal respiratory pattern is interrupted by occasional deep sighs and pauses. If continued dislocation of the diencephalon occurs, Cheyne-Stokes respirations may develop. Progression to central neurogenic hyperventilation occurs as uncal herniation and vascular compromise of the midbrain develop. Hyperventilation is replaced by a more or less regular breathing pattern, although shallow, as the lower pons and upper medulla become involved. Lower medullary dysfunction is evidenced by respiration which is irregular in depth and rate, and interrupted by deep, prolonged sighs and gasps. These agonal respirations are followed quickly by respiratory arrest as medullary respiratory centers fail. Vasomotor and cardiac function can be maintained for hours or days by assisted respiration.

Reducing Intracranial Pressure

A therapeutic adjunct to osmotic diuretics and glucocorticoids in the treatment of intracranial hypertension is controlled hyperventilation. In 1962 Hayes and Slocum[32] advocated controlled hyperventilation of minute volumes 20 percent to 50 percent above normal to reduce intracranial bulk at surgery. The reduction of intracranial pressure is greater when the intracranial pressure is high and when mass lesions are present.[7] Hyperventilation has negligible effects when intracranial pressure is normal. Although many authorities agree as to the efficiency of hyperventilation in reducing brain bulk, intracranial pressure, and intracerebral blood volume,[52] Rosomoff's experiments in dogs indicate that the reduction may be more apparent than real.[70,71] In his studies 30 minutes of hyperventillation to an arterial pH of 7.59 and a P_aCO_2 of 20 mmHg did not change the volume of brain water or solids. The decreased intracerebral blood volume was countered by a proportional increase in cerebrospinal fluid volume. Nevertheless, controlled hyperventillation may be a lifesaving procedure in patients with severe intracranial hypertension. In such patients, even a small reduction of intracranial volume will cause a profound fall in intracranial pressure and, at the present time, hyperventilation is the most rapid, simple method of reducing intracranial volume.[46,75]

Complications of Hyperventilation

Hyperventilatory treatment of increased intracranial pressure is not without complications, both real and theoretical. Hypoxic cerebral damage secondary to hypocapnic cerebral vasoconstriction and shifts of the hemoglobin dissociation curve is possible. Hyperventilation with room air produces increased lactate-pyruvate ratios indicative of tissue hypoxia.[1] The biochemical changes are reversed if pure oxygen or hyperbaric oxygen is used.[67] Controlled hyperventilation for therapeutic purposes does not appear to produce long-term effects as long as P_aCO_2 is kept above 25 mmHg and adequate oxygen is inspired.[50] However, because most experiments have been performed on young healthy patients, long-term or delayed complications in the patient with a damaged brain cannot be completely excluded.[51]

Neurogenic (Cephalogenic) Pulmonary Edema

Acute pulmonary edema, in the absence of cardiac disease, has been observed with patients with acute increases of intracranial pressure.[21] Neither the etiology nor mechanism of neurogenic pulmonary edema is completely understood. Neither the absolute level of intracranial pressure, nor the rate of change, appears to be the sole catalytic determinant. The increased intracranial pressure probably initiates a sympathetic pressure response with increased venous return, increased peripheral resistance, and increased myocardial contractions. The sudden shift of blood from a high resistance systemic system to a low resistance pulmonary system results in increased capillary permeability, edema, and parenchymal hemorrhages.[28,81] Treatment with alpha-adrenergic blockade or rapid cranial decompression has been less than satisfactory.

Pituitary Surgery

Transnasal, transphenoidal surgery for pituitary lesions has become a popular procedure in many neurosurgical clinics. Following excision of the tumor or the pituitary gland itself, the sella turcica and sphenoid sinus are packed routinely with fat to obliterate any communication between the intracranial subarachnoid space and the nasal cavity. Postoperative use of intermittent positive pressure breathing (IPPB) creates a potential hazard of dislodging the sinus packing and contaminating the subarachnoid cerebrospinal fluid with oropharyngeal pathogens.[40,62] Accordingly, postoperative intermittent positive pressure breathing should be avoided in the patient undergoing transphenoidal surgery of the pituitary gland. Patients should be encouraged to deep-breathe and should receive moisturized air by mask if they need it.

POSTERIOR FOSSA DISORDERS

Cerebellopontine Angle Tumors

Improvements in the binocular surgical microscope, microsurgical instruments, and anesthetic techniques have greatly reduced the mortality and morbidity following surgical excision of cerebellopontine angle acoustic tumors, meningiomas, and metastatic tumors.[59,66] As a result of advanced ventilatory support techniques, intraoperative respiratory deaths are rare. However, air embolus in the sitting position can still occur.[38] Respiratory distress may be present in the immediate postoperative period as a result of vigorous dissection to free a tumor capsule from the brainstem[58] or as a result of damage to the anterior-inferior cerebellar artery.[3] The arterial damage may result in infarction of the lateral pontine tegmental area. The upright surgical position, with the neck flexed, can produce laryngeal edema or atelectasis of the left lung if the endotracheal tube slips into the right main-stem bronchus.[65] These occurrences are additional etiologies for labored respirations observed in the recovery room. Postoperative epidural or subdural hemorrhage, cerebellar hemorrhage, or cerebellar swelling may compromise the brainstem and produce sudden respiratory arrest.[61]

Atelectasis and pneumonia remain a hazard for two to three weeks following surgery. Aspiration pneumonia may occur in ten percent of the patients.[65] Although some of the delayed pulmonary complications are due to a depressed level of consciousness, most are due to damage to the glossopharyngeal-vagal outflow with resulting dysphagia and suppressed cough and gag reflexes.[60] Repeated suctioning is necessary to rid the patient of his own secretions. Vigorous suctioning can cause pharyngeal hemorrhage and further compromise respiratory function.[65] Prolonged dysphagia may necessitate gastrostomy.

Traumatic Hemorrhage

Intracerebellar hematomas and extradural and subdural hematomas of the posterior fossa may produce gradual compression or ischemia of the brainstem. Along with irregular pulse and fluctuating blood pressure, there may be apneustic, cluster or ataxia respirations.[9,16,47,64] Similar patterns of irregular respirations may be seen with direct contusions of the brainstem.[64]

CERVICOMEDULLARY JUNCTION

Foramen Magnum Tumors

In addition to disturbing function of the eleventh and twelfth cranial nerves, neoplasms of the foramen magnum compress the lower medulla and upper cervical spinal cord. Respiratory distress, especially when the neck is flexed,[20] has been reported. Because postoperative bulbar failure with respiratory failure occurs frequently following excision of these anteriorly placed tumors,[10] some neurosurgeons recommend prophylactic tracheostomy.[29]

SPINAL CORD DYSFUNCTION

Spinal Cord Neoplasms

Primary or metastatic spinal cord tumors may compromise the spinal cord by direct compression, blockage of vascular supply or drainage, or extradural encirclement. Early respiratory distress with loss of diaphragmatic excursions may occur with cervical tumors, which are cephalad to the fifth cervical segment. Elevation of the chest by the sternomastoid and trapezius muscles, suboccipital pain, and cervical spasm may be diagnostic of a high cervical mass.[30] Tumors caudad to the fifth cervical segment do not carry the same respiratory risks. Spinal cord compression caudal to the fifth cervical segment compromises intercostal function, but spares diaphragmatic function. With each inspiration the abdomen expands and the chest retracts. With progressive spinal cord compression meteorism may result from intestinal paralysis and increase respiratory distress because excursions of the diaphragm are restricted.[31]

Surgical removal of spinal cord tumors is most dangerous in the cervical area because of possible injury to the phrenic outflow system. Indeed, the majority of deaths during surgery or in the immediate postoperative period have been due to respiratory failure.[24,85] Tachypnea, hypotension and hyperthermia responsive to sympathomimetic agents have been reported following tumor removal in the cervical area.[35] Other autonomic aberrations, including gastric dilatation with respiratory distress, have been reported following surgery for cervical spinal cord tumors.[69]

Syringobulbia and Syringomyelia

Primary alveolar hypoventilation and sleep-induced apnea have been reported with syringomyelia and syringobulbia. There is loss of normal sensitivity to hypercapnea and hypoxemia. The patients present with hypoventilation, lethargy, headache, and papilledema.[26,34]

Spinal Cord Injuries

There are no accurate figures reflecting the overall incidence of spinal cord injury in the United States. However, approximately 10,000 unfortunate individuals are rendered quadriplegic or paraplegic each year.[83] Most injuries involve the cervical spine, especially the atlantoaxial junction and lower three cervical vertebra. The damage to the contained spinal cord ranges from concussion to complete transection.

Following injury to the cervical spinal cord, changes in respiratory function may be acute, subacute or chronic. Most injuries which result in physiologic or anatomic transsection of the spinal cord cephalad to the fourth cervical segment are fatal because of acute respiratory failure. Immediate paralysis of the diaphragm and intercostal muscles leaves little time for intubation or tracheostomy. Physiological transsection caudal to the fourth cervical segment immediately paralyzes the abdominal and intercostal muscles of respiration, but the diaphragm is spared. Respiratory distress is evidenced by air hunger, paradoxical movements of the thorax and abdomen during inspiration, and the use of accessory muscles of respiration. Such patients, if not intubated or tracheostomized, often develop respiratory arrest.[41] The cause of death is an ascending myelopathy which destroys the phrenic outflow system. This intra-axial longitudinal extension of edema or hematoma usually occurs within 48 to 72 hours of injury. This devastating consequence can be avoided by careful observation of respiratory function or "prophylactic intubation." Chronic ventilatory support of a quadriplegic patient using an implanted radiofrequency generator has been reported by Glenn.[27]

Subacute respiratory paralysis has also been reported following tong application and realignment in atlantoaxial dislocations and lower cervical fractures.[2,13] The mechanism may involve further compromise of the cervical spinal cord already compressed by an extramedullary hematoma or ruptured disc material.

Of the patients who survive acute or subacute respiratory arrest, more than 75 percent will suffer the complications of pneumonia, atelectasis or pulmonary embolus.[57] All patients with physiological transsection of the cervical spinal cord caudal to the phrenic outflow, have paralyzed intercostal and abdominal respiratory muscles. Since the intercostal group of muscles, rather than the diaphragm, are the major muscles of respiration,[6] patients sustaining injuries to the spinal cord between the sixth cervical segment and the first thoracic segment demonstrate inherent ventilatory deficits. Diaphragmatic breathing is adequate at rest, but requires large expenditures of energy when tidal volumes must be increased to support increased metabolic demands. Metabolic demands are usually increased in paraplegic patients. Vital capacity can be increased by excessive use of trapezium and sternomastoid, however, oxygen tensions and thoracic compliance are reduced in most patients.[53] Increased parasympathetic activity, due to the loss of thoracolumbar sympathetic outflow, increases bronchial secretions. The inability to clear these bronchial secretions because of the low intrathoracic pressures developed during coughing promote atelectasis and pneumonitis.[76] Glossopharyngeal or "frog breathing" may improve the efficiency of coughing.[54] Improvements in tracheostomy care, flexible illuminated bronchoscopes, and improved ventilators have greatly improved the prognosis of quadriplegic and paraplegic patients.[8]

Anterior Cervical Operations

Anterior cervical discectomy and fusion is recommended by many neurosurgeons for cervical disc disease and cervical spine fractures. Since the anatomical structures met in this approach are many, there is a diversity of minor complications following the procedure. However, few complications involve the respiratory system. Postoperative hemorrhage deep to the sternomastoid muscle may produce airway obstruction and require evacuation of the hematoma.[11] Laryngeal or tracheal swelling due to surgical trauma may cause respiratory distress.[63] Temporary intubation is preferred over tracheostomy since the latter procedure may promote infection of the bone graft used at the time of fusion. Laceration of the pleura with pneumothorax has occurred.[14,17] Treatment consists of closed chest thoracotomy with underwater suction. One spinal cord injury with loss of intercostal breathing has been reported.[14] The recurrent laryngeal nerve, where it lies in the sulcus between the trachea and esophagus, may be damaged by retraction or dissection. Paralysis of the intrinsic muscles of the larynx with low, hoarse speech and respiratory stridor has occurred.[14,68] Silicone rubber injections of the arytenoid cartilage has produced improvement.

Stereotaxic Cordotomy

Stereotaxic interruption of the lateral spinothalamic tract to relieve intractable pain has become a common neurosurgical procedure. A portion of the ascending fibers in the lateral spinothalamic tract are destroyed by passing an electrical current along an insulated needle and electrode which has been inserted percutaneously into the spinal cord at the C_2-C_3 spinal foramen. The generated heat at the electrode tip produces a small area of axonal destruction.

In the spinal cord, anterior and medial to the spinothalamic tract, fibers important to normal respiratory function ascend and descend.[5,55,56,84] Permanent injury to the respiratory fibers may occur if the thermal lesion extends beyond the lateral spinothalamic tract. Edematous swelling around the site of thermal destruction can produce temporary dysfunction of neighboring respiratory axons.[56]

Clinically significant respiratory dysfunction is observed in 9 percent of patients undergoing percutaneous high cervical lateral cordotomy.[49] Impairment of normal respiration is higher in patients with pre-existing pulmonary insufficiency. Patients with intractable pain due to metastatic pulmonary malignancy or patients who have undergone pulmonary surgery for malignancy are especially prone to respiratory complications following percutaneous cervical cordotomy. These patients with compromised pulmonary function may decompensate when a percutaneous cervical cordotomy is performed ipsilateral to the lung with normal function.[42] Consequently, percutaneous cordotomy is not recommended for patients whose blood P_aO_2 is below 70, or for patients with an ipsilateral damaged lung, unless the operator has had extensive experience.[55]

Although the postoperative patient may have frank dyspnea, the clinical detection of respiratory embarrassment is usually more elusive. Fatigue, anxiety, confusion, or reduced voice volume may be the only signs of an underlying respiratory problem. Occasionally, the patient is found dead in bed four to five nights after the procedure was performed. The cause may have been "Ondine's curse"* or sleep-induced apnea resulting from damage to involuntary respiratory fibers, but not voluntary fibers, at the time of percutaneous cordotomy.[43]

Respiratory complications following percutaneous cordotomy can be avoided by careful patient selection. All patients should have blood gas determinations before and after cordotomy. Patients with reduced postoperative values should receive oxygen, especially at night, until blood P_aO_2 returns to safe levels.[55] Although most P_aO_2 values return to safe levels within five days, some patients require respiratory monitoring and/or assistance for up to three weeks.[80]

Occasionally bilateral high cervical percutaneous cordotomy is performed to relieve bilateral extremity or midline abdominal pain. Reduced forced vital capacity, reduced forced expired volume, reduced maximal breathing capacity, and reduced maximal midtidal thoracic pressure has been reported in the majority of these patients.[44,49] Patients requiring bilateral cordotomy should undergo a two-stage procedure. The second, contralateral, cervical lesion, should be performed seven to ten days after the first, and two to four spinal segments caudal to the first lesion.[48,49,80]

Open Anterolateral Cordotomy

The operation of open anterolateral high cervical cordotomy is performed through a laminectomy of the upper three cervical vertebrae. After opening the dura, a sharp, pointed knife blade is inserted into the spinal cord at the level of the dentate ligament and swept anterolaterally towards the exiting ventral nerve root, destroying the ascending lateral spinothalamic tract.[25,72] The advancing or sweeping blade tip can section permanently or injure temporarily the respiratory fibers lateral and anterior to the an-

*The mythical Ondine cursed the man who ignored her advances with a loss of involuntary vital functions. Thus, when he fell asleep he stopped breathing and died.

terior gray horn of the spinal cord. Sudden respiratory paralysis has become one of the main hazards of unilateral high cervical section.[73,78] Diminished respiratory excursions have been reported with both unilateral and bilateral high cervical sections.[36]

PERIPHERAL NERVE DAMAGE

Phrenic Nerve

The diaphragm is innervated by the ipsilateral phrenic nerve. The nerve arises from spinal cord segments and anterior motor roots of C_3, C_4 and C_5. The nerve passes ventral to the anterior scalene muscle and traverses the mediastinum to innervate the diaphragm.

The phrenic nerve can be damaged by missile injuries to the neck, stab wounds of the neck, and during surgical exposure of the neck. The phrenic nerve also has been injured as a result of excessive traction of the brachial plexus and with fractures of the cervical spine transverse processes.[79] Dyspnea and local neck or shoulder pain occur with unilateral paralysis. Vague abdominal complaints are occasionally seen with paralysis of the left phrenic nerve.[33] The diagnosis is confirmed by fluoroscopy which reveals elevation and paradoxical movements of the ipsilateral hemidiaphragm.

Recurrent Laryngeal Nerve

The recurrent laryngeal nerve innervates all the intrinsic muscles of the larynx except for the criothyroid. Unilateral interruption of the recurrent laryngeal nerve usually reduces voice volume and decreases the effectiveness of coughing. Bilateral paralysis of the recurrent laryngeal nerves produces hoarseness and inspiratory stridor.[12] Injuries to the recurrent laryngeal nerves have been reported with missile, surgical and mechanical trauma of the neck.[11,79]

DIAGNOSTIC STUDIES

Cerebral Arteriography

Percutaneous femoral artery puncture with transaortic catheter injection of the carotid and vertebral arteries has nearly eliminated respiratory complications during and following cerebral arteriography. However, direct percutaneous puncture of the carotid artery is still performed in many clinics. The incidence of arterial bleeding with the formation of significant hematoma following carotid puncture may reach 19 percent.[23] Uncontrolled extravasation of blood into the paratracheal area can produce respiratory distress. In these cases, the trachea is deviated to one side and there is often an obvious swelling deep to the sternomastoid muscle. The oropharynx, which offers little resistance, may be the site of obstruction rather than the cartilaginous trachea.[22] Intubation is usually effective. Occasionally tracheostomy and/or evacuation of the hematoma is required.[19] Respiratory distress secondary to pneumothorax, jugular vein laceration, and retropharyngeal abscess following carotid arteriography has also occurred.[37]

REFERENCES

1. Alexander, S., Cohen, P., et al.: Cerebral carbohydrate metabolism during hypocarbia in man. *Anesthesiology* **26**:624, 1965.
2. Amyes, E., and Anderson, F.: Fracture of the odontoid process. Report of sixty-three cases. *Arch. Surg.* **72**:377, 1956.
3. Atkinson, W.: The anterior inferior cerebellar artery. Its variations, pontine distribution and significance in the surgery of cerebello-pontine angle tumours. *J. Neurol. Neurosurg. Psychiat.* **12**:137, 1949.
4. Bailey, P., and Sweet, W.: Effects on respiration, blood pressure, and gastric motility of stimulation of orbital surface of frontal lobe. *J. Neurophysiol.* **3**:276, 1940.
5. Belmusto, L., Brown, E., et al.: Clinical observations on respiratory and vasomotor disturbance as related to cervical cordotomies. *J. Neurosurg.* **20**:225, 1963.

6. Bergsofsky, E.: Quentitation of the function of respiratory muscles in normal individuals and quadriplegic patients. *Arch. Phys. Med. Rehab.* **45**:575, 1964.
7. Bozza Marcubini, M., Rossanda, M., et al.: The role of artificial hyperventilation in control of brain tension during neurosurgical operations. *Br. J. Anesth.* **35**:415, 1964.
8. Bricker, D., Waltz, T., et al.: Major abdominal and thoracic trauma associated with spinal cord injury. Problems and management. *J. Trauma* **11**:63, 1971.
9. Campbell, E., Whitfield, R., et al.: Extradural hematoma of the posterior fossa. *Am. Surg.* **138**:509, 1953.
10. Castellano, F., and Ruggiero, G.: Meningiomas of the posterior fossa. *Acta Radiol.* **Suppl. 104**:1, 1953.
11. Clark, K.: Anterior operative approach for benign extradural cervical lesions. In Youmans, J. (ed.): *Neurological Surgery.* Philadelphia, W. B. Saunders Co., 1973, p. 1213.
12. Cleif, L.: Bilateral abductor paralysis of the larynx; results of treatment by the modified King operation. *Ann. Otol.* **64**:38, 1955.
13. Cloward, R.: Treatment of acute fractures and fracture dislocations of the cervical spine by vertebral-body fusion. A report of eleven cases. *J. Neurosurg.* **18**:201, 1962.
14. Cloward, R.: New method of diagnosis and treatment of cervical disc disease. *Clin. Neurosurg.* **8**:93, 1962.
15. Cohen, P.: Alexander, S., et al.: Effects of hypoxia and normocarbia on cerebral blood flow and metabolism in conscious man. *J. Appl. Physiol.* **23**:183, 1967.
16. Coleman, C., and Thomas, J.: Extradural hemorrhages in the posterior fossa. *Am. Surg.* **10**:985, 1941.
17. Connolly, E., Seymour, R., et al.: Clinical evaluation of anterior cervical fusion for degenerative cervical disc disease. *J. Neurosurg.* **23**:431, 1965.
18. Cushing, H.: *Studies in Intracranial Physiology and Surgery.* London, Oxford University Press, 1925.
19. Curtis, J.: Cerebral angiography. *Br. J. Surg.* **38**:295, 1951.
20. Dodge, H., Love, J., et al.: Benign tumors at the foramen magnum; surgical considerations. *J. Neurosurg.* **13**:603, 1956.
21. Ducker, T.: Increased intracranial pressure and pulmonary edema. Clinical study of eleven patients. *J. Neurosurg.* **28**:112, 1968.

22. Field, J., and De Saussure, R.: Retropharyngeal hemorrhage with respiratory obstruction following arteriography. *J. Neurosurg.* **22**:610, 1965.
23. Fink, M., and Stein, J.: A clinical evolution of carotid angiography. *Confin. Neurol.* **12**:181, 1952.
24. Frazier, C., and Spiller, W.: An analysis of 14 cases of spinal cord tumor. *Arch. Neurol. Psych. (Chicago)* **8**:455, 1922.
25. French, L.A., Chou, S.N., et al.: Cervical Tractomy. In *Henry Ford Hospital International Symposium on Pain.* Boston, Little, Brown, 1966, Ch. 22.
26. Gardner, W.: Hydrodynamic mechanism of syringomyelia: Its relationship to myelocele. *J. Neurol. Neurosurg. Psychiat.* **28**:247, 1965.
27. Glenn, W., Holcom, W., et al.: Total ventilatory support in a quadriplegic patient with radiofrequency electrophrenic respiration. *N. Eng. J. Med.* **286**:513, 1972.
28. Graf, C., and Rossi, N.: Pulmonary edema and central nervous system: A clinicopathological study. *Surg. Neurol.* **4**:319, 1975.
29. Grant, F.: A clinical experience with meningiomas of the brain. *J. Neurosurg.* **11**:479, 1954.
30. Greenwood, J.: Spinal cord tumors. In Youmans, J. (ed.): *Neurological Surgery.* Vol. III. Philadelphia, W.B. Saunders Co., 1973, p. 1518.
31. Guttman, L.: *Spinal Cord Injuries.* Oxford, Blackwell Scientific Publications, 1976, p. 215.
32. Hayes, G., and Slocum, H.: The achievement of optimal brain relaxation by hyperventilation technics of anesthesia. *J. Neurosurg.* **19**:65, 1962.
33. Haymaker, W., and Woodhall, B.: *Peripheral Nerve Injury.* Philadelphia, W.B. Saunders Co., 1953, p. 208.
34. Hewlett, T.: Respiratory care of the neurological/neurosurgical patient. In Barton, G., Gee, G., and Hodgkin, J., (eds.): *Respiratory Care.* Philadelphia, J.B. Lippincott Co., 1977.
35. Horwitz, N., and Rizzoli, H.: *Postoperative Complications in Neurosurgical Patients.* Baltimore, Williams & Wilkins Co., 1967, p. 308.
36. Horwitz, N., and Rizzoli, H.: *Postoperative Complications in Neurosurgical Practice.* Baltimore, Williams & Wilkins Co., 1967, p. 291.

37. Horwitz, N., and Rizzoli, H.: *Postoperative Complications in Neurosurgical Patients.* Baltimore, Williams & Wilkins Co., 1967, p. 337.
38. Hullay, J., and Tomits, G.: Experience with total removal of tumors of the acoustic nerve. *J. Neurosurg.* **22**:127, 1965.
39. Kindt, G., and Youmans, J.: The site of action of carbon dioxide on the cerebral circulation. *Surg. Forum* **70**:419, 1969.
40. Kitahata, L., and Collins, W.: Meningitis as a complication of anesthesia in a patient with basal skull fracture. *Anesthesiology* **32**:282, 1970.
41. Klemperer, W.: Spinal cord injuries in World War II. Operative findings and results in 201 patients. *U.S. Armed Forces Med. J.* **10**:701, 1959.
42. Krieger, A., and Rosomoff, H.: Sleep-induced apnea. II. Respiratory failure after anterior surgery. *J. Neurosurg.* **29**:181, 1974.
43. Krieger, A., and Rosomoff, H.: Sleep-induced apnea. I. A respiratory and autonomic dysfunction syndrome following bilateral percutaneous cervical cordotomy. *J. Neurosurg.* **39**:168, 1974.
44. Kuperman, A., Krieger, A., et al.: Respiratory function after cervical cordotomy. *Chest* **59**:128, 1971.
45. Langfitt, T.: Clinical methods for monitoring intracranial pressure and measuring cerebral blood flow. *Clin. Neurosurg.* **22**:302, 1975.
46. Langfitt, T., and Kassell, N.: Acute brain swelling in meningeal patients. *J. Neurosurg.* **24**:975, 1966.
47. Lehrich, J., Winkler, G., et al.: Cerebellar infarctions with brainstem compression: Diagnosis and surgical treatment. *Arch. Neurol.* **22**:290, 1976.
48. Lin, P., Gildenberg, P., et al.: An anterior approach to percutaneous lower cervical cordotomy. *J. Neurosurg.* **25**:553, 1966.
49. Lorenz, R.: Methods of percutaneous spino-thalamic tract section. In Krayenbühl, H. (ed.): *Advances and Technical Standards in Neurosurgery.* Vol. 3. New York, Springer-Verlag, 1976, p. 136.
50. Lundberg, N., Kjallquist, A., et al.: Reduction of increased intracranial pressure by hyperventilation. A therapeutic aid in neurological surgery. *Acta Psychiat. Scand.* **34,** Suppl. 139, 1959.
51. Lundberg, N., et al.: Non-operative management of intracranial hypertension. In Krayenbühl, H., et al. (eds.): *Advances*

and Technical Standards in Neurosurgery. Vol. I. New York, Springer-Verlag, 1974, p. 42.
52. McComish, P., and Bodley, P.: *Anesthesia for Neurological Surgery.* London, Lloyd-Duke, Ltd. 1971, p. 53.
53. McKinley, A., Auchinlos, J., et al.: Pulmonary function, ventilatory control and respiratory complications in quadriplegic patients. *Am. Rev. Resp. Dis.* **100**:526, 1969.
54. Montero, J., and Feldman, D.: Effects of glossopharyngeal breathing on respiratory function after cervical cord transsection. *Arch. Phys. Med. Rehab.* **64**:650, 1967.
55. Mullan, S.: Percutaneous cordotomy. *J. Neurosurg.* **35**:360, 1971.
56. Mullan, S., and Hosobuchi, Y.: Respiratory hazards of high cervical percutaneous cordotomy. *J. Neurosurg.* **28**:291, 1968.
57. Munro, D.: Cervical cord injuries. A study of 101 cases. *N. Eng. J. Med.* **229**:919, 1943.
58. Northfield, D.: Society of British Neurological Surgeons Symposium on the results of operations on acoustic neuromas. *J. Neurol. Neurosurg. Psychiat.* **13**:277, 1950.
59. Olivecrona, H.: Acoustic tumors. *J. Neurosurg.* **16**:6, 1967.
60. Olivecrona, H.: Analysis of results of complete and partial removal of acoustic neuromas. *J. Neurol. Neurosurg. Psychiat.* **13**:271, 1950.
61. Pennybacher, J., and Cairns, H.: Results in 130 cases of acoustic neurinoma. *J. Neurol. Neurosurg. Psychiat.* **13**:272, 1950.
62. Personal communication.
63. Personal communication.
64. Plum, F., and Posner, J.: *Diagnosis of Stupor and Coma.* Philadelphia, F.A. Davis, 1966, p. 15.
65. Pool, J., and Pava, A.: *The Early Diagnosis and Treatment of Acoustic Nerve Tumors.* Springfield, Ill., Charles C Thomas, 1957.
66. Rand, R., Microsurgery for acoustic tumors. In *Microneurosurgery.* St. Louis, C. V. Mosby Co., 1969, p. 126.
67. Reivich, M., Dickson, J., et al.: Role of hypoxia in cerebral circulatory and metabolic changes during hypocarbia in man: Studies in hyperbaric milieu. *Scand. J. Clin. Lab. Invest.* **Suppl. 102,** IV:B, 1968.
68. Robinson, R., and Smith, C.: Anterolateral cervical disc removal and interbody fusion for cervical disc syndrome. *Bull. Johns Hopkins Hosp.* **96**:223, 1955.
69. The surgery of spinal tumors. *Lancet* **1**:187, 1935.
70. Rosomoff, H.: Distribution of intracranial contents with con-

trolled hyperventilation: Implications for neuroanesthesia. *Anesthesiology* **24**:640, 1963.

71. Rosomoff, H.: Adjuncts to neurosurgical anesthesia. *Br. J. Anesth.* **37**:246, 1965.
72. Schwartz, H.G., and O'Leary, J.L.: Section of the spinothalamic tract in the medulla with observations on the pathway for pain. *Surgery* **9**:183, 1941.
73. Schwartz, H.G.: High cervical cordotomy—techniques and results. *Clin. Neurosurg.* **8**:282, 1962.
74. Shapiro, H.: Intracranial hypertension: Therapeutic and aesthetic considerations. *Anesthesiology* **43**:445, 1975.
75. Shenkin, H., and Bouzarth, W.: Clinical methods of reducing intracranial pressure. *N. Eng. J. Med.* **282**:1465, 1970.
76. Siebens, A., Kirby, N., et al.: Cough following transsection of the spinal cord at C-6. *Arch. Phys. Med. Rehab.* **45**:1, 1964.
77. Speakman, T., and Babkin, B.: Effect of cortical stimulation on respiratory rate. *Am. J. Physiol.* **159**:239, 1949.
78. Stookey, B.: The management of intractable pain by chordotomy. *Res. Publ. Ass. Res. Nerv. Ment. Dis.* **23**:416, 1943.
79. Sunderland, P.: *Nerve and Nerve Injuries.* Baltimore, Williams & Wilkins Co., 1968.
80. Tarsen, J.: Physiologic corroboration in stereotaxic high cervical cordotomy. *Confin. Neurol. (Basel)* **33**:285, 1971.
81. Theodore, J., and Robin, E.: Speculations on neurogenic pulmonary edema. *Am. Rev. Resp. Dis.* **113**:405, 1976.
82. Thomas, C.: Acute increased intracranial pressure and the physiology of mass lesions. In Youmans, J. (ed.): *Neurological Surgery.* Vol. III. Philadelphia, W.B. Saunders Co., 1973, p. 950.
83. Wagner, F.: Recent research on spinal cord injury. *Arch. Neurol.* **27**:465, 1972.
84. Woldring, S., and Owens, G.: Centrifugal respiratory pathway in the spinal cord. *Surg. Forum* **15**:418, 1964.
85. Woods, W., and Pimenta, A.: Intramedullary lesions of the spinal cord. Study of sixty-eight consecutive cases. *Arch. Neurol. Psych. (Chicago)* **52**:383, 1944.

14

SLEEP-RELATED RESPIRATORY DISORDERS

Paul A. Nausieda, M.D., and Steve Weber, Ph.D.

The concept of a "sleep-induced" syndrome is a relatively new one, which evolved over the last two decades. Initiated by studies investigating respiratory disturbances during sleep in the Pickwickian syndrome,[1] studies identified nocturnal respiratory disturbances linked to ongoing sleep events.[2,3] These clinical syndromes, the sleep apneas and hypopneas, have become active areas of interest in a number of branches of medicine and surgery and have stimulated renewed interest in the physiological basis of respiratory control and its modification by the sleep process.

CLASSIFICATION OF SLEEP EVENTS

The sleep process is recognized as a complex behavioral state which is mediated by various brainstem and cortical structures and encompasses alterations in physiologic responsiveness, neuroendocrine control and neurotransmitter activity. From a historical and practical standpoint sleep activity is classified on the basis of the electroencephalographic changes which characterize the sleep state. The information derived from the EEG is augmented by simultaneous monitoring of eye movements (electrooculogram, EOG) and submental muscle activity (electromyogram,

TABLE I
Sleep Behavior in Stages

SLEEP STAGE	EEG	EOG	EMG ACTIVITY	CLINICAL FEATURES
1	Loss of alpha rhythm "flat" background	Occasional slow horizontal eye movements	Present	Dozing state, transitional, between wakefulness and sleep.
2	14/second sleep "spindles" "K-complexes"	—	Present	Asleep, easily arousable
3	1-2 hz activity in 20-50% of record	—	Present	Moderately deep sleep
4	Predominant 1-2 cps activity	—	Present	Deep sleep, difficult to arouse
REM	low voltage fast pattern	Burst of rapid, conjugate vertical horizontal eye movement	Absent	Most dream events, penile erection, reflex inhibition, altered central thermoregulation

EMG). Based on the information derived from these sources, sleep behavior can be subdivided into a series of stages as summarized in Table I and illustrated in Figures 1 through 6.

The conventional system for classifying REM and SWS stages is the Rechtschaffen and Kales (1968)[4] protocol. Widely used by academic sleep researchers and clinical practitioners in polygraphic sleep analysis, it provides a reliable and accurate description of the adult sleep cycle. Sleep in the infant is characterized by different electroencephalographic patterns which mature into the adult pattern in the first few years of life.[5] Sleep in the neonate is routinely classified into three stages: active sleep (AS), quiet sleep (QS) and indeterminate sleep (IS). AS is widely believed to be the neonatal analog of adult REM sleep, as its distinguishing features are highly similar. It is characterized by EMG suppression, eye movements, irregular respiration, body twitches and facial grimacing. The EEG of AS is more variable than that of adult REM sleep and can assume a high-voltage low-frequency configuration, a low-voltage irregular frequency pattern, or a mixed high/low voltage irregular frequency background. QS appears to be the developmental precursor of adult SWS. Lacking the unique sleep EEG waveforms of the adult, neonatal QS is not ordinarily broken down into substages. The EMG during QS demonstrates sustained muscle tonus while EOG activity is absent and respiratory rate is regular. EEG activity is again quite variable, encompassing both the high-voltage low-frequency and the mixed patterns seen during AS in addition to the trace alternant rhythm peculiar to QS. Overall, the neonatal EEG is not a reliable discriminator of sleep states and wakefulness. Respiratory, EMG, EOG, and behavioral parameters are better criteria.

Relative to sleep-related alterations in respiratory function, additional monitoring techniques are employed. In usual clinical practice, air flow is monitored using oral and nasal thermistors and thoracic movement is measured with an external strain guage or via impedance pneumography. Alternatively, intrathoracic pressure may be monitored using an intraesophageal pressure transducer. By combining data derived from these sources it is possible to differentiate

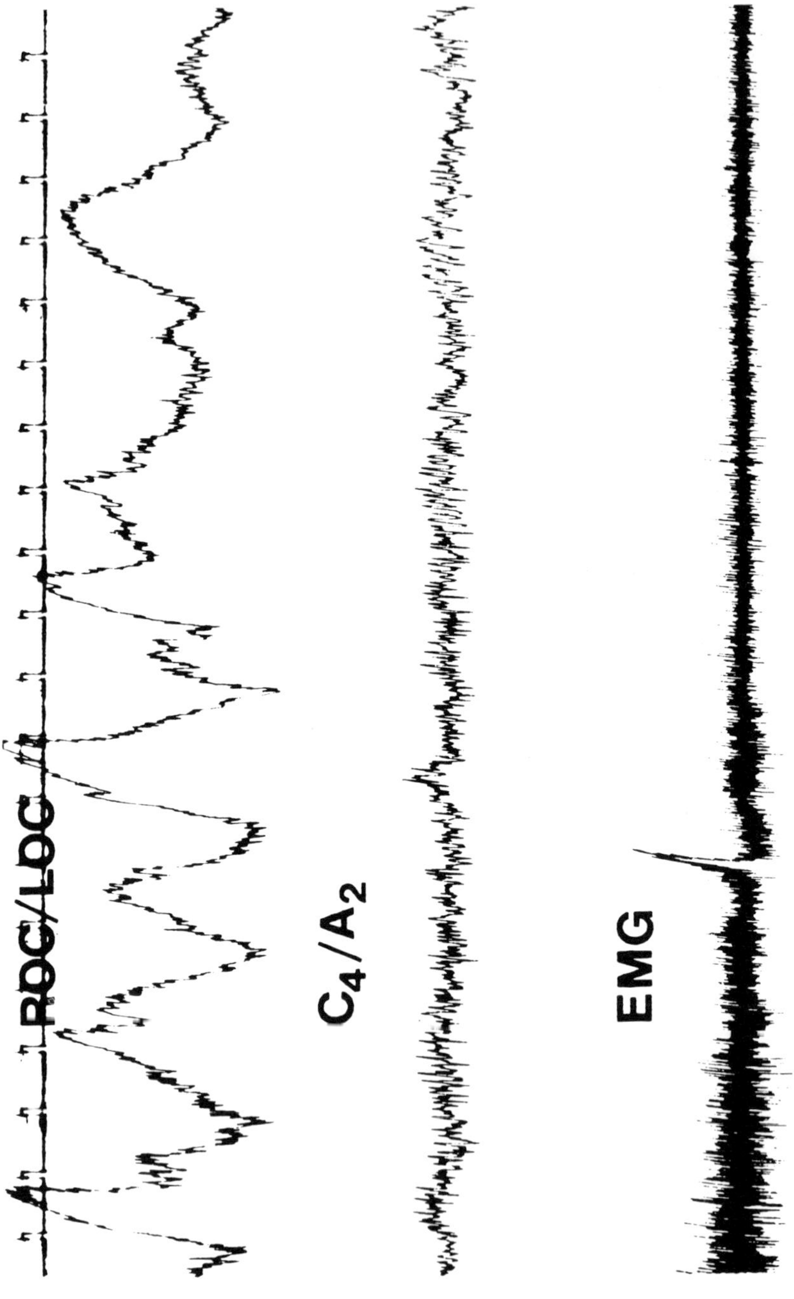

Figure 1. *Wakefulness.* Slow, rolling eye movements characteristic of drowsiness occur in the EOG. Waking alpha rhythm is evident in the EEG, and the EMG demonstrates sustained muscle tone.

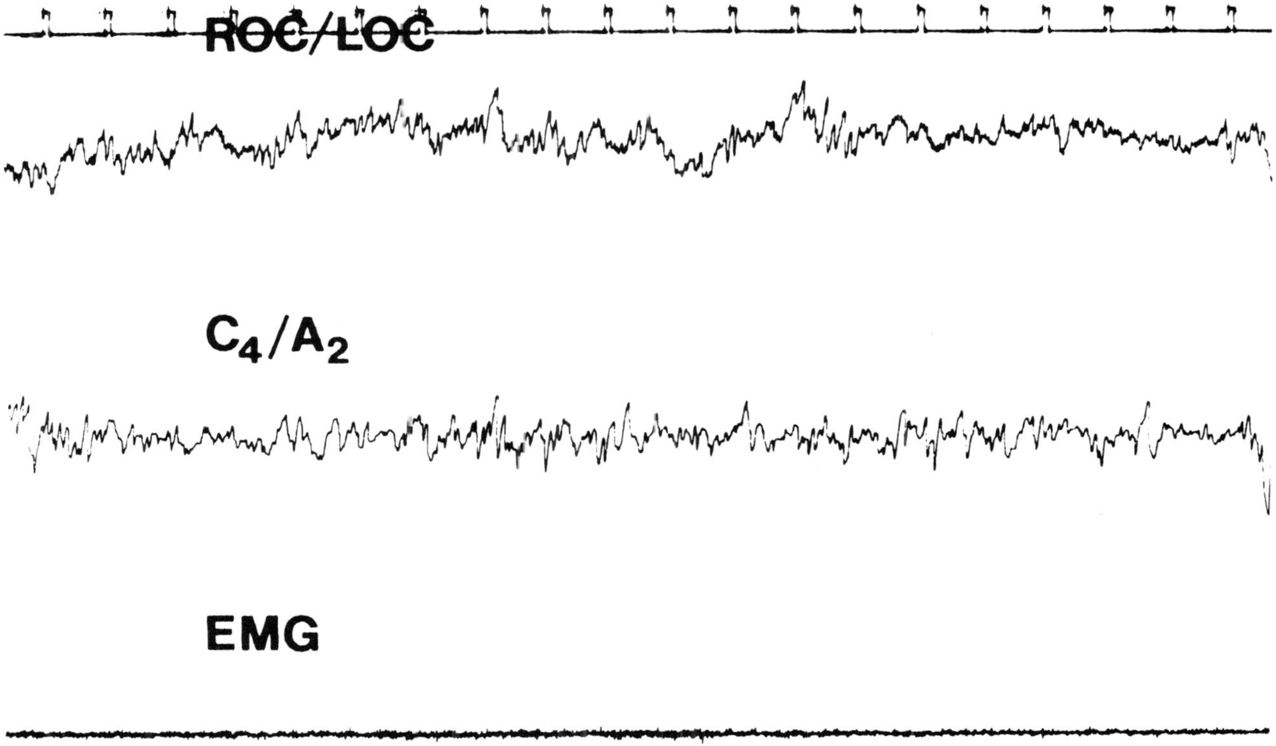

Figure 2. NREM stage 1. Eye movements are not present in the EOG. The EEG assumes a low voltage, mixed frequency pattern with little or no alpha activity. Muscle tone is maintained.

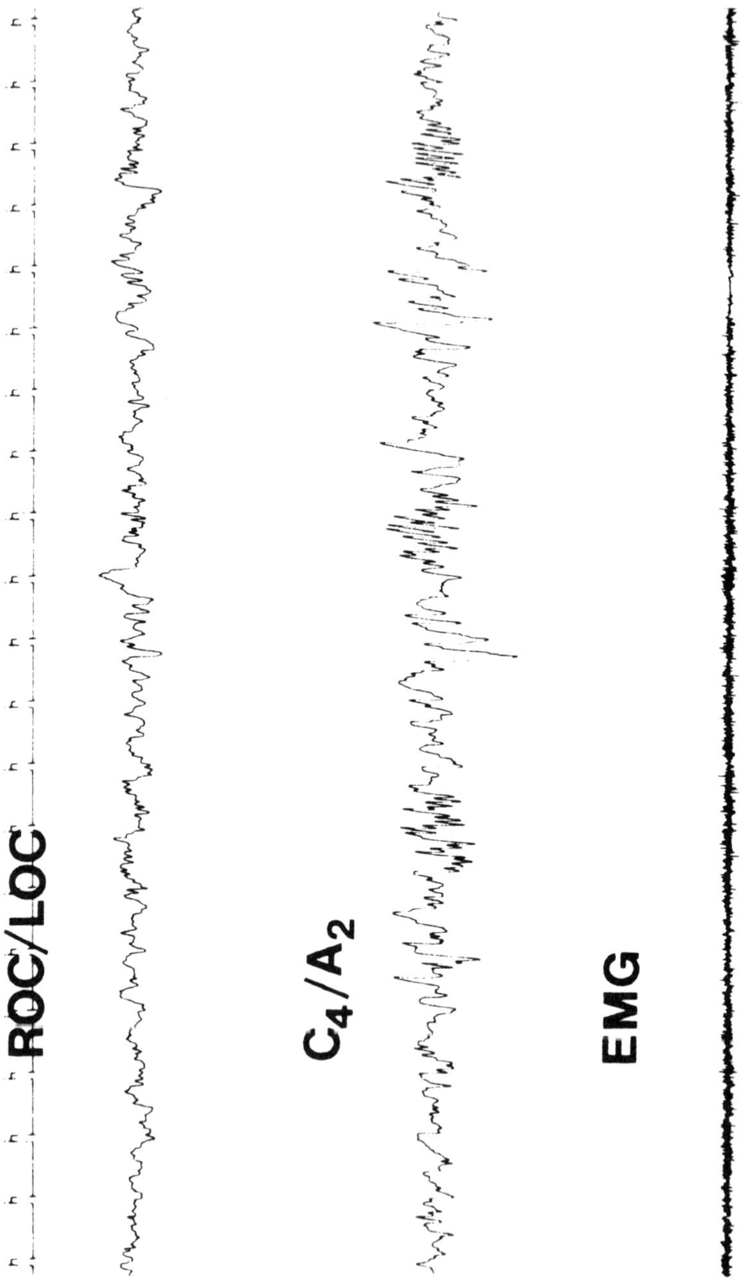

Figure 3. *NREM stage 2.* The EEG contains 14 Hz sleep spindles and high voltage K-complexes which define this stage. Eye movements are absent and EMG activity is tonically present.

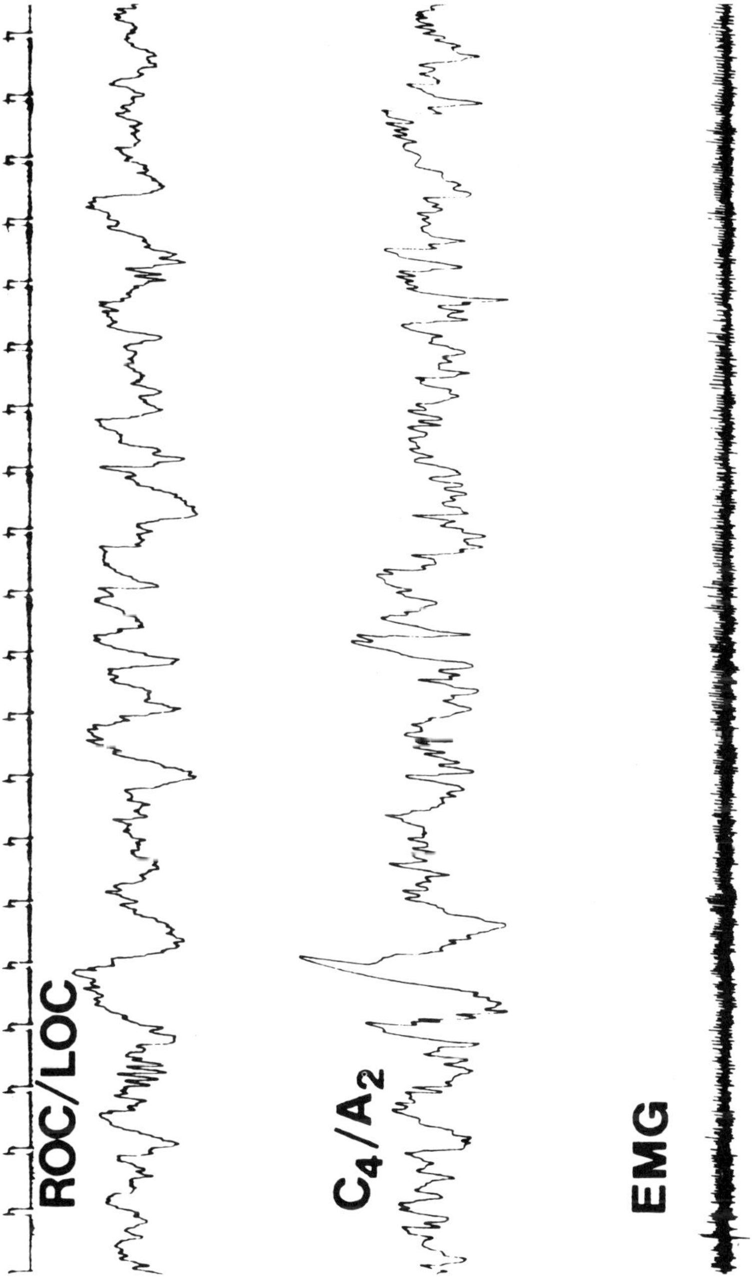

Figure 4. *NREM stage 3.* The EEG shows between 20 to 50 percent high voltage ($< 75\ \mu V$) delta rhythm, with ocular quiescence and sustained EMG tonus.

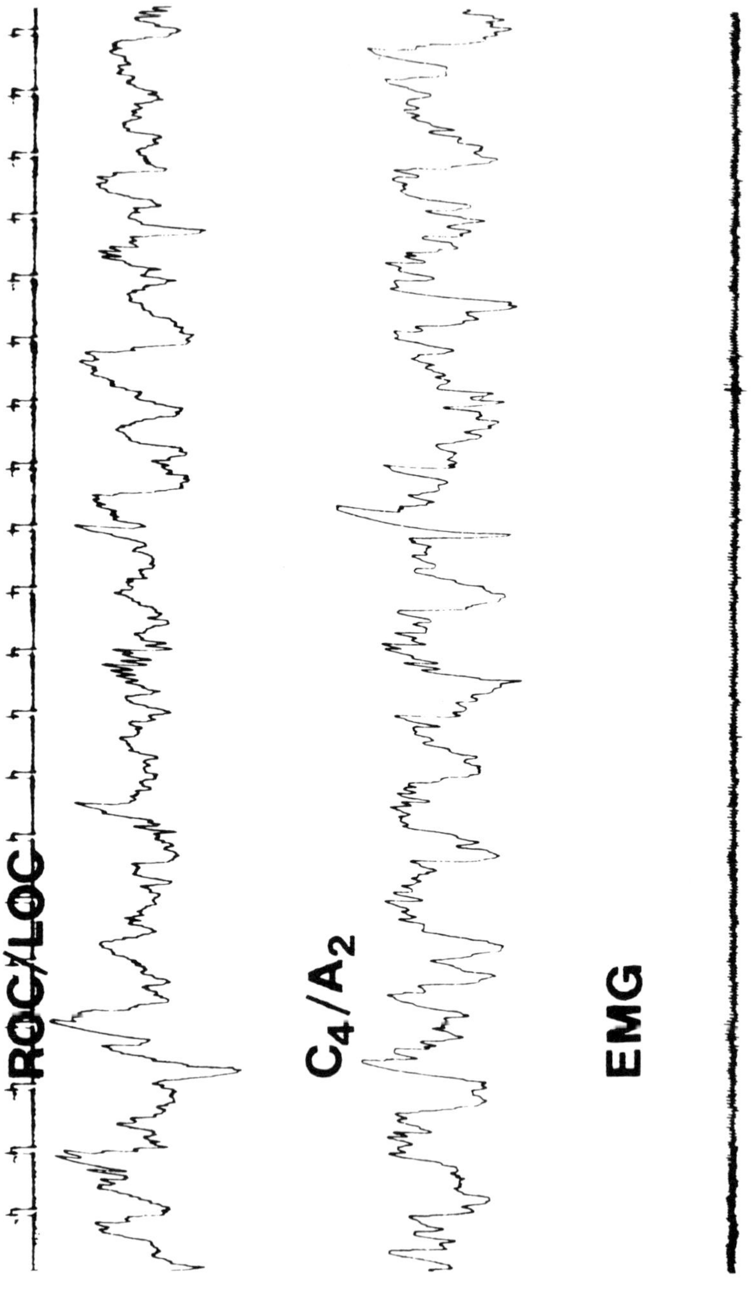

Figure 5. *NREM stage 4.* Delta rhythm occupies greater than 50 percent of the EEG sample, with no eye movements and a relatively high level of EMG activity.

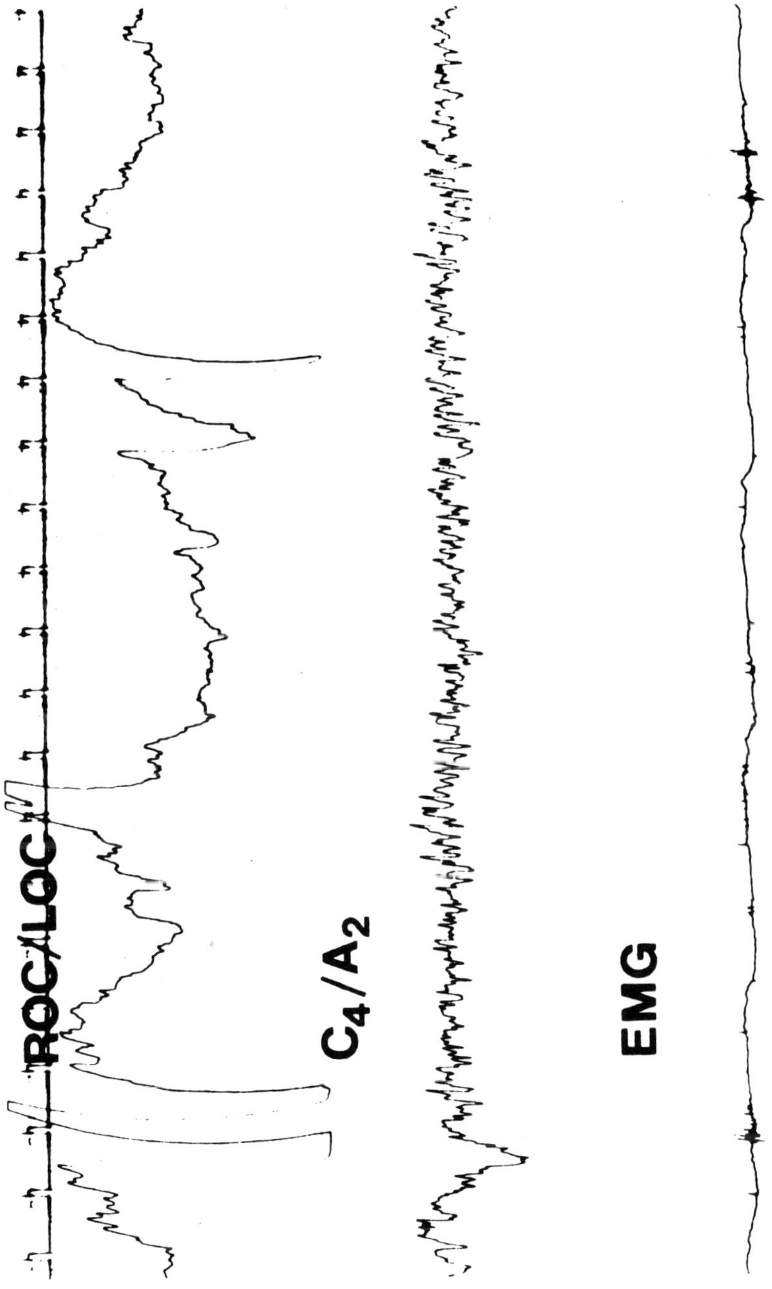

Figure 6. *Stage REM.* The EOG indicates rapid eye movements, while the EEG shows low voltage, irregular frequency activity. The submental EMG is hypotonic.

subtypes of sleep-related apneas and accurately document the duration and frequency of such episodes. Evaluation of the physiological concomitants of these events has been carried out in the past using standard arterial blood gas determinations, catheterization data and expiratory carbon dioxide tension. Inherent in these techniques is the problem of accurately measuring very transient alterations in arterial pH, CO_2 and O_2 concentration, which are easily missed with random sampling techniques. Current use of continual oximetry monitoring has allowed a more dynamic means of following ongoing oxygen saturation and appears to be a less invasive and more sensitive technique. In addition to the above, continual electrocardiographic monitoring is usually carried out and time locked to data collected from other sources. A typical multiparameter polysomnogram is presented in Figure 7. Recorded from a normal adult during stage 2 of SWS, it contains tracings of the EOG, EEG, EMG, O_2 saturation, nasal/oral airflow, thoracic respiratory effort, cardiotachometry and the EEG.

Normally, at sleep onset a progression through the stages of SWS occurs, interrupted by REM periods which occur transiently at intervals of approximately 90 minutes. The temporal progression of sleep stages is commonly termed "sleep architecture" and is graphically illustrated in Figure 8. In addition to the 90-minute REM cycle, two other features are generally evident in the sleep architecture of the normal young adult. First, the majority of SWS stages 3 and 4 appears during the first half of the sleep period. Second, the majority of REM sleep is concentrated in the latter half of the sleep period, due to progressive lengthening of individual REM episodes. The division of sleep into SWS and REM periods is a characteristic feature of sleep at all ages in man and appears to be present in almost all mammalian species as well.

Physiologic data suggests that SWS and REM are distinct behavioral states under the control of separate brain stem control centers. Current studies favor the hypothesis that SWS is mediated by a system originating in the serotonin-containing neurons of the median raphe while REM appears to be modulated by a norepinephrine-containing neuronal population arising in the locus coruleus. Though the precise mechanisms involved are still controversial, the

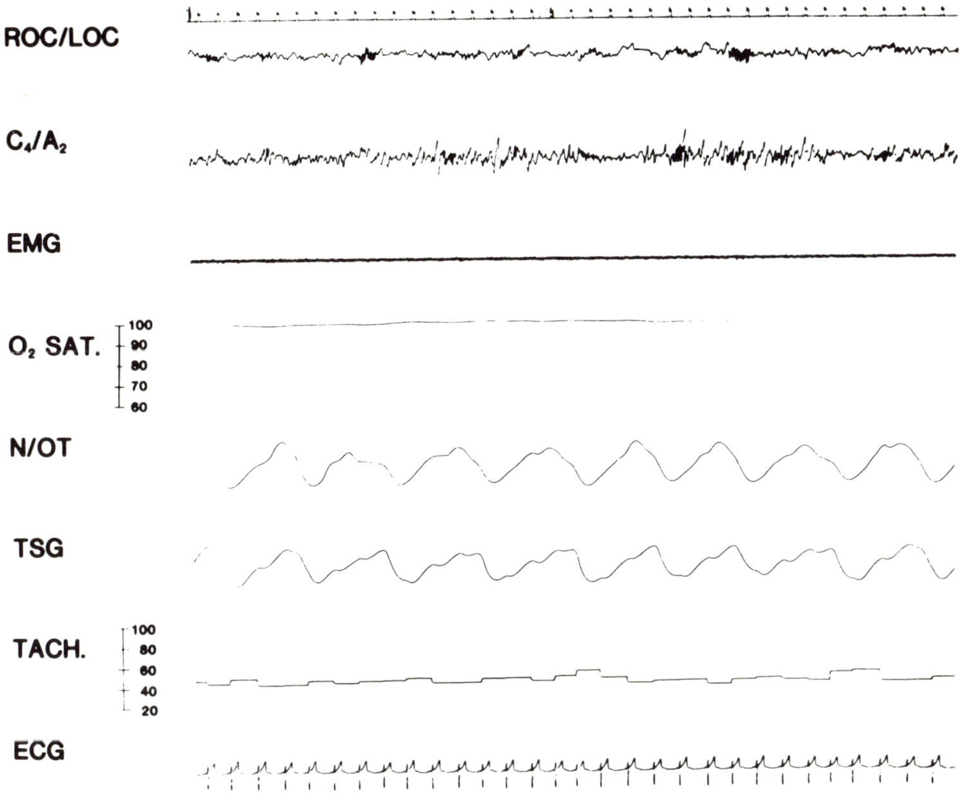

Figure 7. A typical eight-channel polysomnogram recorded from a normal adult male in stage 2 of NREM sleep. Electro-oculogram (ROC/LOC) recorded from right outer canthus referred to left outer canthus; electroencephalogram (C_4/A_2) recorded from the right central lead referred to the right mastoid; electromyogram (EMG) recorded from the submental musculature; arterial oxygen saturation (O_2 SAT.) transduced by an ear oximeter; nasal and oral airflow (N/OT) recorded by a thermocouple mounted in a plastic respiratory mask; thoracic movement (TSG) recorded by a strain gauge; heart rate recorded by a cardiotachometer; electrocardiogram (ECG) recorded from V_5 referred to the left mastoid.

upper airways, which in turn provide feedback information to central control centers via proprioceptors and sensory afferents located in the airway and lungs. In general, the metabolic centers operate on a servo loop principle in the absence of voluntary respiratory drive and are probably the predominant respiratory control mechanism in deeper stages of SWS (Stages III and IV). The role of the voluntary respiratory drive center in sleep remains unclarified but may have a functional role in drowsiness and REM.

Respiratory Dynamics During SWS

The transition from wakefulness to drowsiness to sleep can be viewed as a process of reticular inhibition and a loss of the "stimulant effect" of arousal on automatic respiration.[6] At sleep onset ventilatory volume ($\mathring{V}$) decreases[7,8] and P_aCO_2 rises 4.1 to 6.5 mmHg.[7,9] Arterial oxygen pressure (P_aO_2) drops 3.5 to 9.4 mmHg[10,11] with a lowering of arterial pH by 0.3 to 0.5 units.[12-14]

During SWS ventilatory responses to CO_2 are less than those encountered in the waking state while O_2 drive appears to be unaltered. Using a CO_2 in O_2 rebreathing technique, a progressive decrease in the ventilation-alveolar PCO_2 line ($\mathring{V}/P_ACO_2$) from wakefulness (1.25 liter/min/mmHg) to stage IV sleep (.5 liter/min/mmHg) occurs[8] which can also be demonstrated using steady state CO_2 in O_2 techniques.[15] When these data are considered in conjunction with the decreased $\mathring{V}$ and elevated P_aCO_2 which occur in SWS, it is apparent that a shift in the position of the $\mathring{V}/P_ACO_2$ response line to higher CO_2 pressures must occur in this phase of sleep. Studies of hypoxic drive during slow wave sleep are not as extensive[16,17] but indicate no substantial difference in ventilatory responses to hypoxia in wakefulness and SWS. Similar results have been reported in experimental studies in the rat and dog.[18,19]

Other aspects of the respiratory control system have been studied and include evaluation of pulmonary receptor stimulation, upper airway stimulation, and chest wall stimulation. When evaluated during SWS, the effects of the above maneuvers are found to be similar to those observed during wakefulness, and suggest that afferent influences on respiration remain unaltered during this phase of sleep.[20]

Recent studies have suggested that SWS respiratory control mechanisms are significantly different in a predominately male subgroup of the normal population.[21] In this group a high degree of CO_2 retention is observed which is frequently present in other family members.[22] This tendency appears to be positively correlated with advancing age and obesity, though its significance relative to specific sleep-related respiratory disturbances remains unclear.[21]

As well as the steady state changes in respiratory dynamics reviewed previously, the respiratory events involved in the appearance of periodic breathing (Cheyne-Stokes respiration) in sleep deserve comment. Periodic respiration (Cheyne-Stokes respiration) is frequently encountered in the normal individual during Stages I and II of SWS while Stages III and IV lack this characteristic[2,7,23-25] (Fig. 9). Some authors have suggested that altered vagal outflow or sleep dependent alterations in vagal reflex activity may underly these changes in respiratory rhythm.[26,27] Other studies have demonstrated persistent sleep related alterations in respiratory rhythm in animals following bilateral vagotomy, which suggests that a more complex central respiratory control alteration is probably involved.[28]

The appearance of periodic breathing in Stages I and II and its disappearance in deeper stages of SWS may reflect the fluctuating activity of the cortical respiratory drive system in lighter stages of sleep. Mechanistically it has been suggested that drowsiness is associated with a shift to metabolic respiratory control and accounts for the initial slowing of respiration. Arousal is then triggered by the concomitant shift in blood gases and respiration is accelerated by cortical and reticular influences. This cycle continues until deeper sleep is established and respiration comes under autonomous metabolic control. Periodic breathing can therefore be viewed as a normal physiological variant in drowsiness and light sleep.

Respiratory Dynamics in REM Sleep

As we previously noted, REM sleep is associated with a number of unique changes in central nervous system function including loss of normal thermoregulatory activity and activation of both sympathetic and parasympathetic sys-

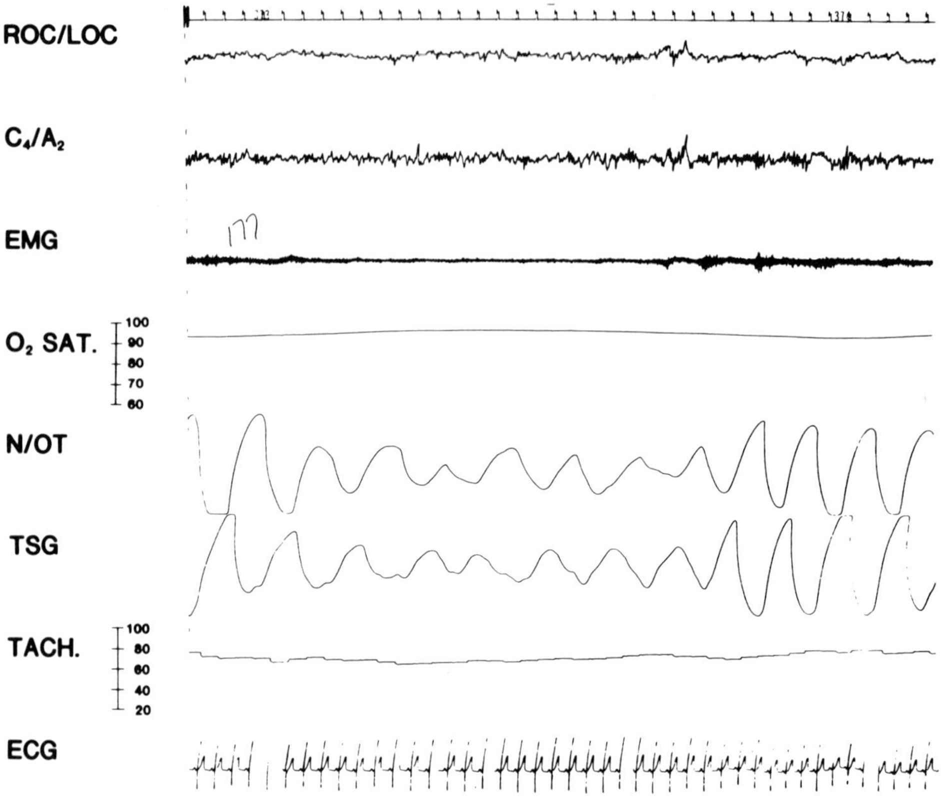

Figure 9. *Periodic Respiration.* During Stage 1, respiratory effort and airflow repetitively wax and wane over an approximately 30 second period. Oxygen saturation changes by 1 to 3 percent in phase with this cycle.

tems. It is not surprising therefore to find that respiratory regulation during this stage of sleep is considerably different from that encountered in wakefulness or SWS.

During REM periods ventilatory volume increases 10 to 15 percent,[8] alveolar ventilation is enhanced and an irregular, rapid respiratory rhythm appears with highly variable tidal volume.[7,23,29,30] Hypercarbic ventilatory drive during REM has not been evaluated extensively in the adult, but has been reported to be decreased to a greater degree than observed in SWS in healthy infants.[31,32] In dogs (which show a sleep morphology similar to man), REM sleep is associated with a 67 to 86 percent decrease in hypercarbic ventilatory drive when compared to SWS. Oddly the irregular respiratory pattern typical of REM sleep is unaffected by alterations in inspired CO_2 and seems to coincide with episodes of rapid eye movements (phasic REM).[33] Other studies in the dog have demonstrated that systemic alkalosis also has little effect on respiration during REM.[34] While the applicability of these data to man remains speculative, it suggests that the sensitivity of the metabolic respiratory center to alterations in CO_2 and pH may be diminished considerably during REM sleep. Philpson has speculated that the aroused EEG patterns seen in REM sleep may activate the cortical respiratory center and explain inhibition of metabolic center control which is implied by the above studies.[20]

Hypoxic respiratory responses have been studied only in healthy infants, and only inferred from the response to 100 percent O_2 inhalation.[35] In these cases responses in REM were similar to those observed in SWS. Studies in dogs suggest that hypoxia in REM leads to an increase in minute volume which is similar to that seen in SWS, suggesting that hypoxic drive is intact.[19] The irregular respiratory pattern of REM sleep, however, does not appear to be influenced by variations in inspired O_2 concentration, suggesting it may be mediated by either the cortical respiratory center or an independent control mechanism.[19] During REM sleep in the dog arousal thresholds to hypercapnea are higher than those in SWS, but lower for hypoxia.[19] The basis of this response is unknown, but has been suggested as a possible explanation for the multiple arousals observed in patients with sleep apnea-related hypoxic episodes.

Studies of the proprioceptive and pulmonary receptor afferent components of the respiratory control mechanism in animals and man have suggested that their regulatory effects are depressed or lost during REM sleep.[20] At the same time, afferent input from the upper airways appears to have an enhanced effect on respiration in the dog and readily elicits periods of apnea,[36] suggesting that selective inhibition of peripheral respiratory control systems may be a characteristic feature of REM sleep.

Summary

Wakefulness is associated with an active cortical respiratory control system and nonspecific arousal-related respiratory stimulation. In the waking state, the metabolic control center acts as a "fail-safe" outflow system for higher drive centers which have a limited capacity to over-ride it (see section on respiratory dyskinesia).

Slow wave sleep reflects the activity of a metabolic control center, while drowsiness is characterized by a fluctuation between cortical and metabolic control. REM sleep, especially during episodes of rapid eye movements, is characterized by suppression of metabolic center controls (with the apparent exception of hypoxic drive and specific sensory afferents) and may reflect a REM-dependent cortical respiratory center activation or a specific unrelated respiratory control mechanism.

Some observations remain difficult to explain in terms of the above constructs. The relative autonomy of REM-related respiration from metabolic respiratory control has been related to the frequent brief episodes of apnea seen in this stage of sleep[20,37,38] Recent studies, however, demonstrate that two-thirds of a "normal" group of male subjects have apnea in REM as well as in Stages I and II of SWS which resulted in a 4 percent or greater decrease in oxygen saturation.[21] The episodes were qualitatively similar to those seen in symptomatic sleep apneics but shorter and less frequent. Increasing age and obesity were positively correlated with the severity of apnea for reasons which remain unexplained.

These data suggest that apneic episodes are a normal phenomenon in a large number of patients and are not restricted to REM sleep. At present, the many explanations for these apneic episodes (which draw heavily on the physiologic alterations characteristic of REM sleep) have failed to offer any explanation for the occurrence of significant obstructive apnea in SWS, or the relative immunity of women from this phenomenon. It is obvious that factors beyond a hierarchical organization of central respiratory control centers need further clarification.

Sleep and Respiration in the Newborn

Recent data suggest that respiratory control mechanisms mature during the first few months of life, and demonstrate unique features in the newborn period which are more pronounced in the face of prematurity. With respect to respiratory responses to hypercapnea and hypoxia, the general pattern observed in adults appears to be present in infancy as well. The unique feature in this age group relates to the frequency of apneic episodes and their possible complications. Normative data in this age group is scanty[39-42] and inconsistent in the definition of apnea, respiratory pauses, and selection biases in "normal" control subjects. Central apneic episodes longer than 10 seconds in duration were frequently observed in low birth-weight prematures (less than 1.4 kg). In premature infants (weight over 1.4 kg) apneic episodes were less frequent and were predominantly obstructive or mixed rather than central. These larger premature infants also demonstrated frequent respiratory pauses (3 to 9.9 seconds in duration). In the small premature, apnea was usually observed in QS, while respiratory pauses in larger prematures were most common during AS. The number of apneic episodes was quite variable between individuals (range 3 to 56 apneic episodes over 20 hours).

Studies in one-to-two-week-old full-term infants[43] indicate that periodic respiration and apneic episodes are normally present at this age but become less frequent with increasing age. While apneic episodes over 15 seconds are rarely seen in the first few weeks of life, such episodes are probably abnormal after three months of age.[40] Studies looking at term infants up to the age of six months have observed a higher incidence of apnea (defined as a cessation of respiration over six seconds) during AS during the first three months of life, which is maximal at birth but declines steadily thereafter.[40] Overall these studies suggest that apnea is a normal finding in the infant and more common with prematurity. Unlike data derived from adult studies, there appears to be no sex difference in the respiratory pattern of infants. The wide variability in data derived from infants makes it difficult to establish a definite "normal" frequency for apneic episodes. Unresolved is the issue of whether multiple, short (two-second) apneic episodes are any more abnormal than infrequent apneas of longer duration. The possible implications of these observations are discussed in more detail in the discussion of sudden infant death syndrome which follows.

PATHOLOGICAL STATES CHARACTERIZED BY SLEEP-DEPENDENT ALTERATIONS IN RESPIRATION

Sleep-induced apnea and hypoventilation are characteristic of a number of recognized "syndromes" and occur in the context of a variety of medical disorders and congenital anomalies. In some cases a common mechanistic factor is involved and we have taken the liberty of grouping some conditions under a single heading. While separation of other entities appears unwarranted, we have chosen to separately discuss clinical syndromes which are rooted in the literature, even where current data suggest a wide overlap with other conditions. Therapeutic approaches have not been discussed in detail, but are included for reference purposes.

Sleep Apnea

This disorder, sometimes referred to as the "hypersomnia-sleep apnea syndrome," is predominantly observed in males who are nonobese, lack detectable pulmonary abnormalities in the waking state, and have no anatomic anomalies of the upper airway on routine examination. The characteristic feature of this "syndrome" is the demonstration of multiple episodes of sleep-related apnea of a central, obstructive or mixed pattern occurring during REM and SWS. Central apnea is defined as a cessation of diaphragmatic and intercostal respiratory effort and is illustrated by the polysomnogram in Figure 10. In obstructive apnea, respiratory effort is sustained, while alveolar ventilation is prevented by obstruction of the upper airway. Shown in Figure 11, obstructive apnea is clearly differentiable from the cen-

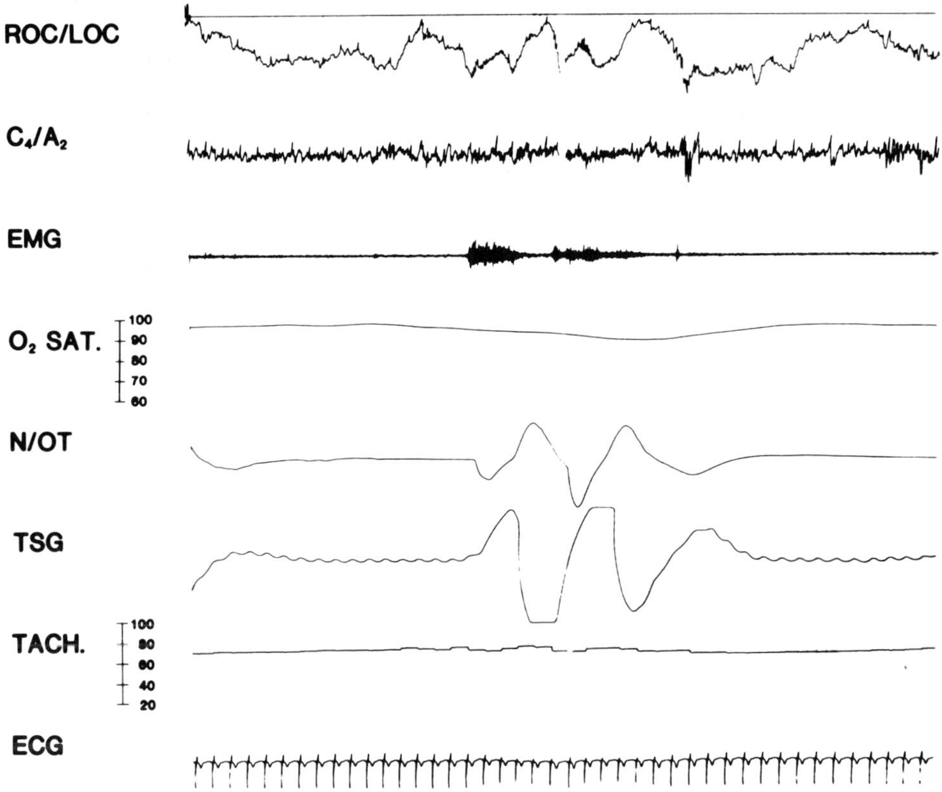

Figure 10. Central apnea. During stage 1, respiratory effort ceases as seen by flattening of the TSG signal (ripples are pulse artifacts). Airflow past the nasal/oral thermocouple stops and oxygen saturation falls to 89 percent. Two adequate respirations are accompanied by a brief run of alpha rhythm in the EEG followed by stage 1 activity and another episode of central apnea.

tral variety by the repetitive activity seen in the thoracic effort tracing. Mixed apneas incorporate polysomnographic features of central and obstructive types. As exemplified in Figure 12, an episode will typically begin as a central apnea of variable duration. Unsuccessful respiratory effort follows, indicating an obstructive component. Eventually the airway opens and ventilation resumes. Since occasional apneic episodes are present in normals, arbitrary limits of normalcy

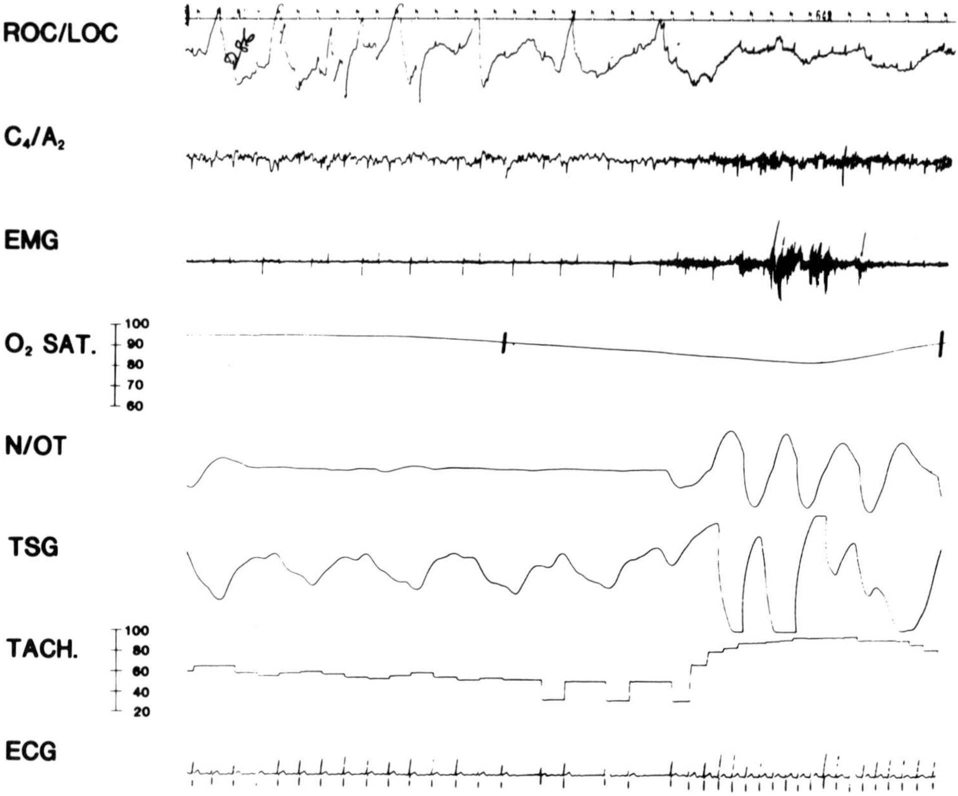

Figure 11. Obstructive apnea. During stage REM, airflow ceases for 21 seconds while unsuccessful respiratory effort continues, indicating obstruction of the upper airway. Oxygen saturation falls to 81 percent. Immediately prior to the resumption of ventilation, the ECG demonstrates 2nd degree A-V block. When ventilation occurs, alpha rhythm appears in the EEG and tachycardia is evident in the ECG.

have been suggested. Guilleminault and co-workers have suggested that patients with more than 30 apneic episodes of 10 seconds or greater duration during seven hours of sleep monitoring are abnormal.[44] In most cases apneic episodes are far more frequent and identification of the abnormality is not a problem. Apneic episodes are associated with oxygen desaturation, hypercarbia and acidosis which tend to be more severe in obstructive and mixed types than in central apnea. Apneic periods have been associated with transient elevations in right heart and pulmonary artery pressure, and systemic systolic arterial pressure is frequently elevated in proportion to the number and severity of the apneic episodes.[44] Polysomnographic records usually demonstrate a loss of deeper levels of SWS and frequent arousals in association with apneic episodes, as seen in the sleep architecture plot of Figure 13. Loud snoring is usually present in affected individuals as well. Some studies have suggested that this disorder may be genetically determined and may

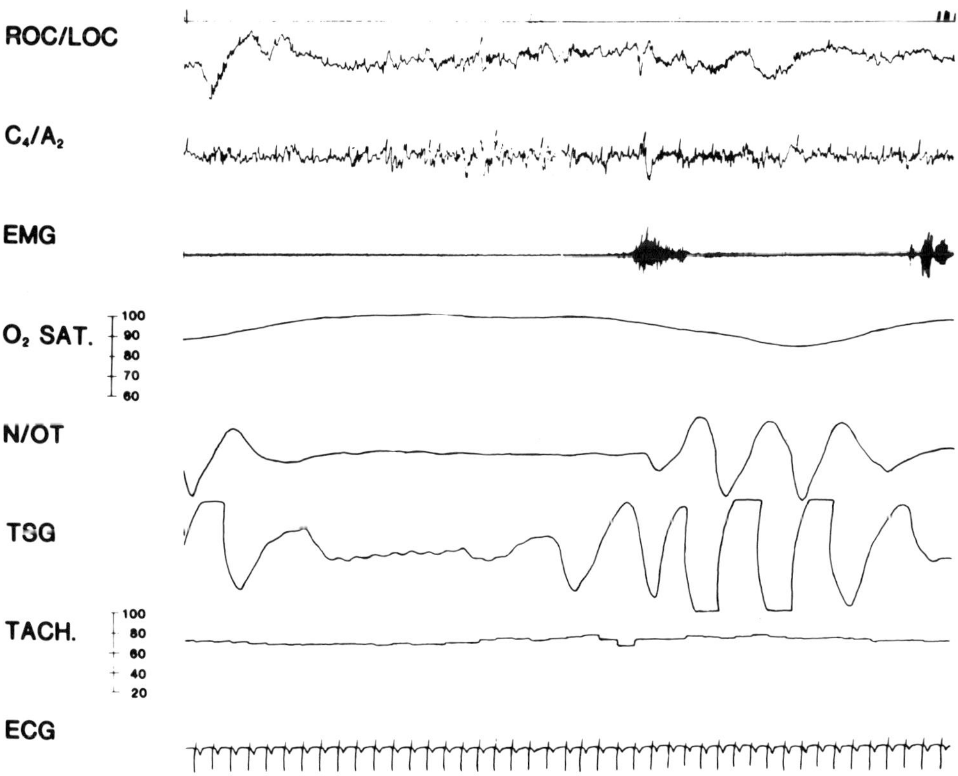

Figure 12. Mixed apnea. A 17-second episode of mixed type apnea during stage 1 begins with a central apnea, cessation of respiratory effort, followed by the appearance of an obstructive component. Two unsuccessful respiratory efforts against an obstructed upper airway occur immediately prior to ventilation. Oxygen saturation falls to 84 percent.

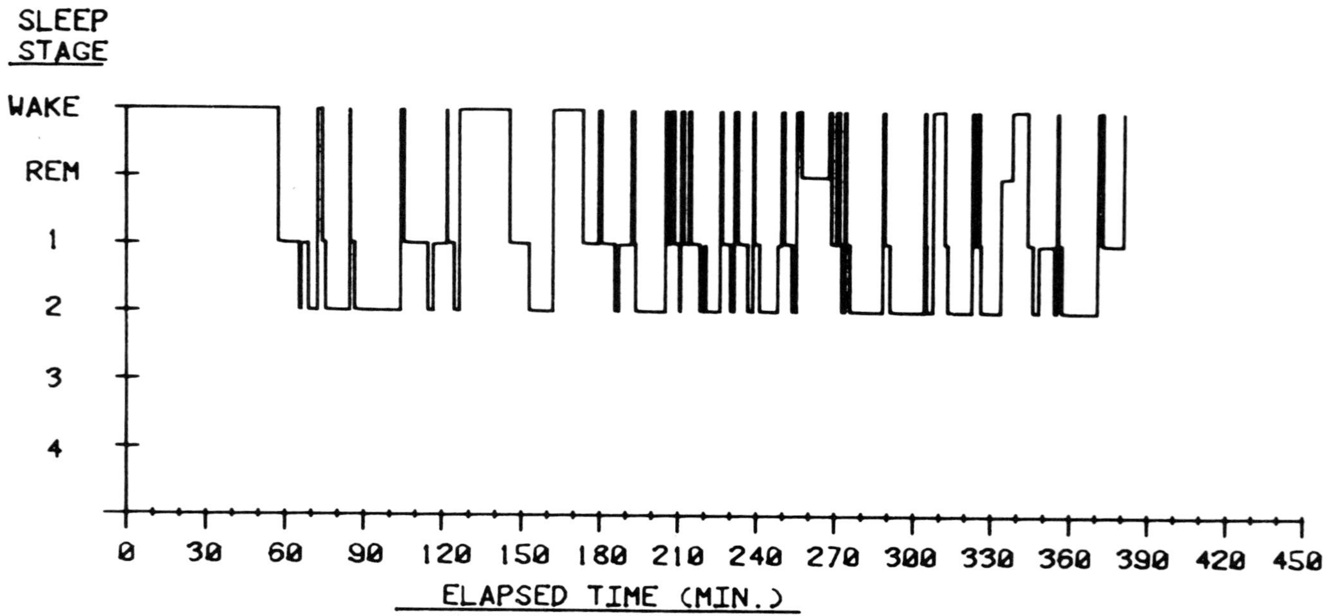

Figure 13. The sleep architecture of an adult male with obstructive sleep apnea syndrome. Stages 3 and 4 are absent, frequent waking arousals occur which fragment the sleep cycle, REM sleep is much reduced as a proportion of the sleep period, and REM periodicity is abolished. The majority of the sleep period consists of NREM stages 1 and 2.

be associated with sudden infant death syndrome in other family members.[45]

Initial studies suggested that a strong association existed between sleep apnea and a host of chronic hemodynamic and behavioral abnormalities including systolic hypertension, pulmonary hypertension, cor pulmonale, hypersomnolence, episodes of amensia, morning headache and insomnia.[44] The view that the syndrome is progressive was supported by some clinical histories and seemed to indicate a need for aggressive treatment even when presenting symptoms were relatively mild. The validity of this assumption has recently come into question.

It is apparent that some patients with sleep-related apnea do not have significant associated symptoms and have no evidence of hypertension or other hemodynamic alterations. Our own experience suggests that selection biases have considerable effect and the severity of symptoms reported initially may reflect the fact that patients in these series were referred primarily for excessive somnolence. As public recognition of the disorder was increased through articles in local newspapers, we saw a number of referrals generated by family members who had observed episodes of apnea in association with excessive snoring. In the majority of these patients, frequent episodes of apnea were observed but other symptoms were relatively insignificant, in spite of the fact that most patients had been lifelong snorers and restless sleepers. Other studies have demonstrated no correlation between the number and duration of apneic episodes and the presence of hypersomnia[46,47] and suggest that sleep-related arterial carbon dioxide retention and polysomnographic abnormalities are not significantly different in apneic patients complaining of or lacking hypersomnia.

It currently appears that clear differentiation between "malignant" and "benign" forms of the sleep apnea syndrome cannot be conclusively made on the basis of routine polysomnographic and respiratory monitoring. Identification of the parameter which is best related to symptomatic deterioration is still a matter of controversy with various authors favoring waking arterial oxygen saturation (P_aO_2)[47] or arterial pH[48] as the critical variables.

The role of other variables such as body weight, intrinsic pulmonary disease or physical habitus to the sleep apnea syndrome is still not entirely clear. The role of obesity is perhaps the most confusing of these issues. On the one hand it is obvious that obesity is not a requisite for the development of symptomatic sleep apnea.[44] Conversely, previously cited studies have demonstrated that hypoventilation and apneic episodes tend to be more prevalent in individuals who are overweight[21] and other groups have reported improvement in symptoms and hemodynamic status in sleep apneics following weight reduction.[49-51] While these studies suggest that excessive weight adversely effects patients with sleep apnea, confusion arises from other studies which have found no benefit from weight reduction.[52]

The issue is further clouded by our lack of understanding concerning the alterations in appetitive drive which seem to be linked to specific hypersomniac states such as the Klein-Levin syndrome (hypersomnia, megaphagia and bulimia).[53] In our own experience it is not uncommon to encounter a history of progressive hypersomnia and concomitant weight gain in patients with documented sleep apnea. It has also been observed that some obese apneics will spontaneously lose weight following therapeutic tracheostomy, suggesting that excessive food intake may be a symptom of sleep apnea as well as a causative factor in its maintenance. If this latter observation is valid it suggests that a vicious cycle may exist in some patients with sleep apnea in which weight gain follows repetitive apneic episodes and then acts as a detrimental factor in maintaining and potentially worsening the apneic episodes.

The role of intrinsic lung disease in this disorder also awaits further clarification. Sleep-related hypoventilation and apnea has been reported in patients with chronic obstructive pulmonary disease[54] and appears to be most prevalent in males. As in the case of sleep apneics with no evidence of intrinsic pulmonary disease, sleep-related respiratory alterations in patients with chronic obstructive pulmonary disease are most common in Stages I and II and REM sleep. From these studies it seems probable that patients with sleep apnea might experience a worsening of the condition in the presence of an independent pulmonary disorder. In this regard we have observed one patient with mild restrictive pulmonary disease who developed severe hypersomnia when treated with low doses of propranolol, and was subsequently found to have sleep apnea. Discontinuation of propranolol led to an improvement of waking pulmonary function, reduced the frequency of apneic episodes and led to an improvement in the original complaint of hypersomnia.

At the present time data suggest that intrinsic pulmonary abnormalities may contribute to the severity of apneic episodes in a patient with preexisting sleep apnea. It seems unlikely that pulmonary disease alone can cause sleep apnea in a patient lacking a primary predisposition to the disorder.

The final variable which may play a role in sleep apnea is that of body habitus. Many sleep apneics have a stocky frame, short neck, and receeding chin (personal observation; see Imes et al.[55] for typical photographs). The association between these physical features and the appearance of sleep apnea is not understood, but raises the possibility that a related anatomic configuration of upper airway (perhaps amenable to surgical correction) may exist in these individuals. Possibly related is the observation that some sleep apneics appear to have position-dependent apnea (personal observation). In such individuals, sleeping in a sitting or decubitus position leads to disappearance of obstructive apneic episodes for unknown reasons. The anatomic changes which occur with positional changes during sleep need clarification before this phenomenon is explained but suggest that relatively critical relationships in the anatomic arrangement of the upper airway may be involved in the ultimate appearance of sleep apnea.

The underlying abnormality in sleep apnea is not completely understood. From a mechanical standpoint, collapse of the upper airway during sleep has been documented radiographically[56] as well as by direct fiberoptic observation, and appears to be the initial event in obstructive apneic episodes. This phenomenon has been related to the diminished EMG activity noted in various muscle groups during REM sleep which is felt to be mediated centrally (possibly via the reticulospinal system). Support for this hypothesis has been derived from experimental studies in the cat documenting increased upper airway resistance during REM sleep associated with decreased muscle activity in the laryngeal adductors.[26] The fact that sleep apnea is rarely confined to periods of REM sleep makes such a theory difficult to accept. While it is possible that patients with sleep apnea exhibit inhibition of muscle tone (upper airway) during SWS periods, proof of such an event is still lacking.

A defect in central respiratory control is easier to accept in the case of central (nonobstructive) apneic episodes though many questions still remain unanswered in respect to its basis. It has been suggested that central apneic episodes are a result of chronic obstructive apnea.[44] This theory is based on the observation that following tracheostomy, obstructive apneic episodes are abolished as is hypersomnia, while episodes of central apnea persist for months.[44] Follow-up of such patients reveals a gradual decline in the number of central apneic episodes, suggesting a reliance on obstructive apnea. The validity of assuming that these observations support the contention that obstructive apneic episodes (or their hemodynamic consequences) somehow alter central respiratory control mechanisms remains open to question. Such a hypothesis also fails to explain the occasional patient who suffers predominantly from central sleep apnea. Since patients with obstructive apnea appear to have diminished responses to hypercapnea, it may be that chronic intermittent hypoxia renders them less sensitive to hypoxic drive as well. From a mechanistic standpoint cessation of wakefulness and a loss of cortical respiratory drive would lead to respiratory failure in the absence of a functional metabolic control center. While amenable to study, data to support this hypothesis are not currently available.

Pathological studies in patients with sleep apnea are scanty and have not clearly identified a related anatomic abnormality of the nervous system which might explain the disorder. One report of gliosis in the raphe nuclei and associated neuronal degenerative changes in the same region in a patient with documented sleep apnea[57] is difficult to interpret in view of the fact that the patient suffered from idiopathic orthostatic hypotension (Shy-Drager syndrome). Even in this case, a careful search for alterations in the medullary pneumotaxic centers failed to reveal any abnormalities.

Other authors have suggested that a search for central nervous system pathology is likely to be fruitless and suggest that sleep apnea "syndrome" is an expression of normal physiologic mechanisms which become "pathological" in the presence of baseline alterations in arterial saturation.[47] In studying the P_aO_2 alterations in hypersomnolent and nonsomnolent sleep apneics, it was found that both groups demonstrated comparable drops in P_aO_2 during sleep. The symptomatic group, however, demonstrated considerably greater desaturation (as determined via the Severinghaus nomogram). From these data it has been suggested that symptomatic sleep apneics tend to have mild hypoxemia at rest, and sleep-related decreases in arterial P_aO_2 therefore tend to fall on a steeper portion of the oxyhemoglobin dissociation curve. This theory is consistent with the observations already cited which indicate that apneic episodes are more prolonged and more frequent in patients with obstructive lung disease or significant obesity, which would both potentially decrease steady state waking arterial oxygen saturation.

Therapeutic approaches have been derived from various theories and all approaches have attracted groups of proponents. Most authors agree that tracheostomy is virtually curative in the sleep apneic with obstructive apnea.[44] The major problem with this form of therapy (aside from the operative complications, cosmetic considerations and inconvenience of such a procedure) has been the establishment of definite criteria for its application. It is clear that sleep apnea may be an asymptomatic disorder. If one believes that it is progressive, however, one could logically argue that all apneics should be treated to prevent potential complications. Our own feeling is that this view is not supported to a degree which warrants surgical intervention in the absence of incapacitating hypersomnia or life-threatening cardiovascular disease (including the presence of significant apnea-related cardiac arrhythmias).

Pharmacologic therapy of sleep apnea has been attempted using a number of agents and has generated conflicting results. Theophylline,[58] protriptylline and pemoline[59] have been reported to improve sleep architecture and reduce the frequency of apneic episodes, presumably through their ability to indirectly increase central monoaminergic activity. While effective in some patients, none of the above agents has been found universally effective. The observation that sleep apnea is predominantly encountered in males has led to attempts at altering hormonal environment by administering progesterone.[48,60] In most trials this form of therapy has been of no benefit.

From the above discussion it would seem worthwhile to urge weight reduction in those patients with associated obesity and maximize pulmonary function in those patients with underlying pulmonary disease before embarking on more heroic forms of therapy. Symptomatic therapy of mild daytime somnolence with low doses of various central stimulants (such as d-amphetamine) is frequently useful though it has little effect on nocturnal apneic episodes.

HYPERSOMNIA-SLEEP APNEA SYNDROME IN ASSOCIATION WITH CONGENITAL OR ACQUIRED ANOMALIES OF THE UPPER AIRWAY

In this group of disorders, summarized in Table II, structural abnormalities of the upper airway appear related to the development of sleep apnea and associated symptoms including hypersomnia and varying degrees of cor pulmonale and alveolar hypoventilation. In those cases where all night polysomnographic monitoring was carried out, apneic episodes of a mixed or obstructive pattern were observed during SWS. Sleep was frequently interrupted by spontaneous awakenings, and relative REM suppression was usually

TABLE II
Conditions Associated With Sleep Apnea

CONGENITAL	
	Prader Willi syndrome[67]
	Pierre Robin syndrome[44]
	Retrognathia[55]
	Micognathia[62]
ACQUIRED	
	Postsurgical micrognathia[62,64]
	Sinusitis, enlarged tonsils and adenoids[65,66]

observed. Very little time was spent in Stages III and IV of SWS. In most cases loud snoring was also noted during sleep. In children studied for evaluation of episodic apnea, the development of upper respiratory infections has been associated with an increase in the frequency and duration of sleep apnea episodes suggesting that acquired upper airway obstruction may induce apnea.[42] Varying degrees of alveolar hypoventilation which appears during drowsiness or sleep are reported in this patient population. Since all night records were not obtained in many instances, it is impossible to establish whether alveolar hypoventilation in the absence of sleep apnea may be associated with any of the above conditions.

In those cases where individualized surgical corrective procedures were performed, dramatic reversal of behavioral symptoms has been reported. These include dramatic cases in which cor pulmonale in association with tonsilar enlargement was entirely reversed following tonsilectomy. The lack of evidence of primary intrinsic pulmonary or cardiovascular abnormalities in these patients strongly suggests that mechanical factors resulting in obstructive apnea during sleep are the primary cause of the symptoms ultimately observed. Since not all individuals with the above acquired or congenital abnormalities develop signs and symptoms of sleep apnea, it has been suggested by some authors that an additional risk factor must be present in those patients who develop sleep apnea. The possibility that affected patients represent that segment of the normal population demonstrating a propensity for alveolar hypoventilation during sleep has been raised[44] but remains unsupported by a definitive study.

Pickwickian Syndrome

This entity, first described by Osler,[67] is classically characterized by obesity, hypersomnolence, periodic breathing, hypoventilation and cor pulmonale. Other variants are characterized by obesity and hypersomnia and varying degrees of cardiorespiratory dysfunction. The primary abnormality in this disorder was debated for many years and various proponents favored a central nervous system abnormality while others stressed the role of obesity in its pathogenesis. Massive obesity has been related to ventilation-perfusion abnormalities, early closure of dependent airways and right-left shunting resulting from upward displacement of the diaphragms.[68,69] The resultant hypercapnea and hypoxemia was felt to somehow alter the sensitivity and function of the central nervous system and give rise to altered levels of consciousness and periodic respiration. Authors favoring a primary alteration in central respiratory control pointed out the lack of behavioral symptoms in patients with hypercapnea arising from other pulmonary disorders and the rarity of the syndrome in these individuals and suggested that factors other than simple obesity were operative in Pickwickian patients.

When Pickwickian patients were evaluated for sleep disturbances it became apparent that episodes of sleep apnea were characteristic in this group.[1,70-72] These observations led many authors to conclude that the Pickwickian syndrome was a subgroup of sleep apnea and did not exist as a distinct entity.[44]

Currently it is very difficult to know whether all Pickwickian patients do in fact suffer from primary sleep apnea. Recent papers have discussed sleep apnea as a complicating factor in Pickwickian syndrome (with the implication that the Pickwickian syndrome is a disorder in its own right) but stressed the role of obesity and poorly defined "central abnormalities" in respiratory control in the management of such patients.[73]

If the Pickwickian syndrome is a distinct entity it is clear that it is difficult to distinguish from sleep apnea. Until distinctive features are found which would support a separation of the Pickwickian syndrome from other forms of sleep apnea, it seems more parsimonious to consider this disorder an historical one amenable to the same therapeutic approaches used in primary sleep apnea.

Primary Alveolar Hypoventilation

This syndrome, characterized by erythrocytosis, pulmonary hypertension, and hypoventilation is a relatively rare disorder thought to rely on an abnormality of central metabolic respiratory control. Previous reports have observed the condition following bulbar poliomyelitis,[75] medullary infarction,[76,77] and bilateral cervical cordotomy.[78] In other cases the disorder arises spontaneously and is occasionally found to resolve.[48] Ondine's Curse[79] constitutes the classic form of the disorder.

In classic form the disorder arises in the absence of any detectable pulmonary abnormality. Respiratory drive in response to hypercapnea and hypoxia is lost, though isolated loss of hypercapneic drive may occur.[48] Hypoventilation during exercise is also routinely encountered.[80] Obstructive apneic episodes during sleep are notably absent in most cases.[48,80,81] During sleep, patients with primary alveolar hypoventilation exhibit a marked reduction in ventilatory effort with resultant carbon dioxide retention, hypoxemia and acidosis. Hypoxic neurologic sequelae or death may result.

Artificial ventilation during sleep has been employed in some cases and current interest surrounds use of phrenic nerve stimulators.[81] The basis of this disorder in patients lacking clear cut neurological injuries is unknown. The marked discrepancy in respiratory drive between the waking and sleeping state has been related to the presence of higher cortical drive mechanisms which are inactivated during sleep though the interaction of these systems in patients with incomplete forms of the disorder remains unknown.

Using the previously developed model of central respiratory control, the hypoventilation syndromes appear to result from a total or partial failure of the metabolic respiratory control system. Thus, waking respiratory function is normal and under the control of cortical respiratory drive and nonspecific arousal-related stimulation, but becomes abnormal when these centers are inhibited by sleep. In the case of patients with bilateral transcutaneous cordotomy, loss of peripheral afferent input may contribute to the observed failure of metabolic respiratory control.

Sudden Infant Death and Near-Miss Sudden Infant Death Syndromes

Unexplained, presumably respiratory deaths occur in approximately 10,000 seemingly healthy infants a year. Prematurity and the presence of nonspecific upper respiratory infections are frequently associated.[82] While many etiologies have been suggested, considerable data now support the hypothesis that these syndromes represent an extreme of normal respiratory events in the sleeping infant.[41,42,60,83]

Because of the nature of the disorder, sudden infant death syndrome is not amenable to direct study and mechanisms operative in this condition have been inferred from studies in infants with prolonged apneic episodes (near-miss sudden infant death syndrome). In these studies infants with episodic apnea and cyanosis or recorded apneic episodes greater than 15 to 20 seconds in duration were viewed as a population "at-risk" for SIDS.[41,42,84] Physical examination in these patients was universally normal. In all studies patients were found to have multiple apneic episodes during sleep. Central apnea was most prevalent and most frequently associated with periods of AS.[42] In infants with audible stridor during sleep or in the presence of upper respiratory congestion, obstructive or mixed apneic episodes were more frequent. In premature infants apneic episodes were usually of a central type and tended to be more common in periods of QS. In comparison with normals, subjects with near-miss SIDS have been reported to be less sensitive to CO_2 inhalation, and exhibit higher sleeping alveolar carbon dioxide partial pressures.[41] In all reports, a number of subjects subsequently died, presumably from respiratory failure, confirming earlier reports that near-miss SIDS is associated with a 20 percent or greater chance of SIDS. Whether central apneas or obstructive apneas are specifically related to fatal respiratory complication remains controversial. Since the percentage of AS sleep is considerably higher in the infant, occupying approximately 50 percent of total sleep time, it has been suggested that the physiological alterations characteristic of this stage of sleep rather than the type of apnea observed represent the critical variable.[20]

The role of genetic factors in SIDS and near-miss SIDS has been stressed in recent publications which demonstrate impaired hypercarbic ventilatory drive and impaired ability to increase respiratory effort in the presence of inspiratory resistance in parents of children dying from apparent episodes of SIDS.[85] This study and the occurrence of SIDS in family members of some patients with sleep apnea syndrome[45] suggest that inherited patterns of respiratory control may be a potential risk factor.

Autopsy studies frequently demonstrate intrathoracic petechiae, pulmonary artery hypertrophy, right ventricular hypertrophy and evidence of extramedullary hematopoeisis. In most cases the central nervous system is normal. A finding of gliosis involving the midline raphe in the absence of neuronal drop-out in one case is of unknown significance.[86] Recent reports indicate that the brain stem auditory evoked-potentials are abnormal in 40 percent of "near-miss'" infants, though the validity of this observation as a predictor of SIDS is unknown.[96]

Since SIDS is encountered in the first year of life, treatment is aimed at supporting the patient through this period. Various approaches have been suggested including home use of an apnea monitor in conjunction with parental training in CPR,[84] or therapy with caffeine.[87,88] Increased surveillance in infants with "near-miss" apneas who develop upper respiratory infections also seems warranted in the context of data currently available.

Nocturnal Asthma

Nocturnal episodes of symptomatic bronchoconstriction are not uncommon phenomena and have been hypothesized to rely on the presence of allergens in the bed,[63] variations in serum corticosteroid levels[89] or the effects of recumbency. None of these theories appears to be an adequate explanation[20] and a relation to sleep events appears more likely. While neither the sleep stage nor the mechanisms involved has been reported, experimental studies in the dog suggest that REM sleep may alter smooth muscle tone in the tracheobronchial tree (probably on the basis of autonomic alterations).[90] The possibility that modification of sleep architecture (e.g., states of REM rebound) might correlate with episodes of nocturnal asthma may offer novel approaches in this disorder.

High-Altitude Polycythemia

In a population of high-altitude dwellers a small number of individuals are encountered with polycythemia (erythrocytosis). In addition to hematologic abnormalities, these patients also frequently complain of impaired thinking and severe headaches (chronic mountain sickness).[91,92] In some cases, diastolic hypertension, pulmonary hypertension and right ventricular hypertrophy have been encountered.[93] Symptoms and hematologic abnormalities resolve following phlebotomy or relocation to lower altitudes.

While some affected individuals suffer from intrinsic pulmonary disease, and are theoretically more susceptible to the effects of ambient hypoxia, other individuals lack evidence of pulmonary dysfunction. Both groups demonstrate blunted hypoxic drive with resultant hypoventilation in the waking state though the basis of this deficit in individuals lacking pulmonary disorders has remained a point of controversy.[91,92]

Recent studies have demonstrated that sleep-related hypoventilation and sleep architecture disturbance are characteristic features of patients with high-altitude polycythemia[94] and differentiate this group from control subjects. From these data it has been suggested that sleep-related hypoventilation may be a critical feature in the pathophysiology of this disorder, especially in symptomatic patients with insignificant arterial desaturation in the waking state. The primary respiratory control abnormality which renders such individuals susceptible to this complication of high-altitude living remains unclear and requires further study.

Therapy with medoxyprogesterone has been associated with long-term reversal of hematologic abnormalities, symptomatic improvement, and a drop in diastolic blood pressure.[95] In some patients serial electrocardiograms demonstrate reversal of right-axis deviation during the course of therapy, interpreted as a reflection of reduced pulmonary artery pressure. Enhanced hypoxic drive was observed in medoxyprogesterone-treated subjects with normal lungs but not in those with intrinsic pulmonary disease. Therapy was not found to have any effect on CO_2 drive in either group.[95] The basis of symptomatic improvement in patients lacking improvement in hypoxic drive remains unclear.

CONCLUSION

The number of "sleep-related" respiratory syndromes has grown larger each year and generated increased interest in the role of sleep in a host of previously unexplained clinical disorders. The discovery of primary sleep-related respiratory disturbances points up the problems in assuming that the routine history and physical examination provides adequate information for the diagnosis and understanding of all pathological conditions. Unconscious events in the course of normal sleep may initiate physiologic events which ultimately produce diurnal behavioral and physiologic pathology. In clinical practice, evaluation of sleep events may be a "dark side of the moon" in need of further investigation.

REFERENCES

1. Gastaut, H., Tassainari, C.A., and Duron, B.: Etude polygraphique des manifestations épisodiques (hypniques et respiratoires), diurnes et nocturnes, du syndrome de Pickwick. *Rev. Neurol.* **112**: 568–579, 1965.
2. Lugaresi, E.: Polygraphic aspects of sleep in man. *Bull. Physiopathol. Respir.* **8**: 1071–1074, 1972.
3. Duron, B., Tassinarini, C.A., and Gastaut, H.: Analyse spirographique et électromyographique de la respiration au cours du sommeil controllée par l'EEG chez l'homme normal. *Rev. Neurol.* **115**: 562–574, 1966.
4. Rechtschaffen, A., and Kales, A.: A manual of standardized terminology, techniques and scoring system for sleep stages of human subjects. Pub. #204, Public Health Service, Washington, D.C., U.S. Govt. Print. Off., 1968.
5. Anders, T., Emde, R., and Parmelee, A.: A manual of standard terminology techniques and criteria for scoring of states of sleep and wakefulness in newborn infants. Los Angeles, UCLA Brain Information Service/BRI Publication Office, 1971.
6. Bellville, J.W., Howland, W.S., Seed, J.C., and Houde, R.W.: The effect of sleep on the respiratory response to carbon dioxide. *Anesthesiology* **20**: 628, 1959.
7. Bulow, K., and Ingvar, D.H.: Respiration and state of wakefulness in normals, studied by spirography, capnography and EEG. *Acta Physiol. Scand.* **51**: 230–238, 1961.
8. Bulow, K.: Respiration and wakefulness in man. *Acta Physiol. Scand.* **59** (Suppl): 209, 1963.

9. Wurtz, R.H., and O'Flaherty, J.J.: Physiological correlates of steady potential shifts during sleep and wakefulness. I. Sensitivity of the steady potential to alterations in carbon dioxide. *Electroencephalogr. Clin. Neurophysiol.* **22**: 30–42, 1967.
10. Guazzi, M., and Freis, E.D.: Sino-aortic reflexes and arterial pH, Po_2 and Pco_2 in wakefulness and sleep. *Am. J. Physiol.* **217**: 1623–1627, 1969.
11. Robin, E.D., et al.: Alveolar gas tension, pulmonary ventilation and blood pH during physiologic sleep in normal subjects. *J. Clin. Invest.* **37**: 981–989, 1958.
12. Birchfield, R.I., Sieker, H.O., and Hyman, A.: Alterations in blood gases during natural sleep and narcolepsy. *Neurology* **8**: 107–112, 1958.
13. Birchfield, R.I., Sieker, H.O., and Hyman, A.: Alterations in respiratory function during natural sleep. *J. Lab. Clin. Med.* **54**:216–222, 1959.
14. Sieker, H.O., Heyman, A., and Birchfield, R.I.: The effects of natural sleep and hypersomnolent states on respiratory function. *Ann. Intern. Med.* **52**: 500–516, 1960.
15. Newson-Davis, J., Loh, L., and Nadal, J.: The effects of CO_2 on the breathing pattern in awake and sleeping man (abs.). *Bull. Eur. Physiolpathol. Resp.* **12**: 237, 1976.
16. Reed, D.J., and Kellogg, R.H.: Effect of sleep on hypoxic stimulation of breathing at sea level and altitude. *J. Appl. Physiol.* **15**: 1130, 1960a.
17. Reed, D.J., and Kellogg, R.H.: Effect of sleep on CO_2 stimulation of breathing in acute and chronic hypoxia. *J. Appl. Physiol.* **15**: 1135, 1960b.
18. Pappenheimer, J.R.: Sleep and respiration of rats during hypoxia. *J. Physiol. (Lond.)* **266**: 191, 1977.
19. Phillipson, E.A., Sullivan, C.E., Read, D.J., Murphy, E., and Kozan, I.F.: Ventilatory and waking responses to hypoxia in sleeping dogs. *J. Appl. Physiol. Respir. Environ. Exercise Physiol.* **44**: 512, 1978.
20. Phillipson, E.A.: Respiratory adaptations in sleep. *Ann. Rev. Physiol.* **40**: 133–156, 1978.
21. Block, A., Boysen, P., Wynne, J., and Hunt, L.: Sleep apnea, hypopnea and oxygen desaturation in normal subjects. *N. Eng. J. Med.* **300**: 513–517, 1979.
22. Arkinstall, W.V., Nirmel, K., Klissouras, V., and Milic-Emili, J.: Genetic differences in the ventilatory response to inhaled CO_2. *J. Appl. Physiol.* **36**: 6–11, 1974.

23. Duron, B.: La fonction respiratoire pendant le sommeil physiologique. *Bull. Physiopathol. Respir.* **8**: 1031–1057, 1972.
24. Gillam, P.M.S.: Patterns of respiration in human beings at rest and during sleep. *Bull. Physiopathol. Respir.* **8**: 1059–1072, 1972.
25. Webb, P.: Periodic breathing during sleep. *J. Appl. Physiol.* **37**: 899–903, 1974.
26. Orem, J., Netick, A., and Dement, W.C.: Breathing during sleep and wakefulness in the cat. *Respir. Physiol.* **43**: 14–22, 1977.
27. Hathorn, M.K.S.: The rate and depth of breathing in newborn infants in different sleep stages. *J. Physiol. (Lond.)* **243**: 101–113, 1974.
28. Phillipson, E.A., Murphy, E., and Kozar, L.F.: Regulation of respiration in sleeping dogs. *J. Appl. Physiol.* **40**: 688–693, 1976.
29. Goodenough, D.R., et al.: The effects of stress films on dream affect and on respiration and eye-movement activity during rapid eye movement sleep. *Psychophysiology* **12**: 313–320, 1975.
30. Hobson, J.A., Goldfrank, F., and Snyder, F.: Respiration and mental activity in sleep. *J. Psychiat. Res.* **3**: 79–90, 1965.
31. Jouvet, M.: Paradoxical sleep—a study of its nature and mechanisms. In Akert, K., Bally, C., and Schade, J.P. (eds.): *Progress in Brain Research Mechanisms,* Vol. 18. Amsterdam, Elsevier, 1965, pp. 20–62.
32. Bryan, H.M., et al.: CO_2 response and sleep state in infants. *Clin. Res.* **24**: (Abs.) A689, 1976.
33. Phillipson, E.A., Kozat, L.F., Rebuck, A.S., and Murphy, E.: Ventilatory and waking responses to CO_2 in sleeping dogs. *Am. Rev. Respir. Dis.* **115**: 251, 1977.
34. Sullivan, C.E., Kozar, L.F., Murphy, E., and Phillipson, E.A.: Primary role of respiratory afferents in sustaining breathing rhythm. *J. Appl. Physiol. Respir. Environ. Exercise Physiol.* **45**: 11, 1978b.
35. Fagenhotz, S.A., O'Connell, K., and Shanon, D.C.: Chemoreceptor function and sleep state in apnea. *Pediatrics* **58**: 31, 1976.
36. Sullivan, C.E., Murphy, E., Kozar, L.F., and Phillipson, E.A.: Waking and ventilatory responses to laryngeal stimulation in sleeping dogs. *J. Appl. Physiol.: Respir. Environ. Exercise Physiol.* **45**: 681, 1978a.
37. Aserinsky, E. Periodic respiratory pattern occurring in con-

junction with eye movements during sleep. *Science* **150**: 763–766, 1965.
38. Aserinsky, E.: Physiological activity associated with segments of the rapid eye movement period. In Evants, E., Kety, S., and Williams, H. (eds.): *Sleep and Altered States of Consciousness.* Baltimore, Williams and Wilkins, 1967, pp. 335–350.
39. Stein, I., White, A., Kennedy, J., Merisalo, R., Chernoff, H., and Gould, J.: Apnea recordings of healthy infants at 40, 44 and 52 weeks postconception. *Pediatrics* **63**: 724–730, 1979.
40. Hoppenbrouwers, T., Hodgman, J., Harper, R., Hofman, E., Sterman, M., and McGinty, D.: Polygraphic studies of normal infant during the first six months of life: incidence of apnea and periodic breathing. *Pediatrics* **60**: 418–425, 1977.
41. Shannon, D., Kelly, D., and O'Connell, K.: Abnormal regulation of ventilation in infants at risk for Sudden-Infant-Death Syndrome. *N. Eng. J. Med.* **297**: 747–750, 1977.
42. Guilleminault, C., Peraita, R., Souquet, M., and Dement, W.: Apneas during sleep in infants: Possible relationship with sudden infant death syndrome. *Science* **190**: 677–679, 1975.
43. Parmelee, A.H., Stern, E., and Harris, M.A.: Maturation of respiration in premature and newborn infants during the first three days of life. *Neuropaediatr.* **3**: 294, 1972.
44. Tuilleminault, C., Tilkian, A., and Dement, W.C.: The sleep apnea syndromes. *Ann. Rev. Med.* **27**: 465–484, 1976.
45. Strohl, K., Saunders, N., Feldman, N., and Hallet, M.: Obstructive sleep apnea in family members. *N. Eng. J. Med.* **299**: 969–973, 1978.
46. Orr, W.C., Imes, N.K., Martin, R.J., et al.: Sleep apnea in symptomatic and asymptomatic groups. *Clin. Res.* **26**: 38A, 1978.
47. Orr, W., Martin, R., Imes, N., Rogers, R., and Stahl, M.: Hypersomnolent and nonhypersomnolent patients with upper airway obstruction. *Chest* **75**: 418–422, 1979.
48. Bubis, I., and Anthonisen, N.: Primary alveolar hypoventilation treated by nocturnal administration of O_2. *Am. Rev. Respir. Dis.* **118**: 947–952, 1978.
49. Karacan, I., et al.: Disturbed sleep as a function of sleep apnea: too much sleep but not enough. *Tex. Med.* **73**: 10 49–56, 1977.
50. Fisher, J.G., de la Pena, A., and Donovan, N.W.: Initial treatment of mixed deep apnea syndrome in an obese patient by starvation. *Sleep Res.* **5**: 168, 1976.
51. Fisher, J.G., et al.: Starvation and behavior modification as a

treatment in obese patients with sleep apnea—a follow-up. *Sleep Res.* **7**: 222, 1978.

52. Guilleminault, C., and Dement, W.C.: Sleep apnea syndromes and related sleep disorders. In Williams, R.L., and Karacan, I. (eds.): *Sleep Disorders: Diagnosis and Treatment.* New York, John Wiley and Sons, 1978, pp. 9–28.
53. Critchley, M.: Periodic hypersomnia and megaphagia in adolescent males. *Brain* **85**: 627–656, 1962.
54. Wynne, J.W., Block, A.J., Hemenway, J., et al.: Disordered breathing and oxygen desaturation during sleep in patients with chronic obstructive pulmonary disease. *Chest* **73** (Suppl.): 301–303, 1978.
55. Imes, N., Orr, W., Smith, R., and Rogers, R.: Retrognathia and sleep apnea. *J.A.M.A.* **237**: 1596–1597, 1977.
56. Schwartz, B., and Escande, J.: Etude cinematographique de la respiration hypnique Pickwickienne. *Rev. Neurol.* **116**: 667–678, 1967.
57. Guilleminault, C., Tilkian, A., Lehrman, K., Forno, L., and Dement, W.: Sleep Apnea Syndrome: states of sleep and autonomic dysfunction. *J. Neurol. Neurosurg. Psychiat.* **40**: 718–725, 1977.
58. Shkurovick, Z.M., et al.: The effects of theophylline on the sleep apnea syndrome. *Sleep Res.* **5**: 188, 1976.
59. Schmidt, H., and Clark, R.W.: Hypersomnia, narcolepsy-cataplexy syndrome, and sleep apnea: Treatment with protriptyline and pemoline. *Sleep Res.* **6**: 179, 1977.
60. Lyons, H.A., and Huang, C.T.: Therapeutic use of progesterone in alveolar hypoventilation associated with obesity. *Am. J. Med.* **44**: 881–888, 1968.
61. Hall, B.D., and Smith, D.W.: Prader-Willi Syndrome. *J. Pediat.* **28**: 686–693, 1972.
62. Tammeling, G., Blokzi, E., Boonstra, S., et al.: Micrognathia, hypersomnia, and periodic breathing. *Bull. Physiopathol. Respir.* **8**: 1228–1238, 1972.
63. Weitzman, E., Pollak, C., Borowjecki, B., et al.: The hypersomnia-sleep apnea syndrome: Site and mechanism of upper airway obstruction. In Guilleminault, C., and Dement, W. (eds.): *Sleep Apnea Syndromes.* New York, Allan R. Liss Corp., 1978a.
64. Weitzman, E., Pollack, C., and Borowiecki, B.: Hypersomnia-sleep apnea due to micrognathia. *Arch. Neurol.* **35**: 392–395, 1978b.
65. Djalilian, M., Kern, E., Brown, H.V., Facer, G., Stickler, G.,

Weidman, W., and O'Connell, E.: Hypoventilation secondary to chronic upper airway obstruction in childhood. *Mayo Clin. Proc.* **50**: 11–14, 1975.

66. Monashe, V.D., Farrehi, C., and Miller, M.: Hypoventilation and cor pulmonale due to chronic upper airway obstruction. *J. Pediat.* **67**: 198–203, 1965.
67. Osler, W.: *The Principles and Practice of Medicine,* 8th Ed. New York, Appleton, 1918.
68. Don, H.F., Craig, D.B., Wahba, W.M., et al.: The measurement of gas trapped in lungs at functional residual capacity and the effects of posture. *Anesthesiology* **35**: 582–590, 1971.
69. Bates, D.V., Macklem, P.T., and Christie, R.V.: *Respiratory Function in Disease,* 2nd Ed. Philadelphia, W.B. Saunders, 1971, p. 100.
70. Duron, B., Tassinari, C., Laval, P., and Gastaut, H.: Les pauses respiratoires survenant au cours due sommeil chez Thomme. *C. R. Soc. Biol.* **161**: 634–639, 1967.
71. Lugaresi, E., Cocagna, G., Berti Geroni, G., Petrella, A., and Mantovani, M.: La "maledizione di Ondine" il disturbo del respiro de, sono nell' ipoventilazione alveolare primaria. *Sist. Nerv.* **20**: 27–37, 1968.
72. Kuhlo, W., Doll, E., and Franc, M.: Exfolgreich Behandlung eines Pickwick Syndrome durch eine dauertracheal Kanüle. *Dtsch. Med. Wochenschr.* **94**: 1286–1290, 1969.
73. Whitcomb, M., Altman, M., Clark, R., and Ralstin, J.: Central and obstructive sleep apnea. *Chest* **73**: 857–860, 1978.
74. Sutton, F.D., Jr., Zwillich, C.W., Creagh, C.E., et al.: Progesterone for outpatient treatment of Pickwickian syndrome. *Ann. Intern. Med.* **83**: 476–479, 1975.
75. Plum, F., and Swanson, A.G.: Abnormalities in central regulation of respiration in acute and convalescent poliomyelitis. *Arch. Neurol. Psychiat.* **80**: 267–285, 1968.
76. Devereaux, M.W., Keane, J.R., and Davis, R.L.: Automatic respiratory failure associated with infarction of the medulla. *Arch. Neurol.* **29**: 46–52, 1973.
77. North, J.B., and Jennett, S.: Abnormal breathing patterns associated with acute brain damage. *Arch. Neurol.* **31**: 338–344, 1974.
78. Krieger, A.J., and Rosomoff, H.L.: Sleep-induced apnea: Part I. A respiratory and autonomic dysfunction syndrome following bilateral percutaneous cervical cordotomy. *J. Neurosurg.* **39**: 168–180, 1974.
79. Severinghaus, J., and Mitchell, P.: Failure of respiratory cen-

ter automatically while awake. *Clin. Res.* **10**: 122, 1962.

80. Solliday, N.H., Gaensler, E.A., Schwaber, J.R., and Parker, T.F.: Impaired central chemoreceptor function and chronic hypoventilation many years following poliomyelitis. *Respiration* **34**: 177, 1974.
81. Hyland, R.H., Jones, N.L., Powles, A.C.P., Lenkie, S.C.M., Vanderlinden, R.G., and Epstein, S.W.: Primary alveolar hypoventilation treated with nocturnal electrophrenic respiration. *Am. Rev. Respir. Dis.* **117**: 165, 1978.
82. Valdes-Dapena, M.A.: Sudden, unexpected and unexplained death in infancy—a status report, 1973. *N. Eng. J. Med.* **289**: 1195–197, 1973.
83. Steinschneider, A.: Prolonged apnea and the sudden infant death syndrome: Clinical and laboratory observations. *Pediatrics* **50**: 646–654, 1972.
84. Kelly, D., Shannon, D., and O'Connell, K.: Care of infants with Near-Miss Sudden Infant Death Syndrome. *Pediatrics* **61**: 511–514, 1978.
85. Schiffman, P.L., Westlake, R.E., Santiago, T.V., and Edelman, N.H.: Ventilatory control in parents of victims of sudden infant death syndrome. *N. Eng. J. Med.* **302**: 486–491, 1980.
86. Guilleminault, C., Ariagno, R., Forno, L., Nagel, L., Baldwin, R., and Owen, M.: Obstructive sleep apnea and near-miss for SIDS: 1. Report of an infant with sudden death. *Pediatrics* **63**: 837–843, 1979.
87. Aranda, J., Mazzarelli, M., Tamas, L., Jasper, M., and Milic-Emeli, J.: Effect of caffeine on control of breathing. *Pediat. Res.* **11**: 530, 1978.
88. Aranda, J., Cook, C., Gorman, W., Collinge, J., Loughman, P., Outerbridge, E., Aldridge, A., and Neims, A.: Pharmacokinetic profile of caffeine in the premature newborn infant with apnea. *J. Pediat.* **94**: 663–668, 1979.
89. Soutar, C.A., Costello, J., Ijaduola, O., and Turner-Warwick, M.: Nocturnal and morning asthma relationship to plasma corticosteroids and response to cortisol infusion. *Thorax* **30**: 436, 1975.
90. Sullivan, C.E., Zamel, N., Kozar, L.F., Murphy, E., and Phillipson, E.A.: Regulation of airway smooth muscle tone in sleeping dogs. *Am. Rev. Respir. Dis.*, in press.
91. Severinghaus, J., Bainton, G., and Carcelen, A.: Respiratory insensitivity to hypoxia in chronically hypoxic man. *Respir. Physiol.* **1**: 308, 1966.

Botulism, neuromuscular impairment from, 51-53, 125
respiratory distress and, 128-129
Brain stem, apneusis and, 164
hiccups and, 217
infection of, 42, 62-63, 232
respiration and, 2-8, 294, 297-298
sleep and, 294, 297-298
yawning and, 228-229
Breath-holding, 258-259
Breathing. See also *Intermittent positive pressure breathing.*
apneustic, 164-165
ataxic, 166-167
physiology of, 244-246
Bronchus, innervation of, 5

C

CAT scanning. See *Computerized axial tomography.*
Cardiac arrhythmia, AIPN and, 97-98
diphtheria and, 100-101
porphyria and, 102-103
sleep apnea and, 313
Central nervous system, infectious disease and, 41-64
in childhood, 259-260
motor neuron degeneration and, 71-81
respiratory dysfunction and, 157-172, 187-196
Central neurogenic hyperventilation, 162-164, 169-170
Cerebral cortex, infectious disease and, 42, 62-64
respiratory dysfunction and, 158-159
Cerebrovascular accident, respiration and, 167-169
Cerebrovascular disease, respiration and, 157-172
Cervicomedullary junction, surgery of, 272-273
Charcot, motor neuron disease and, 71
yawning and, 229
Chemoreceptors, respiration and, 6-7
Chest, pain, respiratory dyskinesia and, 28-30
tightness, stiff person syndrome and, 34
Cheyne-Stokes respiration, 159-162, 168-169
sleep and, 299
Children, respiration and neurologic disease and, 253-263
Chlorpromazine, hiccups and, 221-222
Chorea, respiratory distress and, 22-30
Clonazepam, myoclonus and, 233
Clostridium tetani, respiratory distress and, 60
Complications, hyperventilation and, 270
neuromuscular infection and, 47
respiratory, neuromuscular disease and, 113-156
percutaneous cordotomy and, 276-277
Computerized axial tomography, brain abscess and, 63
spinal abscess and, 62
Congenital malformations, respiration and, 254-256
Cordotomy, open, anterolateral, 277-278
percutaneous, for pain relief, 276-277
Corynebacterium diphtheriae, respiratory distress and, 54-56, 125, 127

Corticosteroids, myasthenia gravis and, 131-132
Cough, neurologic pathways in, 10

D

Depression, mental, postencephalitic Parkinson's disease and, 22
Dermacentor andersonii, respiratory distress and, 53, 125, 127-128
Diaphragm, amyotrophic lateral sclerosis and, 73-74
  anatomy of, 212-213
  diphtheria and, 100-101
  function, ALS and, 78-79
  inspiration and, 8-9
  neuromuscular disease and, 85-88, 120-123
  weakness, 144, 146
Diazepam, epilepsy and, 178-179
  myoclonus and, 233
  stiff person syndrome and, 34
  tetanus and, 60
Diphtheria, respiratory dysfunction and, 100-101
Diphtheritic polyneuropathy, respiratory distress and, 54-56, 125, 127
Discectomy, cervical, complications of, 275-276
Drugs. See under individual agents.
Dysarthria, Huntington's disease and, 23
Dysphagia, Huntington's disease and, 23
  neuromuscular weakness and, 134-138
  Wilson's disease and, 24
Dyspnea, Parkinson's disease and, 16, 17
  Shy-Drager syndrome and, 31-32
Dyspnea (Continued)
  stiff person syndrome and, 34
  tardive dyskinesia and, 28-29
Dystonia, laryngeal, neuroleptics and, 26
Dystrophy(ies), Duchenne, respiratory therapy and, 146-147
  muscular, respiration and, 115, 120

E

ECG. See *EKG.*
Edrophonium, myasthenia gravis and, 130-131
Efferent mechanisms, respiration and, 7-10
EKG, abnormalities, AIPN and, 97-98
Electroencephalography, multiple sclerosis and, 192-193
  sleep and, 285 *et passim*
Electromyography, diaphragm function and, 79, 87-88
  myopathies and, 119
  sleep and, 285 *et passim*
Electrooculography, sleep and, 285 *et passim*
Emphysema, Parkinson's disease and, 18
Encephalitis, Von Economo's, 20
Epilepsy. See also *Fit*; *Myoclonus*; *Seizures.*
  respiratory dysfunction and, 174-185
Expiration, forced, chest size and, 8-9
Extrapyramidal system, respiratory dysfunction and, 15-30

F

Fazio-Londe's disease, 260-261

Fit, "grand mal," respiration and, 174, 175
Flow rates, Parkinson's disease and, 18-19
Foramen magnum, surgery of, 272-273
Functional residual capacity, ALS and, 77

G

Gaucher's disease, 262
Gilles de la Tourette syndrome. See *Tourette's syndrome.*
Goodpasture's syndrome, Wilson's disease and, 25
Guillain-Barré syndrome, *C. Diphtheria* symptoms and, 54-55
  respiratory distress and, 56, 125, 127
  tick paralysis symptoms and, 54
Guillain-Barré-Strohl syndrome. See *Acute inflammatory polyradiculneuropathy.*
Guillain-Mollaret triangle, myoclonus and, 232

H

Haloperidol, respiratory distress and, 26, 30
Heart. See also *Cardiac.*
  disease, hiccups and, 217, 219
  rate, AIPN and, 96-97
    porphyria and, 102-103
Heimlich maneuver, dysphagia and, 138
Hemorrhage, intracranial, postoperative, 272
Hepatic porphyrias, hereditary, respiration and, 101-103
Hering-Breuer reflex, 245
  vagus nerve and, 5
Heroin, respiration and, 201-203
Herpes zoster, phrenic nerve and diaphragmatic paralysis and, 57, 99
Hiccups, 211-225
  neurologic pathways and, 10
Huntington's disease, respiration and, 22-24
Hydantoin, toxicity, 175-176
Hypersomnia-sleep apnea syndrome, 304-314
  airway anomalies and, 314-320
Hyperventilation. See also *Central neurogenic hyperventilation.*
  intracranial pressure and, 269-270
Hypotonia, respiration and, 147-150
Hypoventilation, alveolar, AIPN and, 94-95
    signs of, 22, 88
    sleep and, 316-317
  postencephalitic, Parkinson's disease and, 21-22
Hypoxia, sleep and, 301

I

Infants, respiration and neurologic disease and, 243-253
    sleep and, 303-304
Infection, neurological, respiration and, 41-70
Intensive care unit, respiratory failure and, 124-127
Intermittent positive pressure breathing, pituitary surgery and, 271
Intracranial pressure, reduction of, 269-270
Isaac's syndrome, respiratory distress and, 104-105
Isoniazid, toxicity, 181-182

L

Laboratory findings, poliomyelitis and, 58
Laryngeal nerve, injury of, 278
Larynx, myoclonus and, 230-233
Leigh's encephalopathy, 261
Levodopa, respiratory function and, 19, 29
Lung, abscess, epilepsy and, 176
  capacity, Parkinson's disease and, 18-19
  neuromuscular disease and, 43, 47-49
    vs. lung disease signs, 84-85

M

Maple syrup urine disease, 261-262
Mechanical ventilation, AIPN and, 95
  amyotrophic lateral sclerosis and, 73
  botulism and, 129
  neuromuscular infection and, 51-54, 56
Medulla oblongata, ataxic breathing and, 166
  CSR and, 161
  MS and, 188-189
  salicylates and, 204-206
Medullary center, respiration and, 2-4, 297-298
Meninges, infection of, respiratory distress and, 63
Meningitis, aseptic, respiratory distress and, 57
Metaclopromide, hiccups and, 221-222
Midbrain, CSR and, 161
Moebius syndrome, respiration and, 255-256
Morphine, respiration and, 198-201
Motor neuron disease, respiratory dysfunction and, 71-81, 117
Multiple sclerosis, respiration and, 187-196
Muscle(s), abdominal, neuropathy of, 89-90
  atrophy, respiration and, 115, 116-117
  biopsy of, 119-120
  bulbar, neuropathy of, 90, 117
  intercostal, neuropathy of, 88-89
  motor neuron disease and, 71-81
  pulmonary, respiratory dysfunction and, 83-112
  respiratory, 8-10
  skeletal, infectious disease and, 41-43, 49-51
  spasm, stiff person syndrome and, 34
  tone, stiff person syndrome and, 34
  weakness of, acute, 124-134
    chronic, 134-150
Myasthenia gravis, respiration and, 118, 129-133
Myoclonus, anoxia and, 179-180
  respiration and, 230-233
Myopathies, respiration and, 118-120. See also under *Muscle(s)*.

N

Naloxone, narcotic overdose and, 200-201, 202
Narcotics, respiration and, 197-203
Nerve(s). See *Autonomic nervous system; Central nervous system; Motor neuron disease; Peripheral nervous system;* and individual nerves.
Neuroleptics, respiration and, 25-30

Neuromuscular disease. See under *Peripheral nervous system*
Neuromuscular junction, infectious disease and, 41-43, 51-54, 125
Neuropathy. See under individual nerves and nervous systems.
Neurosurgery, respiratory complication of, 277-284
Neurotoxins, respiration and, 197-209

O

Obesity, sleep apnea and, 310, 315-316
Ondine's Curse, 167, 189, 247
  cordotomy and, 277, 317
Opisthotonos, tetanus and, 59
Oropharynx, myoclonus and, 230-233
Oxygen, hyperbaric, seizures and, 182

P

Pain, percutaneous cordotomy and, 276-277
Palate, myoclonus and, 230-233
Parkinson's disease, dopaminergic therapy and, 16
  respiration and, 16-22, 27, 28
    postencephalitic, 19-22
Pediatric. See *Children; Infants.*
Peripheral nervous system, infectious disease and, 42, 54-57
  respiration and, 8-10, 83-112, 117-118
  trauma to, 278
Pharyngitis, diphtheritic polyneuropathy and, 54-55
Phenytoin, epilepsy and, 175-176, 178-179, 182
Phrenic nerve, anatomy of, 212-213
  block, hiccups and, 223
  dysfunction, 103-104
  injury of, 178
  tests, neuromuscular disease and, 87
Physical examination, neurologic infection and, 44
  neuromuscular disease, and, 86-87
Pickwickian syndrome, 315-316
Pituitary gland, surgery of, IPPB and, 271
Pneumonitis, hemorrhagic, Wilson's disease and, 25
Pneumotaxic center, respiration and,
2-4, 7, 31
Poliomyelitis, paralytic, respiration and, 57-59, 117
Polycythemia, high altitude, respiration and, 319-320
Pompe's disease, 262
Porphyria, acute intermittent. See *Hepatic porphyria, hereditary.*
Posterior fossa, surgery of, complications, 271-272
Posthyperventilation apnea, 158-159
Prednisone, trichinosis and, 51
Pulmonary edema, narcotics and, 201-202
  neurogenic, 270-271
  noncardiogenic, 47-49, 64
  postictal, 173-175
Pulmonary function. See also *Breathing; Respiration; Ventilation.*
  neuromuscular disease and, 120-123
  Parkinson's disease and, 16-22
  studies. See also under *Tests* and individual studies.

Pulmonary function (Continued)
ALS and, 74-79
lung vs. nerve and/or muscle disease, 84-85
neurologic infection and, 45-46
neuromuscular disease and, 122-123
poliomyelitis and, 59
Pulmonary interstitial fibrosis, 147

R

REM sleep, respiration and, 285 *et passim*
Reserpine, respiratory dyskinesia and, 29
Respiration, neuroanatomy of, 1-13
Respiratory acidosis, salicylates and, 205
Respiratory alkalosis, tardive dyskinesia and, 29
Respiratory arrest, spinal cord injury and, 274-275
Respiratory centers, neurologic, 1-4, 297
Respiratory control, testing, neurologic infection and, 46
Respiratory dysfunction, movement disorders and, 15-39
Respiratory dyskinesias, 19, 25-30
Respiratory rate, postencephalitic Parkinson's disease and, 20-21
Respiratory reflexes, 211-242
Respratory tract, infection of, Parkinson's disease and, 17-18
Reye's encephalopathy, 63, 257-258
Roentgen examination, of diaphragm, neuromuscular disease and, 86
Roentgen examination (Continued)
ALS and, 73
Pott's disease and, 62

S

Salicylates, respiration and, 203-206
Scanning. See also *Computerized axial tomography.*
radionuclide, brain abscess and, 63
Scoliosis, pulmonary function and, 116, 138-143
Seizures in children, 259
respiratory disease and, 173-185
Shingles, diaphragmatic paralysis in, 56-57
Shy-Drager syndrome, respiration and, 30-33
Singultus. See *Hiccups.*
Sleep, respiratory disorders and, 285-328
respiratory studies during, 46
Sneezing, 233-236
Sphincterotomy, cricopharyngeal, dysphagia and, 137
Spinal cord, dysfunction, respiration and, 273-278
efferent pathways in respiration and, 8-10
infectious disease and, 42, 57-62
Spine, cervical, surgery of, 275-276
Spirometry, ALS and, 74
neuromuscular disease and, 122
Stiff person syndrome, respiratory function and, 33-35
Stroke, respiration and, 157
Succinylcholine, muscle weakness and, 129
"Sudden death" syndrome, neuroleptics and, 26-28
Sudden Infant Death Syndrome, 247-250
sleep and, 317-319

Supratentorial disorders, respiration and, 269-271
Surgery, for scoliosis, 140-143
Swallowing. See *Dysphagia.*
Syringobulbia, alveolar hypoventilation and, 273
Syringomyelia, apnea and, 273

T

Tardive dyskinesia, respiration and, 25-30
Tests. See also *Pulmonary function, studies.*
  blood gases. See under *Blood gases.*
  diaphragmatic function, 85-88. See also under *Diaphragm.*
  diffusing capacity, ALS and, 78
  flow volume loop, ALS and, 75-77
  lung volumes, ALS and, 77
  multiple sclerosis and, 189-193
  phrenic circle, hiccups and, 216
  pulmonary mechanics, ALS, and, 77-78
  Read rebreathing, 92
  serum enzymes, myopathies and, 119
  stable pressure, ALS, and, 75
  transdiaphragmatic pressure, 87
  ventilation control. See under *Ventilation.*
Tetanus, respiratory distress and, 59-60, 99
Thalotomy, pulmonary function and, 19
Theophylline, apnea and, 247, 251-252
  Ondine's Curse and, 247
Thiabendazole, trichinosis and, 50
Thorax. See also *Chest.*
  muscles of, respiration and, 8-10
Thymectomy, myasthenia gravis and, 132
Tick paralysis, respiratory distress and, 53-54, 125, 127-128
Total lung capacity, ALS and, 77
Tourette's syndrome, respiration and, 33
Trauma, birth-related, respiration and, 257
  CNS, pulmonary edema and, 48-49
  spinal cord, respiration and, 274-275
Trachea, innervation of, 5
Tracheostomy, AIPN and, 96
  Shy-Drager syndrome and, 32
  sleep apnea and, 313
Trichinosis, respiratory muscles and, 49-51
Tuberculosis of vertebral column, respiratory distress and, 61
Tumors, intracranial, in children, 262-263
  of cerebellopontine angle, surgery of, 271-272
  of foramen magnum, surgery of, 272-273
  of spinal cord, surgery of, 273

V

Vagotomy, effects of, 7
Vagus nerve, respiration and, 5, 7
Valvalva maneuver, AIPN and, 97
Ventilation, assisted. See *Mechanical ventilation; Tracheostomy.*
  control of, ALS and, 78
  studies, Parkinson's disease and, 18-19
Vocal cord, paralysis, 252-253
Von Economo, respiratory distress and, 62

W

Wilson's disease, respiratory function and, 24-25

X

X-ray. See *Roentgen examination.*

Y

Yawning, 224, 226-230